AI and Machine Learning for Cancer Care:

Precision Medicine and Beyond

Manvi Mishra
https://orcid.org/0000-0001-6764-3789
Shri Ram Murti Smarak College of Engineering and Technology, Bareilly, India

Piyush Kumar
Shri Ram Murti Smarak Institute of Medical Sciences, Bareilly, India

Himanshi Khattar
Shri Ram Murti Smarak Institute of Medical Sciences, Bareilly, India

Mohammad Zubair Khan
https://orcid.org/0000-0002-2409-7172
Islamic University of Madinah, Saudi Arabia

IGI Global
Scientific Publishing
Publishing Tomorrow's Research Today

Vice President of Editorial Melissa Wagner
Director of Acquisitions Mikaela Felty
Director of Book Development Jocelynn Hessler
Production Manager Mike Brehm
Cover Design Jose Rosado

Published in the United States of America by
IGI Global Scientific Publishing
701 East Chocolate Avenue
Hershey, PA, 17033, USA
Tel: 717-533-8845 | Fax: 717-533-7115
Website: https://www.igi-global.com E-mail: cust@igi-global.com

Library of Congress Cataloging-in-Publication Data

Names: Mishra, Manvi, 1985- editor | Kumar, Piyush, Dr., 1974- editor | Khattar, Himanshi, 1994- editor | Khan, Mohammad Zubair, 1976- editor
Title: AI and machine learning for cancer care : precision medicine and beyond / edited by: Manvi Mishra, Piyush Kumar, Himanshi Khattar, Mohammad Zubair Khan.
Description: Hershey, PA : IGI Global Scientific Publishing, [2026] | Includes bibliographical references. | Summary: "This book explores the ethical, regulatory, and social implications of these technologies, addressing challenges such as data privacy, algorithmic bias, and equity in healthcare"-- Provided by publisher.
Identifiers: LCCN 2025028222 (print) | LCCN 2025028223 (ebook) | ISBN 9798337343129 hardcover | ISBN 9798337343136 paperback | ISBN 9798337343143 ebook
Subjects: LCSH: Cancer--Treatment--Technological innovations | Artificial intelligence--Medical applications
Classification: LCC RC270.8 .A384 2026 (print) | LCC RC270.8 (ebook)
LC record available at https://lccn.loc.gov/2025028222
LC ebook record available at https://lccn.loc.gov/2025028223

British Cataloguing in Publication Data
A Cataloguing in Publication record for this book is available from the British Library.

To our family, for their endless love, patience, and unwavering support; to our teachers, for igniting the light of knowledge and guiding our journey; and to our students, whose curiosity, dedication, and enthusiasm continue to inspire us every day.

Table of Contents

Detailed Table of Contents

by traditional diagnostic methods. This chapter aims to present a comprehensive exploration of how machine learning techniques can revolutionize the process of breast cancer detection and classification. It delves into a wide array of ML algorithms, data acquisition techniques, feature extraction, model evaluation metrics, and real-world implementation challenges, providing a solid theoretical and practical foundation for researchers, practitioners, and students. The vision is to create a holistic and accessible resource that not only informs but also inspires further innovation in the use of ML for breast cancer detection.

Brain tumors represent abnormal growths of cells—either benign or malignant—within the confined space of the human skull. These growths can lead to severe health complications and long-term psychological and physical consequences, greatly diminishing a patient's quality of life. The survival rate for individuals diagnosed with malignant brain tumors decreases significantly over time if early interventions are not implemented. This study investigates advanced hybrid architectures, namely CNN-UNet, ResNet-UNet, EfficientNet-UNet, and EfficientNet integrated with Vision Transformers. A comprehensive comparative analysis of these hybrid architectures is conducted to recognize the most efficient model. The results indicate that EfficientNet-UNet architecture achieved superior performance on the BraTS dataset with an accuracy of 99.47%, while EfficientNet-Vision Transformer on the Nickparvar dataset from Kaggle reached an accuracy of 97%. These findings highlight the efficiency of advanced hybrid deep learning models in detecting brain tumors from multimodal MRI images.

Breast cancer is a kind of malignant tumor that mostly found in women which grows around the tissue of breast. During the process of diagnosis the cancer cells and non cancer cells are been identified and their count is made. If the count of cancer cells is greater than non cancer cells then the patient undergoes the treatments. The early detection of breast cancer can save the life of patient. Now a day's AI is playing a vital role in classifying cancer and non cancer cells in a accurate way. Many of the earlier researchers had performed the work of classifying them but, most of them lack in the accuracy. To have good accuracy a new method EBCS (Early Breast Cancer Screening) is proposed which consists of four steps or phases- preprocessing, classifying, performance evaluation and providing clear understanding to human.. To implement the four steps python programming is been used and cancer data set was extracted from Breast Cancer Wisconsin (Diagnostic) data set. The proposed method EBCS gave an accuracy of 99 percentage and complexity is also reduced.

Lung cancer is the leading cause of cancer mortality, with deaths due to the disease anticipated to exceed 4.6M new cases and 3.5 million lives each year by 2050. AI-based radiomics tools can potentially analyze the levels of pixel distribution and identify hidden biomarkers related to tumor aggressiveness. However, clinicians are reluctant to adopt these methodologies due to the lack of transparency in the DL models, known as the "black-box" phenomenon. The chapter "From Black Box to Glass Box: Interpretable AI for Lung Cancer Radiomics" aims to facilitate the transition of AI-based applications from laboratories to clinics. The protocol for AI-enhanced radiomics is systematically described. The core focus is on enhancing transparency through explainable AI (XAI) techniques. AI designs should be transparent (glass boxes) and have the purpose of assisting clinicians rather than replacing them. The roadmap to success and excellence in the diagnosis and treatment of lung cancer is clear, with data-driven insights.

Machine learning (ML) is transforming radiation oncology by enhancing precision, efficiency, and personalization. Key applications include: (1) Treatment planning—U-Net and nnU-Net achieve >85% Dice scores for tumor segmentation, while GANs optimize dose distribution; (2) Predictive modeling—Radiomics and genomics predict treatment response/toxicity, though data heterogeneity challenges reproducibility; (3) Personalized therapy—Biomarker-driven adaptation and digital twins enable dynamic adjustments. Challenges include data scarcity, model validation, and interdisciplinary collaboration, with federated learning proposed for privacy-preserving data sharing. ML automates workflows, improves outcomes, and addresses resource disparities, but requires standardized protocols, robust validation, and ethical frameworks for equitable adoption. Future directions include federated learning advances, multi-center trials, and prospective studies to translate research into practice.

Cancer is the second-leading global cause of death (>10M/year), posing complex economic and social burdens. Current treatments—conventional (chemo, radio) and advanced (targeted, immuno)—are limited by high cost, toxicity, lack of precision, and unpredictable patient response . An urgent paradigm shift requires leveraging Artificial Intelligence (AI) and Machine Learning (ML). AI/ML drives breakthroughs in the entire oncological care pathway: enabling precise diagnosis, robust prognosis, and individualized prediction of therapeutic response via multi-omics analysis. The future of oncology must be defined by AI-powered precision to solve the problem of variable efficacy and achieve universal access to effective care.

Foreword

I am delighted to write the Foreword for this significant new book, *AI & Machine Learning for Cancer Care: Precision Medicine & Beyond,* edited by *Manvi Mishra, Piyush Kumar, Himanshi Khattar, Mohammad Khan.* This comprehensive edited 10 -Chapters volume explores the transformative role of Artificial Intelligence and Machine Learning in modern oncology, addressing some of the most pressing challenges and emerging opportunities in cancer diagnosis, treatment, and patient management.

The book presents an in-depth examination of advanced AI- and ML-driven methodologies applied across diverse domains of cancer care, including medical imaging, predictive analytics, precision oncology, clinical decision support systems, drug discovery, and outcome assessment. By integrating computational intelligence with clinical insights, this work showcases cutting-edge techniques designed to enhance accuracy, efficiency, and personalization in cancer care delivery.

This volume is a collaborative scholarly achievement, drawing upon the expertise of accomplished authors, editors, reviewers, and advisory board members recognized for their academic and research excellence in artificial intelligence, data science, biomedical engineering, and oncology. The result is a definitive reference that successfully bridges theoretical foundations with real-world clinical applications, while also addressing ethical considerations, data privacy, and interpretability of AI models in healthcare.

I congratulate the editors and contributing authors, reviewers on this remarkable achievement, which is poised to benefit researchers, clinicians, academicians, students, and industry professionals alike.

I highly recommend this book as an indispensable resource for those seeking to understand and contribute to the rapidly evolving field of AI- and ML-enabled cancer care, and for advancing intelligent, evidence-based, and patient-centric healthcare solutions.

Anuj Kumar Sharma

Dr. APJ Abdul Kalam Technical University Lucknow, India

Preface

INTRODUCTION

The book *"AI and Machine Learning in Cancer Care: Precision Medicine and Beyond"* is an in-depth exploration of the transformative potential of machine learning (ML) and artificial intelligence (AI) in modern cancer care. The book delves into how advanced algorithms are revolutionizing the diagnosis, treatment, and management of cancer across various medical disciplines, aiming to shift the focus from one-size-fits-all treatments to more personalized, precise interventions.

In this comprehensive work, experts from diverse medical fields, including radiation oncology, gynaecology, anaesthesiology, radiology, pathology, microbiology, and community medicine, come together to share their insights into the ways ML is reshaping cancer care. Each chapter focuses on a specific specialty, providing a clear understanding of how ML technologies are being leveraged to improve patient outcomes.

The book covers the applications of ML in radiation oncology, where AI helps design customized radiation plans and optimize tumor targeting. It delves into the advancements in Gynaecological cancer care, where predictive models are enhancing early detection and personalized treatments for ovarian, cervical, and endometrial cancers.

In anaesthesiology, machine learning is being applied to predict complications and optimize anaesthesia protocols, improving the safety and recovery of cancer patients undergoing surgery. Radiology, with its reliance on advanced imaging technologies, benefits from ML algorithms that enhance tumor detection, staging, and monitoring, driving more accurate and efficient diagnoses.

Machine learning is also transforming pathology by enabling precise analysis of tissue samples, aiding in tumor classification and prognosis prediction. By integrating molecular and genomic data, AI is paving the way for more tailored therapies that increase the chances of treatment success.

In microbiology, the book explores how ML models are identifying microbial markers that may influence cancer development and response to treatments, shedding light on the microbiome's role in oncology. The book also discusses the intersection of community medicine and ML, emphasizing population health approaches that enhance cancer screening, prevention, and education, particularly in underserved communities.

Throughout, *Machine Learning in Cancer Care* explores the ethical, regulatory, and social implications of these technologies, addressing challenges such as data privacy, algorithmic bias, and equity in healthcare. The book ultimately presents a vision of a future where ML and AI are seamlessly integrated into cancer care, improving early detection, treatment personalization, and overall patient outcomes.

Written for oncologists, researchers, clinicians, and healthcare professionals, the book serves as a valuable resource for those looking to understand the rapidly evolving role of machine learning in the fight against cancer. It offers a unique, interdisciplinary perspective that bridges the gap between technology and medicine, highlighting the vast potential for innovation in cancer care.

Machine learning in cancer care stands at the forefront of one of the most significant transformations in modern healthcare. As cancer remains one of the leading causes of death globally, the demand for faster diagnosis, accurate risk prediction, personalized treatment, and effective long-term management has never been greater. In this landscape, machine learning has emerged as a powerful catalyst for change.

Today, hospitals and research institutions worldwide are integrating ML-driven tools into routine oncology workflows—ranging from imaging interpretation and molecular profiling to treatment planning and patient monitoring. Breakthroughs in deep learning, big data analytics, and precision medicine are enabling clinicians to uncover patterns that were previously invisible, leading to earlier detection, more targeted therapies, and improved survival rates.

Governments, healthcare systems, and pharmaceutical companies are increasingly investing in AI-driven cancer solutions, recognizing their potential to address critical gaps such as clinician workload, variability in human interpretation, and limited access to specialists in underserved regions. At the same time, global initiatives in digital health and cancer research are accelerating the development of ethical, transparent, and equitable AI frameworks.

In the world today, ML in cancer care sits at the intersection of medicine, technology, and public health. It reflects a broader shift toward evidence-based, data-intensive healthcare—where decisions are guided not just by clinical experience, but by powerful computational insights. As such, the topic is not only scientifically relevant but also socially urgent, shaping the future of cancer diagnostics, treatment, prevention, and healthcare delivery.

The intended audience for *AI and Machine Learning in Oncology: Transforming Cancer Diagnosis and Treatment* includes a broad range of stakeholders at the convergence of AI and cancer care. It is designed for oncologists and clinicians integrating AI into diagnosis, treatment planning, and patient monitoring; medical researchers and bio informaticians applying ML to genomics and biomarker discovery; and AI/ML engineers developing imaging and predictive models. The book also serves healthcare administrators, policymakers, pharmaceutical and biotech professionals, academicians, students, and patient advocacy organizations focused on ethical, regulatory, and equitable adoption of AI-driven oncology solutions.

The book balances technical depth with clinical relevance, making it accessible to both technical experts and healthcare professionals aiming to harness AI for trans-formative cancer care.

CHAPTER OVERVIEWS

Chapter 1: Precision medicine represents a new generation of healthcare that tailors therapies to specific patient subgroups based on disease susceptibility and treatment response, moving beyond the traditional "one-size-fits-all" approach. These treatments are customized using individual omics profiles along with social, behavioral, and environmental factors. While the concept existed earlier, the Precision Medicine Initiative gained momentum with advances in artificial intelligence and machine learning. Key enablers include AI, big data, pharmaco-omics, and the integration of population and preventive medicine. Big data derived from electronic health records, encompassing clinical, omics, and imaging biomarkers, is effectively analyzed using machine learning techniques.

Chapter 2: Radiomics is a game changer in oncology since it is able to transform routine medical images into quantitative data to discover tumor heterogeneity, biology, and treatment response, which cannot be detected using visual interpretation. Radiomics, with regard to CT, MRI, PET, ultrasound, and mammography extremes, provides non-invasive information to help in cancer detection, determine correct subtypes, risk assessments, and monitoring therapy. The results of the lung, breast, brain, liver, and pancreatic cancer biopsies all lead us to believe that the predictive accuracy is high, and most of the models have AUC values that surpass 0.90, indicating that radiomics is a useful complement to the conventional diagnostics test.

Chapter 3: The early diagnosis of cancer goes a long way in improving treatment outcomes and the survival rates. Conventional methodological approaches to diagnostics have limitations concerning their accuracy, speed, and accessibility.

Artificial intelligence (AI) has increased the effectiveness of available diagnostics techniques through offering improved solutions in early detection of cancer on different malignancies. This review article discusses the field of AI models in the detection of early cancer, with special focus on the developments in machine learning (ML), deep learning (DL), and other sophisticated methods.

Chapter 4: It is a fact that breast cancer is one of the most common types of cancer amongst women in any part of the world (World Health Organization [WHO]). Early diagnosis and prevention, although, is a serious problem despite the progress reached in medical science. Conventionally, diagnosis is majorly dependent on radiologists and pathologists, hence the possibility of human error and lag time but due to the emergence of Artificial Intelligence (AI) and Machine Learning (ML) a revolution is underway in oncology.

Chapter 5: Brain tumors are the leading cause of cancers deaths worldwide; in adults they arise due to the uncontrolled division of cells. The brain is an essential organ composed of neuronal cells, along with supporting tissues such as cells known as glial cells and meninges that surround them. Damage to these brain regions is permanent and may lead to severe illnesses, including possibly fatal brain tumors. Abnormal growth of cells in the human brain leads to the formation of certain cancers. The National Brain Tumor Society (NBTS) predicts that by 2025, around 18,330 fatalities will occur due to malignant brain tumors, and over 93,000 Americans will have been diagnosed of serious brain tumors. Several obstacles arise during patient treatment, since the survival rate for malignant brain tumors is 35.7%, according to a survey done over the last five years

Chapter 6: Breast cancer refers to a kind of malignant lump that mostly found in women which grows around the tissue of breast. During the process of diagnosis the cancer cells and non-cancer cells are been identified and their count is made. If the count of cancer cells is greater than non-cancer cells then the patient undergoes the treatments. Detecting breast cancer early can save the life of patient. Now a day's AI is playing a vital role in classifying cancer and non-cancer cells in an accurate way. Many of the earlier researchers had performed the work of classifying them but, most of them lack in the preprocessing, imbalance problem was not considered, latest AI tools were not considered for classification, accuracy is not same for all dataset or repository, accuracy is also low, not scalable with large volume of data and none of the previous papers or work considered about AI adoption, AI challenges, AI impact, cost benefit analysis, ethical and privacy issues, policy making, traditional and AI based differences for breast cancer detection.

Chapter 7: Lung cancer is the leading cause of cancer mortality, with deaths due to the disease anticipated to exceed 4.6M new cases and 3.5M lives each year by 2050. AI-based radiomics tools can potentially analyze the levels of pixel distribution and identify hidden biomarkers related to tumor aggressiveness. However, clinicians are reluctant to adopt these methodologies due to the lack of transparency in the DL models, known as the "black-box" phenomenon. The chapter "From Black Box to Glass Box: Interpretable AI for Lung Cancer Radiomics" aims to facilitate the transition of AI-based applications from laboratories to clinics. The protocol for AI-enhanced radiomics is systematically described. The core focus is on enhancing transparency through explainable AI (XAI) techniques. AI designs should be transparent (glass boxes) and have the purpose of assisting clinicians rather than replacing them. The roadmap to success and excellence in the diagnosis and treatment of lung cancer is clear, with data-driven insights.

Chapter 8: Implementing machine learning (ML) in radiation oncology is a disruptive change in the treatment of cancer, bringing more precision, efficiency, and personalisation. This paper provides a critical analysis of ML applications across three main fields: treatment planning, predictive modelling, and personalised therapy. Automated segmentation algorithms, such as U-Net and nnU-Net are both highly accurate (Dice coefficients above 85%) at identifying tumours and organs-at-risk in treatment planning, whereas AI-based dose optimisation algorithms, such as generative adversarial networks (GANs), simplify the treatment planning process and enhance dose distribution. Radiomics and genomics can be used in predictive modelling to determine treatment response and toxicity, but issues such as data heterogeneity and reproducibility remain.

Chapter 9: Cancer remains one of the biggest health challenges for humanity, affecting millions of individuals and families annually. The World Health Organization and the International Agency for Research on Cancer estimates suggest that cancer is responsible for over 10 million deaths annually, making it the second-highest cause of death, behind only cardiovascular diseases, with about 18 million mortalities every year. These numbers indicate the impact of cancer on the economy and human health, not merely through loss of lives, but also through long periods of patient treatment, health systems, and psychological impact on patients and caregivers. Furthermore, cancer is not a single disease but comprises hundreds of types and subtypes, each having different symptoms and treatments. These challenges make cancer a major risk factor for humanity, requiring serious efforts from all stakeholders, including healthcare professionals, researchers, local governments, and international organizations.

Chapter 10: Oncology is being transformed by machine learning (ML) in diagnostics, prognostics, and therapy strategies. The chapter covers ML's usage in cancer care, medical imaging, molecular profiling, and treatment optimisation. Complex algorithms, such as convolutional neural networks (CNNs), can match or exceed human diagnostic accuracy, while radiogenomics uses imaging and genomic data for non-invasive diagnoses. Despite these advances, variability of data, interpretability of the model, and ethical considerations like patient privacy and algorithm bias still hinder clinical use. Moral considerations like data security, justice, and good governance are also stressed. The chapter concludes by suggesting scalable, interpretable models and representative datasets to decrease biases. By addressing these challenges, ML can transform oncology by offering accurate, fair, and successful cancer treatment.

CONCLUSION

We believe that this book provides readers with an in-depth understanding of the critical advancements shaping the future of cancer care. Designed for clinicians, academicians, researchers, healthcare technologists, and policymakers, it offers valuable insights into emerging diagnostic, therapeutic, and data-driven approaches that address key challenges and unlock new opportunities in oncology. We express our sincere gratitude to the contributors whose expertise, research, and commitment have been instrumental in bringing this volume to fruition.

Our sincere gratitude goes to the contributors whose expertise and dedication have made this book possible. It is our hope that *AI and Machine Learning in Cancer Care: Precision Medicine and Beyond* will inspire continued research and clinical innovation, contributing to more accurate diagnosis, personalized treatment, improved patient outcomes, and a safer, more ethical integration of intelligent technologies across the cancer care continuum.

Manvi Mishra

Shri Ram Murti Smarak College of Engineering Technology and Research, Bareilly, India

Piyush Kumar

Shri Ram Murti Smarak Institute of Medical Sciences, Bareilly India

Himanshi Khattar

Shri Ram Murti Smarak Institute of Medical Sciences, Bareilly India

Mohammad Khan

Islamic University of Madinah, Saudi Arabia

Acknowledgment

The editors would like to express their sincere gratitude to all those who contributed to the successful completion of this edited volume, *AI and Machine Learning for Cancer Care: Precision Medicine and Beyond.* This book is the result of collective effort, scholarly commitment, and unwavering support from many distinguished individuals.

We are deeply thankful to our esteemed Chairman, SRMS Trust *Shri Dev Murti Ji*, for his visionary leadership, constant encouragement, and steadfast support toward academic excellence and research advancement. Our heartfelt appreciation is also extended to Secretory SRMS Trust *Shri Aditya Murti Ji* for his guidance, motivation, and continued support in promoting innovation and interdisciplinary research.

We extend our special thanks to all contributing authors for their insightful chapters, technical expertise, and commitment to maintaining high academic standards. Their contributions have been instrumental in shaping this book into a meaningful resource on the role of Artificial Intelligence and Machine Learning in modern cancer care.

The editors also acknowledge the support of reviewers, the publishing team of IGI, and all colleagues and staff members who assisted directly or indirectly during the editorial and publication process.

Finally, we express our gratitude to our families and well-wishers for their patience, understanding, and constant moral support throughout this endeavor.

Chapter 1
Machine Learning in Cancer Care

Anita Kushwaha
https://orcid.org/0000-0002-4144-2732
Birla Institute of Technology, Ranchi, India

R. S. Pandey
Birla Institute of Technology, Ranchi, India

ABSTRACT

The new generation of medicine, known as precision medicine, refers to adjusting therapies for a subgroup of people who share a susceptibility to a certain illness or a comparable reaction to a medication. Instead of one size fits all, these medicines are customized to particular patient's needs and also taken into consideration are patient's omics, social, behavioural, and environmental factors particular to him or her and thus the name precision medicines. Precision medicines existed earlier, but recently the Precision Medicine Initiative was launched with greater interest, with the advent of machine learning and artificial intelligence methods becoming popular. Artificial intelligence, big data, machine learning, pharmaco-omics, social and environmental aspects, and then the integration of these with population and preventive medicines are the primary instruments of precision medicine.

INTRODUCTION

The evolution of oncology is one of the most profound discoveries of the current century with the progress of biology and ability to analyze data simultaneously. Attack on cancer has always been slow evolution for decades of surgery, radiation and chemotherapy. These centers of treatments are important but, the beginning of the

DOI: 10.4018/979-8-3373-4312-9.ch001

21st century has been a shift towards data dominated medicine with revolutionizes the methods of analysis, diagnosis and most importantly, treatment of medicine as a set of intertwined complex diseases. To understand cancer is to commit a mistake of epic proportions, for it is made up of more than a thousand different diseases, each of which has its own molecular identity, its own sequence of evolution, and its own methods of treatment. This multitude of forms presents a formidable challenge which, until very recently, was beyond the comprehension and action oriented grasp of a human specialist.

The novel primary catalyst is the constant accumulation of biomedical data. The Human Genome Project and its sequel explosion in high throughput (>1 sequencer/ instrument) sequencing with its genomics, transcriptomics, proteomics, and metabolomics as shown in Figure 1. In this context, radiology and pathology slides have undergone a significant transformation from qualitative diagnostic tools to quantitative diagnostics due to advancements in medical imaging. Each patient becomes a multi-dimensional, high-volume data stream that is far more complicated than any conventional approach can analyze when these datasets (Swanson et al., 2023) are integrated with the rich clinical information included in Electronic Health Records (EHRs).

As Table 1 illustrates, this is where machine learning (ML) and artificial intelligence (AI) become crucial tools. Doctors can mix vast volumes of diverse patient data with the aid of machine learning. It is capable of making predictions and identifying patterns that people would not be able to perform on their own. This aids medical professionals in choosing more effective treatments. In essence, machine learning approaches cancer treatment like a mathematical problem. The most significant outcomes, such as the patient's potential lifespan, quality of life, and response to various therapies, are predicted using computer programs and all of the patient's health data.

Figure 1. Research Domains in Cancer Biology

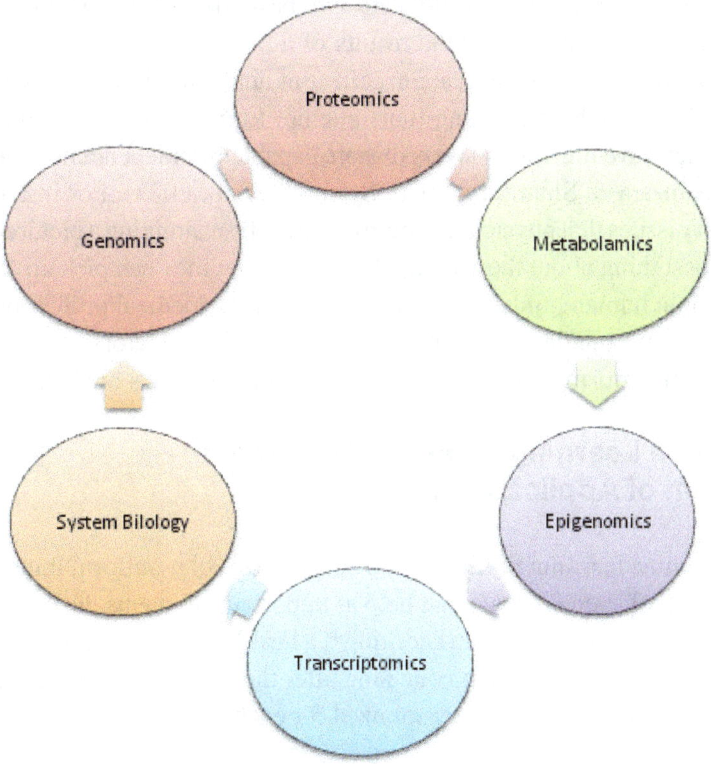

Table 1. Various research domain of cancer research and the methodologies

Genomics	Proteomics	Metabolomics	Epigenomics	Transcriptomics	System Biology
Detection of variants	Protein Function prediction	Biochemical Markers	DNA Methylation	Gene expression changes	Signalling Network
Detection of mutations	Protein Structure prediction	Metabolite abundance	Histone modifications	Profiling of miRNAs	Metabolic Network
Molecular subtyping	Protein-protein interactions	Compound annotations	Alterations in noncoding RNA	Profiling of non-coding region	Simulate cellular regulation
Detection of subtyping	Protein expressions	Unknown constituents	Nucleosome positioning		
Detection of CNVs		Interpretations of Metabolomics			

Doctors can benefit from a variety of machine learning methods [see algorithms 1, 2, 3]. Certain older algorithms do well with basic data that can be entered into tables, such as a patient's age or the results of a blood test. Deep Learning technologies, which are more recent, are excellent at analyzing images, such as scans or X-rays. These machine learning tools attempt to mimic how the human brain functions. They have numerous layers that are capable of independently identifying patterns (Shamsara & Shamsara, 2020; Swanson et al., 2023). For instance, they might identify issues that physicians would overlook by examining a picture of bodily tissue. The best thing about these computer tools is that they can pick up on what to look for without human guidance. This has altered how medical professionals treat cancer. Before, most patients got similar treatments. Now, doctors can look at each person's specific information and create a treatment plan that's made just for them.

The Machine Learning Toolkit in Oncology: A Spectrum of Applications

Using machine learning in cancer care isn't just one big, uniform thing. Instead, it's like a bunch of specific tools that help at important moments during a patient's whole experience. This starts from checking if a healthy person might get cancer, all the way to keeping an eye on someone long after their treatment.These tools make things more accurate, faster, and customized for each person.

A. Early Detection, Prevention, and Risk Stratification

The saying that detection saves lives is true when it comes to cancer. Nowadays Machine Learning is proving to be beneficial in detecting cancer in its earliest and most treatable stages. Machine Learning is capable of predicting the onset of tumours in the future. Take, for example, breast cancer. The challenge of false positives from mammograms such as anxiety and harmful procedures is an utter nuisance to those in the medical field. The project "Guard Her Health" is using Machine Learning models and clinical data to achieve an accuracy of over 98% to improve the suffering of false positives in breast cancer incorrectly diagnosed cases. Other strong Deep Learning models paired with Resnet 50 and throwaway models become the standard for lowest accuracy with the addition of innovative techniques of quantum transfer learning.

To address high mortality rate related to lung cancer, Medical Machine Learning models are starting to address the problems posed by the medical field's datasets which are incomplete, noisy and highly unbalanced. Implementing advanced pipelines that combine multiple techniques, from using Recursive Feature Elimination with SVMs to select the most relevant features and applying later a tuned XGBoost model, is starting to tackle classification problems with a great deal of success. Likewise, in skin cancers, especially Deep learning models (Kann et al., 2021) using Convolutional Neural Networks, have started to perform equally with dermatologists for the classification of dermoscopic images which is one of the more crucial tasks for the early detection of life-threatening melanomas in the case of blood cancers such as leukaemia,

B. Diagnosis and Classification

As soon as there is a suspected cancer, the next step is to obtain a most accurate diagnosis possible. ML is effective at this type of classification, whether through images or through molecular profiles. In pathology, Deep Learning methods or neural networks are used to scrutinize high-resolution whole-slide images (WSIs) of tissue biopsies to detect cancerous regions, predict tumour grade (including Gleason grading for prostate cancer), as well as predict tissue morphology based mutations — a discipline termed as computational pathology. This will lessen the workload of pathologists, while at the same time exposing deeper patterns that are not easily discernible to the human eye.

With regard to complex omics data, ML is crucial at the molecular level. Consider how supervised (e.g. Neural Networks) and unsupervised (e.g. K-means clustering) approaches in bioinformatics have elucidated and validated a set of 21 genes linked to the metastatic spread of prostate cancer to the nearby lymph nodes from TCGA(gene sequence) data. Such analysis offers deep diagnosis as well as in-depth understanding into tumor progression. In addition, advanced DL models such as Multimodal Convolutional Autoencoders (MCAEs) that can integrate and process data from multiple omics layers (e.g. gene expression, miRNA expression, and copy number variations) are able to perform pan-cancer classification, distinguishing 33 tumor types with high precision.

C. Prognosis, Treatment Selection, and Drug Discovery

Besides giving a diagnosis, machine learning has made it easier for people to answer the questions, "What is my outcome of the diagnosed condition?" and "What is the most effective treatment for my condition?" Algorithms can response to and track patient data to develop and integrate tailored models to a patient's entire clinical, biological, and data history documenting system. This is the true beginning of precision medicine.

AI positively influences the drug development and clinical trial processes. New therapeutic drugs are discovered faster now because of KaGML. KaGML models can accurately predict drug-target interactions and design novel drug candidates because they use knowledge from diverse biomedical databases such as DrugBank and Gene Ontology. These models represent molecules and proteins as graphs. In clinical trials, AI and Machine learning are already being applied to streamline trial design, data automation, and most importantly, improve geographic and demographic diversity in recruitment, addressing equity gaps in clinical research.

The Human Imperative: Navigating the Challenges of Clinical Integration

Taking a high-performing algorithm from a research lab and turning it into a bedside tool for patients involves multiple steps. Trust in machine learning and its implemented ML cancer systems center it's functionality around its uncover issues. The objectives of the system should be tailored towards enhancing the human clinically expertise and judgement rather than replacing it.

A. The "Black Box" Dilemma and the Rise of Explainable AI (XAI)

The main hurdle that is quickly becoming the limitation to clinical acceptance of Machine Learning, particularly complex Deep Learning models, is their black-box nature. It provides the prediction with almost 100 percent certainty, but it cannot justify why it gave that prediction. In the absence of a model explanation, a clinician will not fully trust it, and hence he cannot assume responsibility for any clinical decision. This has led to the emergence of the Explainable AI (XAI) domain that focuses on making model reasoning transparent. Although vital insights are now offered by tools like SHAP (SHapley Additive exPlanations) and Grad-CAM, the leukemia risk prediction model, for instance, through SHAP values, elucidates that platelet counts and gender weigh the heaviest on the interpretation, which is both clinically plausible and actionable. In contrast, Grad-CAM produces "heatmaps" over medical images, demonstrating the concrete pixels or regions that were targeted by the CNN in making its diagnosis, thus providing the radiologist/pathologist a means of verifying the focal point of the model. Symbolic Knowledge Extraction (SKE) is a large field that goes well beyond this attempt to somehow extract the defiant logic of a neural network (Shamsara & Shamsara, 2020) into a set of human-readable "if-then" rules at the highest level of interaction.

B. The Data Foundation: Quality, Bias, and Equity

Machine learning models do matter (Kourou et al., 2021), especially with regard to the purpose of training their interaction which is once again asserting the purpose of their relation to the goal of training. One has to appreciate that the data sets in medicine are a disjointed patchwork that is low quality, unfinished, and the biases, the quality of which is the most troubling. It is sad to say, but the discrimination and inequalities which lead to a bias wrongly termed clinically centralized genomic databases which are mostly populated with participants and subjects. The models which were trained on texts from those databases cross ethically problematic thresholds lacking an nuanced understanding of how ethnicity and race shapes lived experience. A discrimination, lacking inclusive, is a collaborative bottleneck. The sociological has to be responsive to the diversity of the context that is studied. The tools which are already set and validated in primary regions like Pakistan for leukemia, and Taiwan breast cancer, are troubling in the populations which are set to benefit from the tools.

Even if an algorithm is brilliant, it is not yet a finished medical device (Shaikh & Rao, 2022). Any AI tool designed to treat patients has to be subjected to a torturous line of validation, approval, and proof of compatibility with complicated clinical workflows, including but not limited to, an FDA check. This process is designed to determine the safety, accuracy, and reliability of the system. It is astonishingly easy to fool Machine Learning systems with, what is known as, adversarial provesophie, where changes to a variable, say an image, are so slight, so imperceptible, the system categorizes it so drastically rivaling the ground truth. That is, models optimally tuned for safety-critical disciplines like cancer diagnosis.

C. The Path Forward: Augmenting, Not Replacing, the Oncologist

As we stand on this technological inflection point, we need to be clear about the exact role of AI in medicine. The aim is not to develop an artificial physician, but rather to construct potent AI tools that enhance the intelligence and skills of human clinicians. AI tools, no matter how advanced, including the best Large Language Models, remain statistical inference machines (Abbaoui et al., 2024). They can recognize patterns, and do so at astonishing speed and scale, but do not possess the most important human qualities that define the practice of medicine: the ability to care, show empathy, possesses commitment and responsibility, and mental reasoning. A machine can calculate a patient's risk but cannot console the patient. It can classify a tumor, but cannot manage a complicated discourse with the patient's family.

As for the case of ML in cancer care, it's almost like the patient and the doctor is living in two different timelines Together, the AI and the doctor is tackling the arduous tasks of sorting out terabytes of genomic data, whilst the doctor is focusing on appreciating the deep arts of patient care. AI's projected future ought not to be not scorned as a terminal judgement, but rather a relevant accord in the diagnostic puzzle being pieced together by a skilled physician. The case of machine learning in cancer care carries tremendous potential. The potential of machine learning in cancer care is rather daunting. But the promise of machine learning is only achievable through great machine learning, ethical accountability, and keeping humanity in the center .

OVERVIEW OF MACHINE LEARNING CONCEPTS

Defining Machine Intelligence: Learning from Data

Revolutionizing healthcare through technology hinges on a branch of AI (Abbaoui et al., 2024) referred to as Machine Learning (ML). In its simplest form, machine learning is a branch of computing technology that frees itself from any form of programming barrier. An ML system is designed to learn directly from the data, and is not given a specified and rigid set of rules that have been hand coded for them to execute. Machines learn to recognize the tasks assigned to them by means of various forms of data (they learn from data). They recognize and understand the presented information, detect patterns and relationships, and formulate models that enable the system to accomplish tasks that only human intelligence was thought to execute. The learning capability from experiences makes ML a prime candidate for a highly complex challenge in oncology, where data volume and heterogeneity, such as genes, high-resolution medical images, etc.

1. **Supervised Learning:** These days, machines can learn from data, recognize patterns, and even make predictions out of previously unseen patient data. When a model is supposed to be "trained," it is given sample data that has been tagged with outcomes that can be defined. For example, a patient's data can be labeled as 'cancer' or 'no cancer' given a supervised prediction of an outcome. Using supervised data, a model can learn to make predictions by mapping and then generalizing to unseen data. In general, supervised tasks can be understood in two types.
    - **Classification:** An aim of a classifier is to assign a certain tag to a given input. For instance, classifying a skin lesion into one of the seven groups (benign, keratosis, melanoma, etc.), determining the class of a breast cancer as 'benign' or 'malignant', and recognizing a tumor's tissue of origin.
    - **Regression:**Trying to find the optimal dosage of a drug, the probability of cancer recurrence and especially a patient's life expectancy in months heavily revolves around the smooth, efficient prediction of a continuous numerical value.

2. **Unsupervised Learning:** Though supervised learning deals with labeled data sets, this paradigm distinguishes itself using unlabeled data. No instructions are provided, and the algorithm dives headfirst into the data looking for concealed patterns, structures, or relationships. Patterns and relationships in the data often lead to the discovery of relationships that would otherwise not be apparent, such as in the case of clustering that is a primary tool in oncology, where patients are sub typed according to molecular and clinical features. Data discovery techniques are common in medical data to discover novel sub-types of diseases, as in new-onset adult diabetes, to refine prognostication and treatment approaches. Other commonly used tools are dimensionality reduction, a method that deals with complex data sets with genomic data that is high dimensional.
3. **Reinforcement Learning:** This type of learning uses a reward system for a computer 'agent' to evaluate and take a series of actions in an environment and score a maximum reward. The agent learns by trying different actions and getting feedback in the form of rewards or punishments. Less frequent in direct clinical diagnosis, reinforcement learning has been helpful in streamlining real-time treatment strategies and tailoring cancer screening intervals to a patient over time.

A TOUR OF KEY MACHINE LEARNING ALGORITHMS

Different types of 'shallow' and 'deep' architectures in machine learning come in distinct and wide-ranging forms and there are a great many algorithms in the field (Hajjar et al., 2024). The type of algorithm is chosen depending on the type of data and the clinical problem, and on the trade-off between accuracy and explainability.

Traditional "Shallow" Machine Learning Models

These models are designed to work with structured datasets in tabular format whereby the features are explicitly defined (e.g. age, tumor size or gene expression). These models form the basis for the majority of predictive models in medicine.

- **Decision Trees (DTs):**The models form a veritable tree of choices. Each internal node is a feature test (e.g., "Is platelet count <150?), and each branch is an outcome of the test which leads to the prediction at the leaf nodes. Their chief advantage is high interpretability. The sequence of steps taken along the tree provides a simple, rule-based rationale for the prediction.
- **Random Forest (RF):** This method is an extension of individual decision trees. Instead of a single tree, during training a Random Forest builds a deci-

sion forest, and during inference, outputs the class which is the mode of the classes (classification) or the average prediction (regression) of all the trees. This reduces overfitting which is a problem with single decision trees, and usually improves accuracy, which is how it was used to predict the risk of breast cancer and leukemia.

- **Support Vector Machines (SVMs):** An SVM is an impressive classification method that achieves its purpose through constructing an optimal hyper plane and separating classes of data points in a high dimensional space. The support vectors are the data points that are closest to the hyper plane. SVMs are particularly efficient in their field resolving classification problems that have distinct separation margins. Their applications have varied, spanning from breast cancer recurrence predictions to gene expression data analysis.
- Logistic Regression (LR): Logistic regression is a classifier that predicts the likelihood of a case's outcome (e.g., a malignant or benign diagnostic, (yes or no outcome), going beyond its nomenclature as a regression approach. It is commended for its simplicity of use and its ability to clearly explain the many elements of a model, particularly the coefficients of variables, which can show the degree of importance of specific risk factors. It also assesses the probability of an outcome.
- K-Nearest Neighbors (KNN): This simple, instance-based approach classifies new data points based on the plurality class of the point's "k" nearest neighbors in the feature space. It is often used as a baseline and in several cancer classification problems due to its simplicity.

Deep Learning: The Architecture of Intelligence

A shift from traditional machine learning to something more sophisticated is represented by deep learning (DL). Artificial neural networks (ANNs), which are more complex and made up of multiple "neurons" connected to one another on various levels, are the source of models. These networks are capable of learning hierarchical feature representations from unstructured data, including text, audio, and images. The automated extraction of features reduces or even eliminates feature engineering which is quite tedious and time intensive. This has become a game changer in the analysis of medical data.

- CNNs, or convolutional neural networks: In medical image analysis, convolutional neural networks handle the most demanding jobs. These networks are specifically designed to handle data that resembles a grid. They use "convolutional filters" that find relevant features by moving across a picture in several layers. While complex structures like tumor forms are identified and examined in the advanced levels, outlines and patterns are among the primitive aspects that are discovered and examined. When it comes to processing histopathology slides, categorizing skin lesions, diagnosing lung nodules in CT scans, and detecting breast cancer in mammograms, CNNs excel.

- Recurrent Neural Networks (RNNs): RNNs are specifically designed for sequential data, such as genetic or time-series clinical data from EHRs. RNNs can be used for context-sensitive tasks like predicting the course of an illness because of its "memory" modules. They can also be used to evaluate time-ordered clinical-activity sequences.
- **Graph Neural Networks (GNNs):** Given the interconnected nature of biomedical data, GNNs can effectively model such data as graphs (networks of nodes and edges). This is particularly useful for drug discovery, where molecules can be represented as graphs consisting of atoms and bonds, or for modeling protein-protein interactions. The Knowledge-augmented Graph Machine Learning (KaGML) paradigm uses GNNs in a novel way by incorporating external knowledge graphs for improving predictions, a notable enhancement for precision medicine.
- **Transformers and Vision Transformers (ViT):** Initially built for working with natural language, the Transformer architecture employs a feature known as "attention" to assess the significance of manifold aspects of the input information. This architecture has been changed to accommodate vision tasks as Vision Transformers (ViTs), which have outstandingly performed image classification tasks, even in determining breast cancer, by transcending local dependencies and capturing global relations across an entire image.
- **Generative AI and Large Language Models (LLMs):** Recent advancements in deep learning include training large neural networks on large text and image datasets available on the Internet. ChatGPT and other large language models (LLMs) can produce human-like text, summarize text documents, and write computer code. In the healthcare domain, LLMs have the potential to summarize clinical documents and other scientific literature. However, their usefulness can be undermined by a serious defect; they have the propensity to "hallucinate" and produce detailed, convincing answers that are completely inaccurate. Because of this, LLMs cannot be used alone in important clinical situations. There must be systems that attach real grounding verification to LLMs outputs, such as the CER system designed for biomedical LLM fact-checking.

The Practical Workflow: From Raw Data to Clinical Insight

To ensure a clinical ML model (Dankwa-Mullan & Weeraratne, 2022) is accurate, robust, and reliable, its development must follow a clearly defined, methodical pipeline

1. **Data Collection and Preprocessing:** To start with, one needs to obtain high-quality datasets. Raw data is usually noisy, with a great deal of pre-processing to be done, such as addressing missing values, normalizing numerical features to a common scale, or encoding categorical variables (for example, converting 'male'/'female' to machine-readable format). For imaging data, one more pre-processing methods may include resizing, contrast stretching, and artifact removal.
2. **Data Augmentation:** Obtaining large and well annotated datasets can be challenging in medicine. One way to address this is to use data augmentation to artificially expand the training set by creating modified copies of data (i.e., rotating or flipping an image). This helps the model to be more robust and counters overfitting, when the model memorizes the training data without learning to generalize.
3. **Feature Selection and Engineering:** Choosing the most predictive features is pivotal for classical ML models. Techniques such as Recursive Feature Elimination (RFE) improves model performance and interpretability by systematically selecting the most significant variables from a large pool.
4. **Model Training and Validation:** Training, validation, and testing are the three parts of preprocessed data. The model finds patterns in the training set while it is being trained. The validation set is used to modify the model hyperparameters, such as the number of estimators in a Random Forest. The next stage is to use the enclosed test set to estimate the model's performance in real-world applications. This is a true gauge of the model's efficacy.
5. **Transfer Learning:** Using transfer learning is invaluable for deep learning especially when the available data is limited. This involves taking a model pre-trained on a big dataset such as ImageNet, which consists of millions of general images, and fine-tuning it on a smaller, targeted medical dataset. The model uses the general visual features it learned previously, like edges, shapes, and textures, and modifies them for the medical task, enhancing efficacy.
6. **Evaluation Metrics:** Statistical measures can determine how a model performs. Accuracy (the percentage of correct predictions) seems like an intuitive metric at first but can be misleading on imbalanced datasets (e.g., where 99% of cases are benign). Hence, other measures become vital: precision (the proportion of positive predictions that were actually correct), recall or sensitivity (the proportion of actual positives that were correctly identified), and the F1-score

(the harmonic mean of precision and recall). The AUC-ROC (Area Under the Receiver Operating Characteristic) curve is another widely used metric that summarizes a classifier's performance at all thresholds.

To sum up, the transformative impact of machine learning on the scientific and clinical frameworks for addressing cancer is profound, and the array of machine learning tools at our disposal remains invaluable. Understanding the fundamentals—learning paradigms, algorithms, practical workflows, and assessment metrics—enables us to harness the complete possible transformative impact of machine learning on the future of cancer care to make it more predictive, precise, and personalized for every patient.

HISTORICAL EVOLUTION AND ADOPTION OF AI IN HEALTH CARE

From Aspiration to Application: The Genesis of AI in Medicine

Giving computers human-like intelligence is undoubtedly not a novel idea. The phrase "artificial intelligence" (AI), which refers to the study of enabling robots to do jobs requiring human intellect, was first used at the Dartmouth Summer Workshop in 1956. Early on, the vision was remarkable, including everything from problem-solving to natural language interaction. Joseph Weizenbaum created one of the earliest attempts at conversational AI in 1966 with ELIZA, a program that pretended to be a psychiatrist by substituting keywords. It was an early and promising concept of machine language interaction, even though it was not a learning system by today's standards.

This restriction brought to light the need for more significant changes in the industry: intelligent systems should learn on their own instead of being programmed in a traditional way. Machine learning emerged as a result of this need. In this new paradigm, algorithms develop their own predictive frameworks by learning to identify patterns in data. The first major step toward today's data-centric AI was the application of early machine learning methods like Artificial Neural Networks (ANNs), Support Vector Machines (SVMs), and Decision Trees.

These models offered promising opportunities in patient classification and outcome prediction and opened doors for more advanced innovations. The predictive models themselves, however, faced SKE, as opaque 'black box' models (Azenkot et al., n.d.) triggered a parallel, four-decade pursuit of Symbolic Knowledge Extraction (SKE) methods aimed at converting the sub-symbolic knowledge of trained models into rules.

The Deep Learning Revolution: A Paradigm Shift in the 2010s

AI in healthcare can be understood in two eras: pre-and post-deep learning revolution (Ijaz & Wozniak, 2024) in the 2010s. Although ANNs had been proposed since the 1940s, the absence of the critical data and the massive computing resources to train them hampered their use. The first three factors of "big data" from the internet and digitized medical records, the new advanced parallelized computing offered by powerful Graphics Processing Units (GPUs), and novel deep learning architectures provided the crucial shift.

The development of medical AI technology has fundamentally changed with "deep learning" methods owing to the invention of neural networks consisting of multiple layers. Among the newer architectures, the Convolutional Neural Network (CNN) has made the most impact. As CNNs are modeled after the human visual cortex, they excel in the interpretation of medical imagery. Beginning around 2015, numerous studies documented CNNs capabilities in performing tasks such as breast cancer detection on mammograms, skin lesion classification on dermoscopic images, and lung nodule identification on CT scans with a level of accuracy comparable to, and in some cases exceeding, that of human specialists.

Deep learning advancements were not limited to imaging alone (Carriero et al., 2024). The advent of multi-omics technologies resulted in a data deluge in genomics, proteomics, and metabolomics. Subsequently, the integration of various deep learning models became necessary for unified prediction of cancer subtypes, cancer prognosis, and drug response. The ability to learn from multimodal data—integrating imaging, pathology, genomics, and clinical data—was a remarkable step in attaining a comprehensive, personalized perspective on an individual patient's disease. The volume of publications in this domain witnessed stellar growth between 2015 and 2020, indicating a shift in the perception of AI from a niche academic curiosity to a burgeoning entity within mainstream medical research.

A. The Validation Pathway and Regulatory Hurdles

An AI model has to show its clinical validity to show clinical readiness. This is typically a multi-step process with increasing levels of complexity:

1. **Internal Validation:** Evaluating the model on a held-out test set from the same data source used for training.
2. **External Validation:** Testing the model on completely independent datasets, often from different hospitals or patient populations, to assess its generalizability.
3. **Prospective Testing:** Evaluating the model in a real-time clinical setting, often in a "silent" run-in period, to see how it performs on current patients.

4. **Randomized Controlled Trials (RCTs):** The gold standard, where patients are randomized to receive care with or without the AI intervention to directly measure its impact on clinical endpoints.

Validation pathways can bottleneck progress. A systematic review of the deep learning literature on medical imaging identified thousands of publications reporting strong performance metrics. However, there were only a few prospective studies and a meager two published randomized controlled trials.

In order for an AI tool to be legally marketed as a medical device, it must first obtain regulatory approval from the U.S Food and Drug Administration (FDA). The FDA started approving AI/ML-integrated medical devices in the last decade, with more than 300 devices approved by the early 2020s, most of which are in the field of radiology. These devices serve very narrow, focused functions, like automated lesion segmentation, pulmonary nodule detection, and screening mammogram triage to streamline the workflow of radiologists. The Clinical Laboratory Improvement Amendments (CLIA) certification, which has a lower regulatory threshold than typical U.S. regulations, has become the standard for regulatory approval for laboratory-developed tests (LDTs) including many ML liquid biopsy tests. The different, and still evolving, regulations in the U.S. and the rest of the world, create a perplexing environment for developers and for clinicians.

Computers-aided detection (CAD) Software in mammography also provides a cautionary example for the history of AI adoption. After 1998's FDA approval, CAD software was widely adopted, yet a large observational study later found that in practice, this software had failed to improve the accuracy of mammography. Radiologists' behaviors had changed over the years, and the original evaluation data had older film mammograms that were subsequently removed. This reinforces the importance of post-market surveillance and ongoing evaluation to ensure that the AI tools achieve the anticipated post-market advantages.

Maturation of the Field: Addressing the Human and Ethical Dimensions

The latest AI developments brought in a wave of excitement as new tools were made available for use in healthcare. However, excitement is not as high in advanced stages of tools because of the need of considering the human and ethical side of the technologies. The shift in emphasis has extended from the construction of precise models to the design of dependable AI frameworks.

A. The Imperative of Explainable AI (XAI)

One major issue is the "black-box problem." Clinicians are reluctant to accept a prediction that lacks an explanation. This has led to the development of Explainable AI (XAI)—a branch of AI focused on making model decisions transparent. Techniques such as Grad-CAM, which produces heatmaps illustrating a convolutional neural network's focus areas within an image, and SHAP, which assesses and assigns values to the input variables used in making a prediction, are becoming routine in the validation and interpretation of complex models. Explainability is an essential element of trust and must be provided to the clinicians in order to successfully translate the models into clinical practice.

B. Confronting Bias and Ensuring Health Equity

Addressing the decline of health equity fueled by the integration of AI and ML technologies into the economy is critical. Machine learning models analyze and learn from historical data. If that data is biased, machine learning models will learn those biases. The healthcare industry has chronic problems with data unrepresentativeness and the absence of racial and ethnic minorities, the poor, and other marginalized groups in the clinical trials and genomic databases. Highly biased AI systems will fails to generalize predicts for underrepresented groups and will inequitable distribute the benefits of precision medicine. Solutions to these complex problems must be executed in multiple concurrent ways. Opting varied and inclusive strategies in clinical data generation and the inclusion of marginalized groups in clinical data. Third, fairness in AI or machine learning models needs to be established, through the evaluation of performance metrics across disparate demographic groups. Finally, the inclusion of social determinants of health as variables in predictive AI systems will account for some of inequity gaps in the predictive and outcome models of disparate social and environmental factors.

C. The Human-in-the-Loop: Collaboration and Co-Design

As AI continues to be implemented in various fields of healthcare, there remains a universal understanding; AI will be used as a supplement to human clinicians rather than a replacement. The most successful AI applications in healthcare integrate seamlessly into clinical processes, working as a facilitator in clinician decision-making rather than a replacement. For this reason, there has been a shift to designing systems with Human-Centered Design (HCD) principles, which involve end-users—physicians, nurses, and patients—early in the planning and designing stages. Take the SHARE-C robot for example. Staff and patients of a hospital in

Lebanon were interviewed to inform the robot's design, features, communication style, and other contextual configurations to suit the hospital's cultural and contextual needs. Collaboration of this kind, which is also incorporated into holistic governance and multidisciplinary team structures, is vital for building AI systems that are clinically meaningful in addition to being technically competent.

The history of AI in medicine has gone through cycles of hype and disillusionment, but we feel that the progress of the last decade is different. It is more grounded, driven by data and more acutely responsive to the real-world complexities of medicine. There has been a shift in the focus of our aspirations, moving away from the monolithic universal "thinking machine" to the more practical and incremental creation of specialized, accepted, and explainable instruments that solve precise clinical problems. As the future unfolds, the history of this domain reminds us that the most significant impediment—and therefore, the most significant opportunity— lies not in the sophistication of the algorithms, but in the ethical and judicious integration of the algorithms into the intricate tapestry of human health and the healing process.

RELEVANCE OF MACHINE LEARNING IN PRECISION ONCOLOGY

From One-Size-Fits-All to N-of-One: The Promise of Precision Oncology

Historically, oncology practice has followed a "one-size-fits-all" model. Cancers were largely categorized by the organ they originated from and their histological appearance. Treatment decisions were made based on clinical trials that determined the best average response to treatment for a large and heterogeneous population, which, while life-saving for many, was rather frustrating—one patient might have a remarkable response to a treatment that was completely ineffective, or even harmful, for another patient with an identical diagnosis. The lack of consideration for the biological and pathological variance within and between the different types of cancers, and the different individual patients, was the fundamental flaw of this model.

With the initiation of precision medicine, and more specifically, precision oncology, there is a new paradigm shift in 2011 vision of precision medicine. It is a new and innovative approach that focuses on the unique medical treatment and prevention of an individual. The core concept of precision oncology is that no two tumors are the same. Each one is composed of its own unique set of genetic alterations, epigenetic changes, and dysfunctional molecular pathways. The objective is to transcend the clinical and organ based understanding of cancer to a more robust and medical definition at the molecular and genetic level. This enables a more precise selection of treatment options aimed at the targeted exploitation of the most and least sensitive areas of the tumor to an intensive direct attack, thus preserving healthy tissues.

This ambitious vision has a monumental challenge to overcome: data. Each tumor has a complex set of factors such as a unique genomic profile, transcriptomic signature, proteomic landscape, and interactions with the immune system, all of which contribute to data so vast and complex that it challenges human analysis. This is where the significance of Machine Learning (ML) becomes indispensable. ML is the computing power that converts large, multidimensional and complex data sets in oncology to clinically useful information which makes the promise of precision medicine a reality.

Decoding Complexity: How Machine Learning Powers Precision Oncology

Machine learning translates the raw data of a patient's cancer into a personalized clinical approach a clinician can use. Its significance is not limited to a singular function. It spans the entirety of the precision oncology pipeline—from molecular characterization to the selection of treatments and even to the discovery of drugs.

A. Molecular Characterization and Biomarker Discovery

At the core of precision oncology lies the need to characterize a tumor with precision on a molecular level. Machine learning algorithms are especially good at pattern recognition within complex high dimensional omics data to demonstrate cancer subtype recognition. It also help in predicting the clinical outcome.

- **Discovering Novel Subtypes:** Unsupervised learning techniques like clustering analyze thousands of patients' gene expression or methylation data to uncover new subtypes of cancer. These classifications tend to be more prognostically relevant than older histology-based classifications, facilitating better patient stratification. Machine learning, for instance, has identified new subgroups within adult-onset diabetes, which presents proof of concept for similar applications within cancer.
- **Identifying Predictive Biomarkers:** A key objective of precision oncology is determining which biomarkers (Maurya et al., 2023) predict response to therapy, whether it is a gene mutation, a certain protein, or something else entirely. Through machine learning (ML), one can use clinical trial multiomics data to determine complex, multi-gene signatures that far exceed the predictive capabilities of single-omics markers. ML has been used to create a classifier-trained genomic profile to predict resistance to immunotherapy

in melanoma patients. Also, a comprehensive bioinformatics approach employing various ML techniques (K-means clustering, neural networks, Naïve Bayes) on data from the TCGA enabled the identification of a constellation of 21 genes associated with lymph node metastasis in prostate cancer, which provided diagnostic biomarkers and a bio-mechanistic understanding of the metastasis process.

B. Predicting Treatment Response and Personalizing Therapy

One of the most direct uses of machine learning (ML) in precision oncology is forecasting whether a patient will respond to a given treatment. This helps clinicians stop using the trial-and-error method of treatment selection. They can choose the optimal therapy right away and spare patients the burden, both financially and in side effects, of wasting several ineffective therapies.

- **Guiding Targeted Therapy and Immunotherapy:** Many cancer therapies are effective for only a limited number of patients. Machine learning algorithms can meld varied data streams—imaging, pathology, genomics, and clinical history—in order to construct a "digital twin" of a patient and estimate their probability of responding to a targeted therapy. For instance, in non-small cell lung cancer, researchers have constructed a multimodal model with radiology, pathology, and genomic data to foresee the response to PD-(L) 1 blockade immunotherapy. In another study, researchers designed a Random Forest algorithm that works on multi-feature MRI data from the I-SPY2 clinical trials, and used it to predict, with a high degree of accuracy, the response to neoadjuvant chemotherapy in patients with breast cancer.
- **Radiation Sensitivity Prediction:** ML helps in personalizing radiotherapy. Based on radiomic features (patterns extracted quantitatively from imaging techniques) and genomic information, some models can ascertain whether a tumor is sensitive or resistant to radiation. This can inform whether clinicians should escalate or de-escalate radiation for a particular patient.
- **Computational Pathology for Treatment Selection:** Deep learning models have the ability to assess conventional H&E-stained pathology slides to forecast important predictive molecular characteristics for treatment, for example, microsatellite instability (MSI) and tumor mutational burden (TMB). This "virtual staining" would eliminate the requirement for additional costly molecular testing and would allow large patient populations to be pre-screened for eligibility for biomarker-driven clinical trials, which in turn would expedite new therapeutic innovations.

C. Enhancing Prognosis and Risk Stratification

Classic cancer staging systems, such as AJCC TNM classification, assign patients to large buckets based on tumor size, whether lymph nodes are involved, and if metastasis has occurred. While these systems serve a purpose, they are still a gross underestimation of a patients real risk. The use of ML allows the development of more sophisticated and precise prognostic models.

- **Beyond TNM Staging:** Incorporating diverse elements like clinical information, genomic classifiers (for instance, Decipher score in prostate cancer), and radiomic signatures, ML models help generate a personalized risk score to better predict outcomes such as recurrence and survival. Machine learning has been applied to develop prognostic systems for endometrial cancer that surpass the performance of older methods.
- **Dynamic Risk Profiling:** As cancer develops, machine learning (ML) models, especially those leveraging Recurrent Neural Networks (RNNs), hold the potential to analyze longitudinal data, which includes CT scans and liquid biopsies performed over intervals. This opens the potential to meticulously refine risk profiles, allowing the real-time modification of prognosis and treatment as a patient responds to therapy, and ultimately facilitates more responsive and personalized treatment.

D. Accelerating Drug Discovery and Clinical Trial Design

Machine Learning is useful to all the stages of the therapeutic pipeline especially drug discovery and development. This is a part of the pipeline where time and money required with the conventional approaches are exceedingly high.

- **Target Identification and Drug Design:** The impact of machine learning on preclinical research is profound. AI models have the ability to review biological networks and multi-omics data to discover new drug targets overlooked by conventional approaches. Innovative methods such as Knowledge-augmented Graph Machine Learning (KaGML) stand out. KaGML models treat molecules as graphs and enhance them with biomedical knowledge to predict drug-target interactions and drug-drug interactions. These models can also invent new molecules with tailored therapeutic attributes.
- **Optimizing Clinical Trials:** Artificial intelligence technologies increase the efficiency, effectiveness and equity of clinical trials. Machine learning algorithms can optimize patient cohort selection by targeting individuals who are most likely to respond to the investigational drug, thus improving statistical

power. AI will enhance the accessibility and integration of diverse real-world data captured in electronic health records, allowing for trials that better represent the diversity of the patient population and tackle inequities in healthcare.

Navigating the Path to Clinical Reality: Trust, Ethics, and Governance

In order for ML to achieve its fullest potential in precision oncology, it must be integrated into everyday clinical practice. The movement from research to reality incorporates more than just a technical challenge; it is also a human and ethical challenge centered around the trustworthiness of AI and its applications.

A. The Necessity of Explainable AI (XAI)

Ethics guidelines stipulate that clinicians should not base decisions involving life-altering interventions on "black-box" AI models that fail to shed light on their workings. Therefore, the use ML in precision oncology largely stems from translation. The demand for Explainable AI is rapidly growing. SHAP and comparable technologies have gained popularity in the industry for constructing simple, feature-aware explanations for a model's predictions. As an example, clinicians reviewing SHAP output for a leukemia risk model can see which features (e.g., high platelet counts, male gender) were most important in the model's high-risk prediction for that specific patient. Interpretability is not optional; it is a necessary condition to ensure the accountability, safety, and trust required for clinical adoption.

B. Health Equity and Data Diversity

For precision medicine to truly serve its purpose, it needs to be precise for every individual.One of the foremost ethical challenges is exposure of machine learning models to disparate health inequities. If a machine learning model is built with training data unrepresentative of all the necessary demographics, it is likely to be inaccurate for the model's minority or neglected populations. This is one of the reasons the advocacy for diversity in clinical trials needs to be coupled with developing models using datasets from a particular region. And this to ensure all underserved patients, all demographics, can access the advancements in AI-powered precision medicine oncology.

C. Governance and Robustness

For ML to be clinically adopted, strong governance frameworks prioritizing the accuracy, safety, and dependability of the ML models are essential. Governance frameworks develop models that can withstand adversarial attacks and misdiagnosis. Governance models analyze and verify multi-institutional and real-world data. Constructing adversary-aware models that clinch to the standards of ML governance is needed to facilitate safe clinical deployment.

From One-Size-Fits-All to N-of-One: The Paradigm Shift in Cancer Care

Oncology practice has historically operated under a paradigm that was limited in its reasoning. Cancers were classified and treated simply based on their site of origin—lung, breast, colon—and upon their histological appearance. Treatment was based on clinical trials that captured the best average response for a cohort that was large and heterogeneous. This "one-size-fits-all" construct was blunt in a contest that needed the precision of a scalpel. It left treatments with a peculiar pattern of efficacy, wherein a subset of patients manifested a striking response, while others with a similar diagnosis, faced a complete response, with added toxicity. The major flaw of this construct was the neglect of the considerable biological diversity that exists in various types of cancers, and most critically, the differences among patients.

Shifting from conventional approaches to precision medicine, and especially precision oncology, is not only necessary but also a positive development within the field. Every person, along with their treatment and prevention strategies, should be considered. What makes precision oncology different is the recognition that every tumor is different. Each tumor is governed and shaped by a different combination of dysregulations and unique mutations. The goal is to move past the organ-based classification systems towards a deeper and more comprehensive molecular understanding of a patient's cancer. This will help clinicians to choose customized treatments that are designed to focus on the most sensitive regions of the tumor and protect the healthy tissues adjacent to the cancerous mass.

This ambitious vision certainly has one major obstacle: the data (Varlamova et al., 2024). The very nature of a tumor's individuality—its specific genomic, transcriptomic, and proteomic information as well as its relationship with the immune system—creates a volume of data that is too complex for a human to analyze. This is where the relevance of Machine Learning (ML) comes into play. ML is the only technology available that can automate the required computations needed to convert high-dimensional data from the field of oncology into clinically relevant information. It can make the promise of precision medicine much more realistic. It helps

LSAC MLP to identify the signal amidst all the biological information and diffuse data to produce a more defined model of personalized medicine for a given patient.

Decoding Complexity: How Machine Learning Powers Precision Oncology

You wouldn't know it from the breadth of precision oncology efforts (Zhang et al., 2023), but deep learning plays a singularly important role in transforming disparate complex patient cancer data into actionable patient-specific clinical plans. It deep learns the entirety of the precision oncology (Bhinder et al., 2021) value chain, from deep molecular characterization and therapy selection to gap-driven innovative drug discovery.

A. Molecular Characterization and Biomarker Discovery

Being able to pinpoint and identify the most fundamental and basic building blocks of a tumor formation serves as the core of the foundation in precision oncology. The application of ML algorithms is highly regarded in distinguishing high-dimensional omics data. Moreover, ML algorithms identify and discern patterns that determine the cancer subtype and its potential clinical pathways.

- **Discovering Novel Subtypes:** Techniques for unsupervised learning, particularly clustering, evaluate thousands of patients' gene expression or methylation data in order to identify novel subtypes of cancer (Khandaker et al., 2024). Such classifications, based purely on data, often surpass conventional histological classifications in terms of prognosis, resulting in a more accurate patient stratification and improved insight into the disease's natural history.
- **Identifying Predictive Biomarkers:** Identifying biomarkers such as a gene mutation or a protein expression level that predicts a patient's response to a targeted therapy is a cornerstone of precision oncology. Machine Learning (ML) models can examine data from clinical trials (Ayad et al., 2025; Hajjar et al., 2024) that use multiple approaches to uncover complex multi-gene signatures that are exponentially more predictive than single markers. For example, ML has been applied to predict the resistance of melanoma patients to certain therapies by creating a classifier-trained genomic immunophenotype. In an influential study focused on prostate cancer, the use of various ML methods (K-means clustering, neural networks, and Naïve Baye's) to conduct bioinformatics analyses on TCGA data successfully identified a validated set of 21 genes that were later shown to be associated with the metastatic spread of the disease to the cancer-bearing lymph nodes. The amplification of two

of these genes, SPAG1 and PLEKHF2 (Cutillo et al., 2020), was significantly linked to a decline in patient survival, which indicates that these genes are likely key prognostic biomarkers.

B. Predicting Treatment Response and Personalizing Therapy

Machine learning has the most interesting impact on precision oncology in predicting responses to individual treatments. Clinicians can skip much of the trial-and-error process and start with the most likely effective therapy.

Guiding Targeted Therapy and Immunotherapy: A limited number of patients see benefits from many contemporary cancer medications (Zhang et al., 2023). Machine learning (ML) makes it possible to Process and combine disparate types of data of varying modalities—imaging, pathology, genomics, and other clinical data—to create a personalized comprehensive digital twin. ML predicts whether a patient will respond to a given medication. For instance, in non-small cell lung cancer, a multimodal model comprising radiology and pathology and genomic data has been constructed to predict responses to PD-(L)1 blockade immunotherapy. Likewise, within the I-SPY2 clinical trials, a Random Forest model applied to multi-feature MRI data could successfully predict the pathological complete response to neoadjuvant chemotherapy in patients with breast cancer, thus ML demonstrates the ability to predict success of a given treatment.

The Human Imperative: Trust, Ethics, and the Goal of Improving Survival

In order for machine learning to reach its highest capacity within precision oncology, it needs to be integrated into everyday clinical practice effectively and ethically. This change involves more than just technical difficulties; it involves the human factor of establishing dependable AI and showing its positive impact on outcomes. The complexity and "black box" nature of these models can be problematic. Without the reasoning behind model's prediction, a clinician simply cannot make a life-altering decision based on it. This has led to the development of Explainable AI (XAI), which provides clarity into model decisions and explains AI-generated insights using SHAP, Grad-CAM, and other techniques. Transparency remains a prerequisite for accountability, safety, and the clinical trust required for adoption.

Figure 2. Federated Learning- I (icons from internet sources)

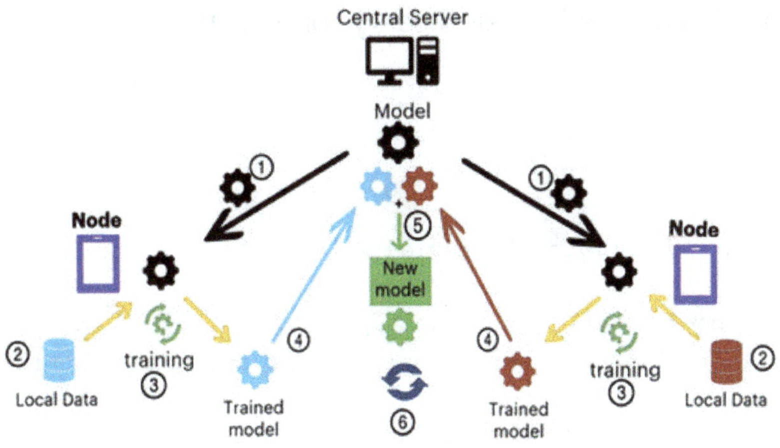

Figure 3. Federated Learning- II (icons from internet sources)

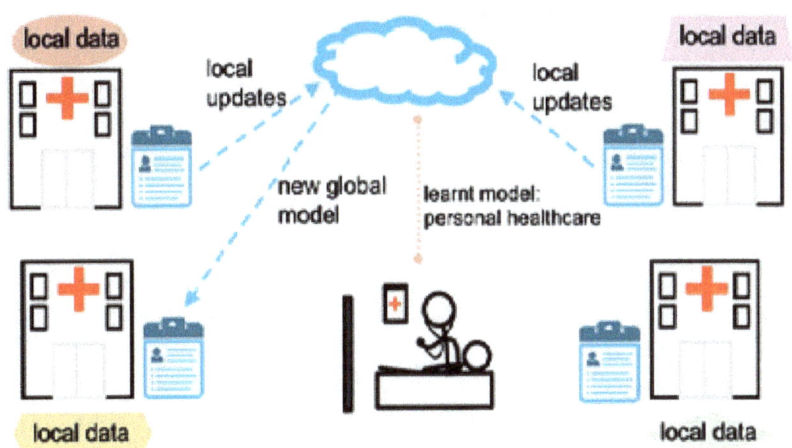

Shared model is trained on server to create generic models, sent to clients.

These are some of the algorithm developed for finding the probability of benign cell to be cancerous:

Algorithms

Algorithm 1: Determine if a cell is benign or malignant

```
   Inputs: cell Datasets
   Outputs: Status of Cancerous cells

   Algorithm: IdentifyCellStatus(data)
   {
   Step1: Accept the cell data as input
   Step2: Initialize counters for malignant and benign attri-
butes. Set both to zero.
          benign_ctr=0,malignant_ctr =0
   Step3: Examine the data for specific characteristics like
cellsize, shape, nucleus attributes,  texture, mitosis-count
and more by executing the algorithm ExamineDataChar(Data, Be-
nign_ctr, malignanat_ctr) mentioned in step 3.1
             Step3.1: Algorithm  ExamineDataChar(data, benign_
ctr,  malignant_ctr)
          {
              For each cell  in Cell dataset
                 {
                    If (the cell's size indicates a benign at-
tribute)
                    Then  "Increment the benign_ctr"
                    If(The cells's shape suggests a Malignant
attribute)
                     Then " Increment the malignant_ctr"
                           //…(similar evaluations of other
characteristics)
          }} End of Algorithmic substeps
   Step 4: Repeat the examination process for additional attri-
butes such as gene expression, celladhesion, immune response
and DNArepair by executing the algorithm FurtherExamineData(da-
ta, benign_ctr,malignant_ctr)
   Mentioned in step 4.1
          Step 4.1: AlgorithmFurtherExamineData(Data, benign_
ctr, malignanat_ctr)
          {
```

```
For each cell in the data
    {
If gene expression pattern towards malignancy
        Malignant_ctr +=1;
    If(cell adhension properties lean towards a benign characteristic)
    Then benign_ctr +=1
        //…(similar evaluation of other attributes)
}} End of algorithms sub-steps.
```

Step 5: Based on the collected attribute assessments determine if a cell is classified as benign or malignanat by executing the Algorithm DisplayCellStatus(benign_ctr, malignant_ctr) mentioned in step 5.1

```
Step 5.1 Algorithm DisplayCellStatus(benign_ctr, malignant_ctr)
{
 If (malignant_ctr >>benign_ctr)
 Then Display("The cell is categorized as malignanat")
Else
        Display("The cell is categorized as benign")
```

Step6: Display the total count of identified benign and malignant attributes by executing the algorithm mentioned in step 6.1.

```
Step 6.1 Algorithm DisplayTotalAttributes(benign_ctr,malignanat_ctr)
{
  Display("total identified benign attributes", benignCounter);
  Display(Total identified malignant attributes",malignant_ctr)
} //…End of Algorithm substeps
```

Step7:end of Algorithm

}//End of IdentifycellStatus Algorithm

Algorithm 2: Probability of a benign cell to be cancerous.

```
Inputs: Cells from Dataset
Outputs: Probability of the cell to be cancerous

Algorithm EstimateCancerLikelihood(cellInfo)
{
        Step1: Input cellInfo  obtained from Dataset.
        Step2:Initialize approximately 20 variables for cell features/parameters.
        Step 3:For each feature in the cell set the following values
                Set its value between 1 and 4. //(1 and 2 for healthy cells, 3 and 4 for Malignant cells)
        Step4: Identifying cell with potential for malignancy.
        Step 5: Identifying cells with potential for healthiness.
        Step 6: Calculating probability of Cell healthiness and Malignancy.
                Step6.1 count parameters with values 1 or 2.
                Step 6.2: Calculate and store the probability percentage of cell healthiness.
                Step 6.3 Count Parameters with values 3 or 4.
                Step 6.4: Calculate and store the probability percentage of complete cell malignancy.
        Step7:Calculate the probability of benign cells turning malignant.
        Step 8:Calculate the probability of malignant cells turning benign.
} //…End of Algorithm
```

Algorithm 3. Probability of a lung cell to be cancerous.

```
Inputs: Lung cells data from Dataset
Outputs: Probability of the lung cell to be cancerous
```

```
Algorithm EstimateLungCellCancerLikelihood(cellData)
{
          Step1: Input cellData retrived from  the dataset.
          Step2:Inilialize 6 variables to represent lung cells
attributes, all initially set to 0.
          Step3:Initialize a variable called cacerLikelihood
and set it to 0.
          Step4: Analyzing the cell parameters and adjusting
cancer Likelihood.
                    Step4.1: If the cell size is over 15
                              Then "increment CancerLikelihood by
1".
                    Step4.2: If cell size between 10 and 15
                              Then "  Increment Cancer Likelihood
by 0.75".
                    Step 4.3: Repeat similar assessment  and
adjustments  for other parameters.
   Step 5:Scaling cancerLikelihood by  afactor.Further Multiply
the variable cancerLikelihood by 25.
   Step 6:Store the calculated cancerLikelihood of the lung
cell in the cancerLikelihood variable.
   } //… End of the algorithm
```

CONCLUSION

Due to the growing capacity to collect, store, and exchange health-related data as well as the proliferation of genetic testing instruments, accuracy, the combination of public health and medicine will be very fruitful. Health risks assessed using a population's electronic health records and information from other data sources, allows for the identification of higher-risk subpopulations so that preventive measures can be directed towards them. Precision medicine will be properly integrated with preventive medicine and public health to avoid chronic diseases, improve quality of life, lower healthcare costs, and close healthcare gaps.

REFERENCES

Abbaoui, W., Retal, S., El Bhiri, B., Kharmoum, N., & Ziti, S. (2024). Towards revolutionizing precision healthcare: A systematic literature review of artificial intelligence methods in precision medicine. *Informatics in Medicine Unlocked, 46,* 101475.

Ayad, S., Al-jamimi, H. A., & ElKheir, A. (2025). Integrating advanced techniques RFE SVM feature engineering and Nelder-Mead optimized XGBoost for accurate lung cancer prediction. *IEEE Access : Practical Innovations, Open Solutions.*

Azenkot, T., Rivera, D. R., Stewart, M. D., & Patel, S. P. (n.d.). Artificial intelligence and machine learning innovations to improve design and representativeness in oncology clinical trials. *American Society of Clinical Oncology Educational Book.*

Bhinder, B., Gilvary, C., Madukar, N. S., & Element, O. (2021). Artificial intelligence in cancer research and precision medicine. *Cancer Discovery, 11*(4), 900–915.

Carriero, A., Gronhoff, L., Volginav, E., Basile, P., & Albera, M. (2024). Deep learning in breast cancer imaging: State of the art and recent advancement in early 2024. *Diagnostics (Basel), 14*(7), 848.

Cutillo, C. M., Sharma, K. R., Foschini, L., Kundu, S., Mackintosh, M., & Mandl, K. D. (2020). Machine intelligence in healthcare: Perspectives on trustworthiness, explainability, usability, and transparency. npj. *Digital Medicine, 3*, 47.

Dankwa-Mullan, I., & Weeraratne, D. (2022). Artificial intelligence and machine learning technologies in cancer care: Addressing disparities, bias, and data diversity. *Cancer Discovery, 12*(6), 1423–1427.

Hajjar, M., Albaradei, S., & Aldabagh, G. (2024). Machine learning approaches in multi-cancer early detection. *Information (Basel), 15*(11), 627.

Ijaz, M. F., & Wozniak, M. (2024). Editorial: Recent advances in deep learning and medical imaging for cancer treatment. *Cancers (Basel), 16*(4), 700.

Kann, B. H., Hosny, A., & Aerts, H. J. W. L. (2021). *Artificial intelligence for clinical oncology. Cell.* Elsevier.

Khandaker, S., & Almanuin, , M. AIslam, , M. MHossain, , KHassan Melon, , M. MJaved, , M. S. (2024). Unveiling early detection and prevention of cancer: Machine learning and deep learning approaches. *Education Administration: Theory and Practice, 30*(5), 14814–14828.

Kourou, K., Exarchos, K. P., Papaloukas, C., Sakaloglou, P., Exarchos, T., & Fotiadis, D. I. (2021). Title. *Computational and Structural Biotechnology Journal, 19*, 5546–5555.

Maurya, S., Tiwari, S., Mothukuri, M. C., Tangeda, C. M., Nandigam, R. N. S., & Addagiri, D. C. (2023). Title. *Biomedical Signal Processing and Control, 80*, 104398.

Shaikh, F. J., & Rao, D. S. (2022). Prediction of cancer disease using machine learning approach. *Materials Today: Proceedings, 50*, 40–47.

Shamsara, E., & Shamsara, J. (2020). Bio-informatics analysis of the genes involved in the extension of prostate cancer to adjacent lymph nodes by supervised and unsupervised machine learning methods: The role of SPAG1 and PLEKHF. *Genomics, 112*(5), 3871–3882.

Swanson, K., Wu, E., Zhang, A., Alizadeh, A. A., & Zou, J. (2023). From patterns to patients: Advances in clinical machine learning for cancer diagnosis, prognosis, and treatment. *Cell, 186*(9), 1772.

Varlamova, E. V., Butakova, M. A., Semyonova, V. V., Soldatav, S. A., Poltavskiy, A. V., Kit, O. I., & Soldatov, A. V. (2024). Machine learning meets cancer. *Cancers (Basel), 16*(6), 1100.

Zhang, B., Shi, H., & Wang, H. (2023). Machine learning and artificial intelligence in cancer prognosis, prediction and treatment selection: A critical approach. *Journal of Multidisciplinary Healthcare, 16*, 1779–1791.

Chapter 2
Role of Radiomics in the Diagnosis of Cancer

Syed Hasan Mehdi
https://orcid.org/0009-0002-6561-7434
Symbiosis Institute of Health Sciences, India

Milind Chunkhare
Symbiosis Institute of Health Sciences, India

Sushant Matre
Symbiosis Institute of Health Sciences, India

ABSTRACT

Radiomics has become a game changer in the field of cancer imaging. Because ordinary medical images can be transformed into measurable mineable information, they thus provide both diagnostic accuracy and precision to treatment planning. Radiomics automatically identifies hundreds to thousands of quantitative features that include tumor shape, texture, intensity, and spatial relationships. AI, especially machine learning and deep learning algorithms, allows automated feature selection, pattern recognition, and predictive modeling that have reliably shown better performance when compared to conventional diagnostics methods. Lung, breast, brain, liver, and pancreatic cancer case studies show remarkable diagnostic performance, with area under the curve values that commonly range above 0.90. Multi-modality radiomics methods have been proven better than single-modality methods. The clinical advantages relate to precision oncology enables, minimized invasive biopsy, reducing the cost of utilizing. However, there are issues such as variability and non-standardization in imaging protocol.

DOI: 10.4018/979-8-3373-4312-9.ch002

1. INTRODUCTION

Cancer is one of the significant causes of mortality and a challenging issue to life expectancy increments in all global countries. Estimates by the WHO in 2019 show that around the world cancer is now the leading or the second leading cause of death before the age of 70 years in 112 of 183 countries and in the remaining 23 countries cancer is the third or the fourth leading cause of death before the age of 70 years. Even though oncology has experienced an impressive array of innovations in the field, the increase in the burden of cancer is caused by such factors as aging populations, environmental exposure, and lifestyle. One of the major factors that can determine the prognosis of the cancer is the stage of the disease where it is identified. The timely and correct diagnosis can ensure a better outcome of the treatment, survival, and fewer costs in the healthcare industry (Osei-Afriyie et al., 2021; Gillies & Schabath, 2020).

Medical imaging plays a crucial role in detecting cancer, determining its stage, designing treatment approach and assessment of response. Conventionally the assessment of the radiological information was performed after a site- based assessment and subjective assessment of the information such as size, shape and contrast enhancement of a tumor., it has the limitation of lacking quantitative depth required for characterization of intra-tumoral heterogeneity. This gap between the visual interpretation and biological complexity is the main reason why radiomics has its justification (Gillies et al., 2016).

Radiomics helps to fill this gap by turning images into mathematically rich datasets which can be used to further characterize tumor heterogeneity than is visible to the human eye. Radiomics is a system that derives a very large number of quantitative characteristics of a standard medical image (such as CT, MRI or PET), using sophisticated algorithms, and statistical methods (Aerts et al., 2014).

By synthesizing insights from previous studies it can be seen that radiomics is not just a technological advancement, but rather a clinically necessary evolution towards precision oncology because Radiomics offers a useful, non-invasive approach to employ high dimensional mineable information in order to describe tumors with a greater level of detail by transforming imaging data. Radiomics can help in the prevention of advanced cancers, the stratification of risk of heavy-hitters and may also have the capability of replacing the molecular/histopathological data in cancer diagnostics. It is also potentially useful to distinguish between malignant lesions and benign lesions, not to mention gauging the agility of the tumor, and even forecasting treatment response (Parmar et al., 2015).

This chapter gives an idea of how radiomics has developed as a cancer detection tool,, the major principals involved in the context of using radiomics to detect cancer, the various current applications of radiomics to the different type of cancer and the problems associated with the validation of radiomics in addition to how it may eventually be integrated in routine workflow within clinical contexts with respect to precision medicine.

2. WHAT IS RADIOMICS?

Radiomics is a revolutionary innovation in the field of radiology and oncology research that helps to capture very large numbers of quantitative features from the radiographs (medical images) based on sophisticated data-characterization algorithms. These radiomic features are able to measure factors like intensity, shape, texture, and patterns in areas of interest, and provide information on the heterogeneity, morphology, and spatial complexity in various regions in the tissues that cannot be perceived by the human eye. Radiomics aims to convert these quantitative characteristics into useful information to diagnose, prognose, and plan the personalized treatment, especially in oncology. Radiomics allows non-invasive assessment of tumors or lesions throughout the volume based on the analysis of imaging data, and complementary or even superior values with respect to traditional clinical measurements or single-point biopsies (Mayerhoefer et al., 2020a).

Radiomics is not only limited to the diagnosis of diseases. Radiomics is also utilized to provide digitally labelled fingerprints of disease, such as disease progression, disease prognosis, and targeted therapy by integrating imaging characteristics with clinical, genomic, and proteomic evidence. Some of these include that radiomics has been effective in differentiations of benign and malignant lesions, survival prediction in lung cancer and phenotype of diseases; hence, when personalized medicine is used. Interestingly, these quantitative biomarkers can be used in patient stratification, virtual biopsies in tissues, and even in demonstrating the responses of the treatment at a much earlier stage than other conventional measures (Hong et al., 2024; Li et al., 2021).

Despite the potential, radiomics is facing various technical challenges which include imaging practices standardization, intense feature segmentation, feature reproduced repercussions, and preexisting reporting principles most radiomic model's translation into clinical routine necessitates concerted labour on harmonization, thoroughly accomplished automatic algorithms, and established report guiding lines. The ability of radiomics to further illuminate how diseases work and direct personalized care will continue to multiply as it continues to merge with artificial intelligence and with omics data, which is why it will have a significant place in the future of precision diagnosis and treatment. one of the biggest difficulties the radiomics research faces is the fact that Radiologists and computer scientists lack communication as their languages are separate (Li et al., 2021).

2.1 Feature-Based Radiomics

One area of radiomics is feature-based radiomics, which relates more precisely to the creation, search, and application of handcrafted quantitative features of medical images to describe tissues or lesions in a non-invasive manner. The assumption behind feature-based radiomics is that medical imaging has highly-quantitative information, which is a reflection of underlying pathophysiology and morphology of tissues and can be systematically represented using mathematical formulae. Instead of limiting to subjective visual analysis, it measures structures by deriving shape, intensity, texture and wavelet transformations features in regions of interest. These collections of features, which can frequently be in the hundreds, enable researchers and clinicians to construct predictive models that may contribute to the objective understanding of tumor biology, disease progression or therapy response or other clinically relevant endpoints (Magnin et al., 2025).

Radiomic features that are systematically categorizable are handcrafted. Basic statistics of the values of intensity, e.g. mean, variance, skew or kurtosis, are described by the first-order features. Shape features include geometrical information such as volume, sphericity or compactness and display the morphology of the lesion. The spatial relationships and heterogeneity of the pixel or voxel intensity can be revealed with the help of texture features, obtained based on complex matrices like gray-level co-occurrence matrix or run-length matrix, which can indicate the difference in the microenvironment of the tissue. Moreover, the higher-order characteristics can be obtained through the application of a filter, e.g. a wavelet filter or Laplacian of Gaussian, which uncovers another layer of information, i.e. concentrating on another frequency band or the scale of the image. These features are extracted, closing the gap between medical imaging and data science, with the result, a dataset (the radiomic signature), which can be subjected to statistical and machine learning methods to provide clinical decision support (Van Timmeren et al., 2020).

Building of feature-based radiomics model is done in a systemic pattern of steps that guarantee the validity and clinical applicability of the biomarkers thus obtained:

- Image Acquisition: The standardized protocols of image acquisition have been used to reduce technical variation between scanners and centers.
- Segmentation: Regions of interest (ROI) typically tumor or suspicious lesions are segmented with manual, semi-automatic or automatic technique. Proper and consistent segmentation is critical as all subsequent processing is dependent on it.
- Image Pre-Processing: Technological variability is minimized by the use of image normalization, resampling to regular voxel size, image denoising

and bias field correction which improve the consistency of features across datasets.

- Feature Extraction: Radiomics features are calculated on pre-processed and segmented ROI with software (e.g., PyRadiomics). Generally generates hundreds of measures of intensity, shape, texture and transformed spaces, which are quantitative in nature..
- Feature Selection and Reduction: This applies to decision-making data that is high-dimensional: data is reduced with respect to its statistical tests (correlation analysis, univariate filtering) and machine learning techniques (LASSO, PCA, recursive feature elimination) to remove redundant, irrelevant or unstable features.
- Model Development: The correct predictors are used to help in the development of a selected feature train predictive or prognostic model using classical machine learning algorithms (logistic regression, support-vector machines, random forests) as per clinical requirements (classification, regression, survival prediction).
- Model Validation: This high level of validation Robustness and generalizability are tested by train-test interval, cross-validation, and ideally, by externally-validated independent cohorts. Accuracy, AUC, sensitivity and specificity are all performance measures.
- Clinical and Biological Interpretation: This associates the features that were chosen with established histopathology, molecular profiles, or biological processes and increases the confidence of predicting models and insights.
- Multi-Modal Integration: Radiomic features are more effective when combined with the clinical, molecular, or other omics data because this design is able to improve and provide multilayered, patient-centered profiles.
- Lastly, external assessment, standardisation, and reporting against guidelines are sought to enable reproducibility and multicentric relationships, e.g. Image Biomarker Standardisation Initiative guidelines (Van Timmeren et al., 2020; Magnin et al., 2025).

2.2 Delta-Radiomics

Delta-radiomics is a sophisticated method which builds upon the traditional radiomics as it examines the variation in the quantitative imaging characteristics over time, specifically between more than two scans of the imaging of the patient at various points of the treatment. This time dynamics analysis is able to measure the dynamic changes in tumor properties, which are more indicative of biological and treatment reactions compared to radiomics of a single time point. Delta-radiomics can predict response to treatment, prognosis, and disease progression in oncology more effectively by quantifying these changes in texture, shape, and intensity features as delta-radiomics (Abbas et al., 2023).

The delta-radiomics analytical pipeline begins with the acquisition of imaging at a series of clinically relevant multiple time points such as baseline scans, post-therapy scans. The second step that is critical is a relative refinement of the regions of interest (ROIs) on each scan e.g. tumors or lesions and guarantees a spatial consistency in the extraction of features across time points. After segmentation, each image is subject of a set of standardized radiomic features comprising the intensity, texture, shape and wavelet features. The computed quantities then compute the delta features, which is the quantification of the absolute or relative changes in these radiomic features between the two or more time points. Following these are procedures of discriminating against invalid features and arriving at robust and prognostically intense delta features, usually by use of machine learning procedures. The last step is to construct predictive/ prognostic models incorporating the chosen delta features with the model performance signed by cross-validation/ independent cohort testing (Nardone et al., 2024).

The combination of temporal changes through delta-radiomics allows for a more complete evaluation of tumor biology which is much better at predictive modeling in oncology. The combination of temporal changes obtained by delta-radiomics produces a more complete evaluation of tumor biology, allowing for much better predictive modeling of oncology (Ahrari et al., 2024).

3. IMAGING MODALITIES USED IN RADIOMICS FOR CANCER DIAGNOSIS

Radiomics uses quantitative computational analysis on numerous medical imaging modalities, each with different diagnostic benefits and technical limitations used to diagnose cancer.

3.1 Computed Tomography

Computed Tomography (CT) is one of the main modalities of radiomics to evaluate lung cancer and liver cancer, among others. Radiomics-based on CT allows exploration of tumor morphology and internal texture, as well as heterogeneity, and such analysis is clinically viable with the standardization of procedures. Nevertheless, feature maps obtained through radiomics can be significantly different than the standard image reconstruction on CT: Although some radiomics feature maps could represent increased lesion contrast and take away the tedious work to less experienced readers by increasing detectability, others can decrease resolution therefore not allowing to repair lesser lesions. The usage of some radiomics feature maps including first-order RootMeanSquared as supplemental to standard CT reads is proposed, not as an alternative to traditional imaging, as the readers would not gain much familiarity with the imaging information in the form of the computer-aided diagnosis tool used to interpret standard CT imaging results (Hertel et al., 2024).

3.2 Magnetic Resonance Imaging

The Magnetic Resonance Imaging (MRI) offers better contrast of the soft tissues and its multiple protocols (e.g., T1, T2-weighted, diffusion-weighted imaging) depict microscopic alteration of tissue essential in cancer evaluation. Radiomics attributes obtained on MRI are helpful in grading brain tumors, forecasting the reaction to medication in breast cancer, and examining malignancies of the pelvis. Research illustrates that many normalization methods influence the ability of radiomics to extract features of MRI, influencing the reproducibility and the effectiveness of the findings across sites. The processing that is performed using Radiomics would frequently on networks like Pyradiomics and DICOM, which read 3D and 2D image data differently respectively, and have different effects when it comes to calculating texture and shape features. These variations in how these computations are carried gives rise to a potential difference in association between features identified and clinical outcome, and therefore standardization would be important (Quang et al., 2024).

3.3 Positron Emission Tomography

Positron Emission Tomography (PET) is most often used in combination with CT (PET/CT) and provides both functional and metabolic information that could be used to determine spatial heterogeneity of the tumor, metabolic activity, and tumor aggressiveness via radiomics. Radiomics using PET enhances staging of malignancies, assessment of metastatic dissemination and respond to therapy by identifying metabolic markers and not only anatomical characteristics (Hertel et al., 2024).

3.4 Ultrasound (USG)

Ultrasound (US) is also accessible, cheap and useful in real time imaging especially in breast, thyroid and liver cancers. In combination with special methods such as elastography, radiomics features extracted on US images achieve good performance advantages in diagnosis. An example of this could be when shear wave elastography (SWE) together with the conventional features of US demonstrated high sensitivity and specificity in the assessment of breast lesions, which was close or even higher than the accuracy of visual assessment criteria, e.g., BI-RADS. In such investigations, the diagnostic accuracy of multi-modality signatures (including the combination of two methods of imaging data, e.g., DCE-MRI and US) was superior to any single imaging modality and this fact proves the complementary character of multi-modality methods (Liu et al., 2022).

3.5 Mammography

Mammography, which has been the basis of screening in breast cancer, routinely creates high-resolution images and it is through it that microcalcification and architectural distortion characteristics can be extracted. Radiomics adds predictive value in risk prediction and subtype of breast cancer and this is clear when there is integration of mammographic data with other modes (Liu et al., 2022).

The modality of imaging directly influences the choice of the features describing the image, feature strength and accuracy of the model. The feature aggregation, normalization, and computational pipeline differences also affect reproducibility, clinical correlation, and generalizability of radiomics finding. One of the major obstacles on its path to becoming a common practice in clinical settings is standardization of radiomics extraction and processing techniques.

Table 1. This table gives an idea about different imaging modalities used in which type of cancer detection

Imaging Modality	Main Cancer Applications	Key Quantitative Features
CT	Lung, liver, gastric, colorectal	Shape, size, density, texture
MRI	Brain, breast, prostate, soft tissue	Texture, diffusion, perfusion, subtyping
PET / PET/CT	Lung, breast, lymphoma	Metabolic activity, heterogeneity
Ultrasound (US)	Breast, thyroid, liver	Texture, boundary, molecular profiling
Mammography	Breast	Microcalcification, texture, density

4. LITERATURE REVIEW

Review of the radiomics literature shows three general trends that can be seen overall and are essential for understanding the clinical relevance of radiomics:

4.1 Convergence on Multi-Parametric, Multi-Modal Imaging

Across CT, MRI, PET, USG, and mammography, the results of studies have consistently demonstrated that combination modalities improve diagnostic accuracy, indicating that radiomics would benefit from complementary information of anatomical and functional data.

4.2 Strong Performance but Limited Generalizability

Most studies report the results of area under the curve (AUC values between 0.724 and 0.997), however external validation is often lacking. This gap highlights the need for harmonization across scanners, protocols and feature extraction tools.

4.3 Shift From Handcrafted to Deep Learning Radiomics

Deep learning models increasingly improve performance over traditional feature-based radiomics by not requiring predefined assumptions but introduce challenges in term of interpretability.

Table 2. ROL Summary Table

Cancer Type	Study Title	Author (Year)	Objective	Dataset	Methods	Key Results	Short Conclusion
Lung Cancer	Radiomics for Prognosis in Locally Advanced NSCLC	Meng Yan et al., 2025	Evaluate tumor + whole-lung radiomics for predicting overall survival	661 LA-NSCLC patients	Cox model + LASSO; intensity/ shape/texture/ wavelet features; KM survival	C-index: 0.71 (train), 0.68 (test)	Combining tumor + lung radiomics improves prognostic accuracy and reflects tumor–host interaction.
Lung Cancer	EGFR Mutation Prediction Using Radiomics + Deep Learning	Ruifeng Xu et al., 2025	Predict EGFR mutation non-invasively	135 NSCLC patients	Radiomic + CNN deep-features; ROC, F1, confusion matrix	AUC: 0.964 (train), 0.724 (external), 0.844 (internal)	Hybrid radiomics–DL system enhances mutation prediction and supports targeted therapy decisions.
Breast Cancer	Mammography Radiomics for Cancer Classification	Aida Karami et al., 2025	Classify mammographic images into normal, benign, malignant	798 mammograms (218 women)	107 radiomic features; PCA + ET/RF/ GBDT	PCA-ET: AUC 0.997, Accuracy 0.960	Radiomics + PCA yields extremely accurate and reliable breast cancer classification.

continued on following page

Table 2. Continued

Cancer Type	Study Title	Author (Year)	Objective	Dataset	Methods	Key Results	Short Conclusion
Breast Cancer	MRI Radiomics for Predicting pCR in TNBC	Rania M. Mohamed et al., 2024	Predict early pathologic complete response to neoadjuvant therapy	163 TNBC patients	DCE + DWI radiomics; logistic regression	AUC: 0.905 (train), 0.802 (test)	MRI-based radiomics helps identify early responders, enabling personalized TNBC management.
Brain Cancer	Radiomics for Cognitive Impairment Detection	Feng et al., 2025	Detect cognitive impairment in WMH patients	108 patients (2 hospitals)	Deep VB-Net segmentation + RF model	AUC: 0.976 (train), 0.937 (internal) , 0.900 (external)	Automated radiomics gives objective, reliable cognitive impairment detection.
Brain Cancer	MRI Radiomics to Predict EGFR T790M Mutation from Brain Metastases	Wu et al., 2024	Predict EGFR T790M status from metastasis MR images	125 NSCLC brain-metastasis patients	480 features; XGBoost + SVM-SMOTE	AUC: 0.89; Key features from T2WI textures	Radiomics accurately predicts mutation status using metastatic lesions.
Liver Cancer	MRI Radiomics for Predicting Post-Hepatectomy Liver Failure	Chen et al., 2021	Predict PHLF using preoperative MRI radiomics	Non-tumor liver region MRI; 1044→24 selected features	Feature elimination + combined model	Radiomics AUC: 0.900, combined AUC: 0.956 (train)	Radiomics with clinical factors markedly improves prediction of postoperative liver failure.
Pancreatic Cancer	Early PDAC Detection on Pre-Diagnostic CT Scans	Sovanlal Mukherjee et al., 2022	Detect PDAC up to 36 months before clinical diagnosis	155 pre-diagnostic CTs + 265 controls	88 features; SVM/ RF/KNN/ XGBoost	SVM: AUC 0.98, Accuracy 92.2%	Radiomics identifies subtle pre-diagnostic changes that human readers miss.

All The studies, shown in (table 2) a common thread can be found: radiomics is consistently showing promising findings for the prediction of imaging biomarkers that are better for the detection of tumour heterogeneity as well as early signs of the disease than the traditional radiologist's assessment. The merging of handcrafted and deep features further enhances performance and multicenter cohorts show moderate generalizability despite imaging protocol variability.

5. INTEGRATION OF RADIOMICS WITH ARTIFICIAL INTELLIGENCE

Radiomics in combination with artificial intelligence (AI) is revolutionizing the context of clinical cancer imaging with the ability to extract, process and interpret tremendous and complex amounts of medical imaging data. The combination is driving greater precision diagnosis, prognostication, and individualized treatment decisions. Machine learning, deep learning and the Omics-AI nexus. The subsequent sections report, in detail, the nature of the roles of machine learning, deep learning and the multi-omics approach in the radiomics-AI nexus.

5.1 Machine Learning in Radiomics

The infrastructure of radiomics-based predictive modeling is based on machine learning (ML), in which statistical methods to learn large volumes of data with quantitative imaging features and clinical outcomes are applied. The major importance of ML to the radiomics workflows is in the selection of features, patterned activations, estimations of prognosis, and decision-support system creation. High-throughput extraction of hundreds or thousands of quantitative features (shape, texture, intensity, and wavelet descriptors of medical images) usually constitutes the first part of the process. Due to a high dimension and redundancy of these features, ML algorithms are important to find a subset of features that will best describe the problem, without over fitting (Zhang et al., 2023).

After the selection of features, supervised ML models, including but not limited to logistic regression, random forests, support vector machines (SVMs) and gradient boosting machines are implemented to classify tumors, predict therapeutic response, or patient risk profiles among others. As an example, ML models have targeted the differentiation of malignant and benign lesions, tumor grading and subtypes, as well as survival and recurrence outcomes. In breast cancer, the radiomics models based on ML have proved to be more accurate than human visual assessments alone in pre- and postoperative multiparametric MRI or ultrasound data to identify benign or malignant lesions. Validity and generalizability of predictive models are part of the critical steps in ML-based radiomics. High-quality feature selection, cross-validation, and external independent testing is necessary to guarantee reliability and clinical applicability. Radiomics is now integrating multiple imaging protocols (CT, MRI, PET, ultrasound) hence multi-modality can enable the combination of features across heterogeneous data sets with the help of multi-modal ML. Moreover, with the use of ML, it is feasible to stratify patient population in clinical study, automize workflow, and use computer-aided diagnostic (CAD) software to achieve real-time decision-making (Majumder et al., 2023).

Validity and generalizability of predictive models are part of the fundamental actions in ML-based radiomics. The quality of feature selection, cross-validation and a non-study test are necessary in order to guarantee reliability and clinical relevance. Radiomics is going to be multi-imaging (CT, MRI, PET, ultrasound) and therewith ML models can be arranged to facilitate the implementation of features in the heterogeneous data sets, unfortunately, called multi-modality. Additionally, the ML enables stratification of the patient population in clinical trials, automatization of workflow, computer-aided diagnostic systems (CAD) to make real-time decision making. Machine learning transforms the field of radiomics, using automation of feature selection and pattern recognition to enable move the field of radiomics beyond descriptive results in imaging analysis and into actionable precision medicine, facilitating accurate, reproducible and scalable clinical decision-making in oncology and beyond (Maniaci et al., 2024).

5.2 Deep Learning in Radiomics

Deep learning as the extension of ML, with convolutional neural networks (CNNs) in particular, does not require such handcrafting in feature extraction. DL models can learn highly integrated, hierarchical representation directly on raw imaging data, and have been reported to perform well in image segmentation, classification and prediction subtasks in radiomics pipelines. Studies show that the DL approaches have the potential to be used to identify tumors and locating boundaries of lesions as well as differentiating multi-class diseases frequently better than solid conventional ML models to the modalities which include CT, MRI, PET, and ultrasound just to mention a few. Advanced computer-aided diagnostics (CAD) systems supporting automated detection to objectively based risk scoring and individualized treatment choice in oncology and beyond are driven by DL-based radiomics. Moreover, explainable AI approaches to visualizing the DL models' outputs and their attention mechanisms are guiding toward overcoming the conventional black box shortcoming, thereby contributing to the clinical acceptability and regulatory acceptance of the next-generation tools. Consequently, DL-radiomics has the potential to make workflow processes efficient, scale to large volumes, and be accurate and observer-independent, critical properties when transferring the technology to the real world for clinical implementations (Guo et al., 2025).

5.3 Multi-Omics Integration

The radiomics data combined with other omics layers- genomics, proteomics and metabolomics- is creating the second chapter of the AI-powered precision medicine. The integration of multi-source data with ML and AI platforms can now generate a variety of disease-centric models with high detail and breadth that have the potential to better stratify patients, predict therapeutic response and prognosis. Recent research points to the fact that by incorporating radiomics and multi-omics, models with significantly higher detection, monitoring and outcome prediction of a broad variety of malignancies are achieved (had been accomplished with liver and brain tumor). This synergy enhances the ability further to non-invasively measure tumor heterogeneity, prospectively track the fluctuations of the molecular and phenotype state, and finally goes to the individualized treatment paradigm by employing population-based methods. As much health data is collected, there will be significance in the vision of personalized, real-time patient management with the integration of disparate inputs across the omics continuum through AI, including imaging results, lab results, and clinical variables (Camps et al., 2025).

6. ECONOMICS OF RADIOMICS AND COST-EFFECTIVENESS OF RADIOMICS

Radiomics, by using high-level computational techniques, enables the extraction of quantitative information from medical images that can be used in diagnosis, prognosis and treatment planning in oncology and other disciplines. The economic impact of radiomics is significant, as it allows more clinical information to be derived from the images that are already taken as part of everyday clinical practice and have the potential to reduce the need for additional imaging and invasive procedures. This can translate into reduced healthcare expenditures, especially through the ability to target surveillance and interventions to high-risk patients to prevent unnecessary follow-ups and treatments to those patients who are unlikely to benefit (Miles, 2020).

Cost-effectiveness analysis (CEA) is a popular tool in radiology that compares different strategies both in terms of cost and effectiveness. The incremental cost-effectiveness ratio (ICER) is an important measure and is calculated by dividing the difference between the cost of two strategies by the difference between the effectiveness of the two strategies, usually in Quality-adjusted year-lives (QALYs). For example, in the area of breast cancer screening MRI mammography (MRM) has been demonstrated to be cost-effective compared to standard mammography for certain patient groups, in spite of higher initial costs, due to the fact that it offers more accurate prognostic information and downstream reduction. Similarly in the intervention of ablation for tumors of the liver, microwave ablation (MWA) has been found to be the dominant strategy as it is linked to lower costs and better outcomes as compared with alternatives (Froelich et al., 2022).

However, formal economic evaluations that specifically addressed radiomics are still limited. The implementation of radiomics into clinical workflows entails investment into infrastructure, training and data management with significant cost. Nevertheless, the potential for cost savings through improved decision-making and less intervention is an attractive proposition from an economic standpoint. As the field further matures, stronger CEA studies are needed that help quantify the long-term economic benefits of the field, in addition to guiding healthcare policy and resource allocation (Zhou et al., 2018).

7. FAIRNESS, BIAS, AND ETHICAL EQUITY

Fairness in radiomics and AI-driven medical imaging includes the concept that all patients, regardless of their background, should receive an equal amount of benefits from medical image technologies and be treated in a fair and just manner. Algorithmic bias simply occurs when the data that are used to acquaint the AI models fail to represent the wider population, which results in differential diagnostic abilities and treatment recommendations to under-represented sections of the population. As an example, an algorithm that was trained on imaging data in urban centers might not work well in rural or underserved communities and lead to the diagnosis being missed or the wrong care being given out (Filippi et al., 2023).

There are various types of bias in AI systems, such as allocational and representational harm (negative stereotype reinforcement). Fairness has to be intentionally obtained by making training data more varied, and by audit algorithms to detect bias over their lifecycle. It involves gathering information about various ethnic, racial and socioeconomic groups, various healthcare settings and across geographic areas (Ahmed, 2025).

Ethical equity in radiomics is also associated with dealing with inequities in the access to advanced imaging technologies and AI tools. Developed countries and developing countries have a significant economic difference, and there is a considerable economic gap within communities themselves that influences the introduction and use of radiomics and AI in healthcare. Such measures as specific funding and allocation of resources, policies that promote data exchange and cooperation between institutions and regions can be considered as strategies that may help to promote equity. The central tenet of ethical adoption of radiomics in clinical practice entails upholding the rights of the patients and non-discrimination (Hanna et al., 2025).

8. RADIOMICS WORKFLOW INTEGRATION (PACS/RIS SYSTEMS)

To achieve a seamless workflow and clinical adoption, radiomics need to be integrated in Picture Archiving and Communication Systems (PACS) and Radiology Information Systems (RIS). PACS and RIS are the key areas of the contemporary radiology department, as they are the ones that handle the storage, retrieval, and distribution of medical images and the data. Radiomics workflows should interface well with these systems such that quantitative imaging features can be extracted, analyzed and reported along with traditional radiological findings. Issues that may arise during integration are standardization of data format, interoperability between various vendors and platforms, and handling of the huge amounts of data produced by radiomics analyses. Also, regulatory and privacy issues arise because radiomics data can include information about patients that is sensitive and should be secured according to the local and international regulations. Effective integration demands a very tight linkage among radiologists, IT experts and programmers to come up with easy-to-use interfaces and data management systems that are robust and take care of all data related to the department of radiology Integration is important as it allows the radiologists to gain access to radiomics-generated insights at the point of their operation, allowing them to make more informed decisions and improve patient outcomes. Moreover, the inclusion into PACS/RIS facilitates routine tasks automation, including image segmentation, feature extraction, which enhances efficiency and eliminates the possibility of human error (Miles, 2020).

9. TRANSLATIONAL AND EXTERNAL VALIDATION.

Moving radiomics models into clinical practice is referred to as a transnational validation such that these models are reliable, reproducible, and relevant in clinical settings. This is achieved by a series of steps such as internal validation (checking the model on the same data that has been used in training), external validation (testing the model on independent datasets of different institutions or populations) and prospective validation (testing the model in real-life clinic situations) (Garau et al., 2020).

The external validation is especially essential when measuring the applicability of radiomics models because it aids to highlight possible bias and limitations that could otherwise remain unnoticed in internal validation. An example is a radiomics model that was used to classify malignant pulmonary nodules and was shown to work well on the training set but performs worse when used on the external datasets where patients have different properties or imaging protocols. External validation of imaging data really depends on harmonization of imaging data and feature extraction strategies as variability in image acquisition and processing could influence the model performance (Bordron et al., 2022).

Although radiomics promises, most of the published models have performed poorly in their external validation and this point demonstrates that rigorous validation protocols and standardized reporting guidelines should be adhered to. The next steps include prospective external validation research on models in clinical practice that will prove their clinical usefulness and regulatory approval. Continued work to enhance the transparency and reproducibility of radiomics studies, including open data sets and open code, can assist in improving the field, and bring radiomics to everyday clinical use (Spaanderman et al., 2024).

10. CLINICAL IMPACT AND ADVANTAGES

Radiomics builds the prospect of a new era of non-invasive, data-driven healthcare, that can effectively change clinical practices and instigates immeasurably positive differences, which is already beginning to be revolutionized in terms of cancer disease detection and treatment.

10.1 Precision Oncology

Radiomics has emerged as a major concept of how oncology should be precise and transform regular medical images into hundreds of measurable features that describe tumor shape, texture, and biology in detailed precision. The procedure defines inter- and intra-tumor heterogeneity to a far more impressive degree than the classical visual examination and cannot be exaggerated in regard of the personal attitude towards patient treatment. Future opportunities: Radiomic signatures would allow clinician predict patient response to treatment, allow a risk assessment whether treatment is improving and select appropriate specific targeted treatment options in such a way that it will be possible to offer each patient the best possible treatment plan. These findings are confirmed by research results, which indicate that the integration of radiomics features with machine learning/deep learning models can more readily outperform traditional image knowledge in the classification of tumors and their associated significance/risk to deliver a greater degree of clinical outcome and responsive management. The prospect that such fusion of radiomics with genomic and clinical data would enhance prediction power even more introduces the possibility of personalized oncolgence-directing decision-support to emerging operationalization, bringing it closer still to the clinical workflow in reality (Quraishi, 2022).

10.2 Predicting Tumor Biology Non-Invasively

The advantages of radiomics include the fact that it can predict tumor biology in a non- invasive manner. Radiomics can be used to deduce critical genomic, proteomic, and immunological tumor traits by extracting imaging biomarkers linked to molecular features (e.g., mutations, rates of proliferation, hypoxia). This facilitates the non-invasive prediction of tumor subtype, grade, aggressiveness, and sensitivity to therapy and may, in relation to or sometimes in lieu of tissue profiling. Consider, radiomics models can differentiate virus- and non-virus-induced head and neck cancers, or HER2 status in breast cancers, and compete with molecular assays. The ability can provide a vital advantage to clinicians seeking to tailor care and treat disease in the areas where biopsy is impractical, hazardous, or otherwise constrained (Russo et al., 2024).

10.3 Reducing Need for Biopsy

Radiomics is a form of virtual biopsy disorders explicitly sensitive to the spatial and temporal heterogeneity of whole-tumor systems and microenvironment, not just the tiny percentage of real-world structures reached through conventional tissue biopsy. This eliminates the necessity of invasive biopsy processes, which are also associated with the possibility of discomfort, hemorrhage, infection, and tumor spreading. In addition, serial imaging, done without the benefit of serial surgery, can be used with radiomics to track the effects of treatment or the progression of a disease, and is therefore of invaluable benefit. The recent retrospective as well as prospective research demonstrates that using radiomics-based model allows to differentiate between malignant and benign nodules, and predict the response to chemoradiotherapy and molecular phenotype, with the patient never taking an invasive examination. Patients with compromised and untreatable tumors, weakness or hard-to-reach anatomies are especially helped by such advances (El-Jammal & Chung, 2025).

11. CHALLENGES AND LIMITATIONS

Although radiomics is revolutionizing the field of oncology, including the diagnostics and planning of treatment, several challenges and restrictions exist that should be considered when resolved into bringing radiomics to the clinical practice.

11.1 Variability in Imaging Protocols

One of the most long-standing obstacles to radiomics research and implementation is the difference in imaging protocol between scanners across institutions. Radiomic characteristics are highly sensitive to acquisition parameters (slice thickness, reconstruction algorithms, image resolution, bolus and contrast enhancement protocols) These inconsistencies can introduce high amounts of noise to the radiomics data and endanger the reproducibility and extrinsic validation of the models built. Given the slight case of a signature created based on thin-slice CT data on a vendor machine as an example, not all vendor-generated data, but particularly 25-bit-thin-slice data, might be robust across all vendor choices based on reconstruction kernels. These deficiencies can be particularly crippling to the types of multi center studies that are required in making generalizations. Standardization of acquisition procedures and ease concurrent pre-processing procedures of images- such as resampling voxels or normalization of intense-but practical acquisition has is being pursued further in light of implementation burdens. Finally, radiomics tools can be reliably integrated into the imperative clinical workflow solely through inflexible standardization (Stefano, 2024; Martin et al., 2022).

11.2 Need for Large Annotated Datasets

Development of strong radiomics models needs vast and adequately annotated data sets that subsume wide-ranging disease manifestation and patient demographics. Unfortunately, such datasets are scarce. Annotation involves precise tumor/ tissue segmentation which requires time and depends on the judgment of experts. Also, quality outcome data (clinical, pathologic and molecular correlates) is Nearly universally discontinuous or unevenly distributed. The privacy rules and internal rules deny data sharing and various other kinds of data which further reduces the chances of sharing resources between various centers to perform adequately powered analysis. Despite the emergent stages the formation of federated learning structures and public repositories as a solution face some technical and regulatory difficulties, even though they are in their early stages. The overfitting and lack of external validity of radiomics studies imply small sample sizes and under annotated results and complicate the development of robust and generalizable models. The extraction of these vulnerabilities will be through effective mixes of multicentric networking, reporting habits and procedures, and innovative technological solutions of pertinent freshness in riskless and successful aggregation and aggregation of the information (Horvat et al., 2024).

11.3 Regulatory and Ethical Concerns

The radiomics-based tools (with or without artificial intelligence) are viewed as high-risk medical equipment in which they operate to form an important decision in diagnosis or selecting the form of therapy. This brings out regulatory and ethical issues that need to be addressed before using it in the clinic. The FDA and EMA, as regulatory authorities, insist on rigorous validation, the explicit description of the mechanism of the models and the guarantee that performance will be the same in the population and upon different platforms. The explainability issue of many machine learning and deep learning solutions and the black-box nature of these complicate this, and further undermine the possibility of clinician trust in the solution, which is further delaying the process. Also, ethical issues concerning the usage of patient information, data privacy, and possible algorithm bias are quite profound. Underrepresented data samples can result in underperformance in these AI models in the underrepresented patient populations continuing the disparity in health care. To guarantee patient trust and comply with regulations, it is necessary to ensure the security and confidentiality of large-scale aggregation of image data, adhere to such frameworks as GDPR and HIPAA, and be transparent in the development and implementation of AI. The legal structures continue to grow in their capabilities to support the special qualities of AI-enabled radiomics, such that interdisciplinary collaboration between the clinicians, technologists, and the regulators remains an ongoing requirement (Horvat et al., 2024).

12. CURRENT RESEARCH TRENDS

Radiomics has become the focus in modern cancer research as there has been a sudden boom in innovations, efforts towards clinical translation, and the discovery of novel imaging biomarkers that are increasingly defining the future of precision oncology.

12.1 Recent Breakthroughs in Radiomics

Over the past few years, radiomics has seen massive advances not only in the innovative feature engineering and mapping to AI, but also with breakthroughs in predictive modelling of therapeutic response and machine discovery of biomarkers. Indicatively, radiomics-based models have enhanced the predictive value of the non-invasive anticipation of cancers to neoadjuvant/targeted therapy in many cancers. Or, as another example, more advanced radiomics models based on MRI are already being developed to predict the response of neoadjuvant chemotherapy in cervical and breast cancer, so patients could be stratified more effectively before treatment begins. There is also an overlap that the field is experiencing with pathomics and genomics, which gains a greater understanding of tumor biology. Radiomics features acquired by CT/MRI have also been shown to reflect underlying molecular/genomic changes e.g. EGFR or HER2 status, or even markers of immunotherapy e.g. PD-L1 expression.

Further, implementation of delta radiomics (features are extracted and compared across serial imaging during treatment) has allowed dynamic tracking of treatment response, allowing clinicians to receive time-sensitive and actionable assessments. The Ref. was considered publicly cited in meta-platform and using deep learning nomograms MRI-based radiomics has been successfully used to predict molecular genotypes including the isocitrate dehydrogenase (IDH) status in gliomas, further developing non-invasive virtual biopsies and precision medicine (Fournier et al., 2021).

12.2 Ongoing Clinical Trials

Radiomics are increasingly understood to be incorporated and assessed in clinical trials as either novel biomarkers or supportive stratification and outcome prediction tools. In neuro-oncology the European Organization for Research and Treatment of Cancer Brain Tumor Group is also incorporating radiomics into clinical trials to assess response and identify prognostic biomarkers in the glioblastoma and other brain tumors. Prospective studies in breast cancer are exploiting the radiomics in terms of MRI to reflect the tumor microenvironment and determine important molecular subsets, which have the potential to complement the conventional efforts of risk stratification. Other multi-institutional research is underway to evaluate the capacity of radiomics signatures to forecast HER2 status HER2 and therapeutic responses in metastatic breast cancer and their potential to forecast responses to immunotherapy in various tumors (Jha et al., 2023).

Ongoing studies are evaluating the predictive value of PET/CT radiomics in identifying early response to radiation treatment and developing radiomics signatures as companion diagnostics to allow real-time patient selection and monitoring. There is a shift in the field towards the unification of multi-omics data with radiomics being used alongside genomic and pathological data streams to create a more circumstantial and executable overview of cancer behavior and response to treatment (Ferro et al., 2024).

12.3 Emerging Biomarkers

Among the most significant advantages of radiomics is the contribution in the new imaging biomarkers finding which may be used as a complement or even an improvement of the traditional tissue-based biomarkers. Radiomics allows three-dimensional, whole-tumor, and longitudinal measure of prognostic-related, treatment response-related, and risk of recurrence associated characteristics. To give a specific example, radiomics signatures based on CT, MRI, and PET images have been established as immune-related gene expression (e.g., CTLA-4 and PD-L1) hypoxia, tumor-stromal ratio, and other clinically relevant phenotypes found in lung, breast, head and neck, bladder, colorectal, and brain cancers.

Particularly, quantitative imaging parameters, including heterogeneity, shape irregularity, edge sharpness, and alteration of tumor density tend to be better predictors of outcome and response to treatment than historical, size-based RECIST parameters. Combining radiomics and transcriptomics with pathomics (multi-omics fusion) has provided biomarkers improving prognostic accuracy, as demonstrated in the recent models predicting immunotherapy response with high AUC values over a radiomics or genomics-only model. Routine imaging enables the ready availability of these emerging biomarkers, and therefore their scale is potentially very large and their practical application to medicines easy to apply clinically and potentially suitable to individual therapy with real time observation of the patient without the need to be invasively tested (Fournier et al., 2021).

13. FUTURE DIRECTIONS

The coming few years will experience the Transformational radiomics innovations in the field and several key directions are shaping the future of clinical and research applications of radiomics.

13.1 Radiogenomics and Integration With Molecular Data

A key trend into which radiomics is now moving is its amalgamation with radiogenomics or the whole genome approach to studying quantitative features of imaging and coupleting with molecular features in order to discover relationships between cancer phenotype and cancer genotype. In this way, investigators have been able to map radiomics signatures on CT, MRI images or PET to the underlying gene mutations, transcriptomic patterns and protein expressions. Such integration is proving to be vital in the identification of the imaging biomarkers that describe such biological functions immunogenicity, angiogenesis, hypoxia and stratification of tumors to targeted therapy or resistance. Recent studies indicate that radiomics-genomic composite models outperform each image modality maximally in prognostic prediction, particularly the recurrence of a disease, and therapy response. Molecular profiling is starting to become a common practice in the clinic. With the onset of these fluctuations, radiogenomics may support intermediations between non-invasive imaging and molecular diagnostics- dosing real-time- sensitive medication and expanding personalized oncology provision (Ibrahim et al., 2021).

13.2 Standardization of Radiomics Pipelines

The standardization of radiomics pipelines is known to be a scourge of the field. A difference in the image acquisition protocol, feature extracting software, and information on the parameters of ITK leads to the fact that imaging radiomics features cannot be replicated or compared across studies. An increasing set of standardization efforts, including the Image Biomarker Standardization Initiative (IBSI), is making the realization of more harmonized definitions of radiomics features, pre-processing methods and annotation criteria across locations and vendors a reality. Radiomics tools also promote the standardization promoting high-quality multi-center clinical trials, regulatory, and electronic health record integrations that are important in encouraging the possible clinical viability of these tools. Such reproducibility may be accomplished via consistency throughout the radiomics pipeline as in the case of image acquisition, feature selection, modeling, and reporting in order to enable repeatable, reproducible, comparable study findings and even vastly scale up bench-to-bedside translation (Boubnovski Martell et al., 2025).

13.3 Automated Radiomics (AUTOML + AI)

AutoML based and AI-based automated radiomics has the potential to revolutionize feature extraction and model building, and decision assistance by introducing scalable artificial intelligence. Automated pipelines can efficiently analyze acquisitions or imaging database, automatically synthesis and select features, and optimize models, without considerable user intervention, to conserve time and effort. This kind of AI consists of convolutional neural nets (CNNs), random forest, and boosting algorithms that have demonstrated their superb capability at automated segmentation, measurement of tumor biology, and real-time clinical forecasting. Experiplaining AI by large language models (LLMs) is a growing field of study and radiomics is being integrated with clinicians in a way where it can assist in surmounting the decision in radiomics-driven predictions. By making radiomics technology a consist of a democratic component within the clinical routine, it becomes less manpower-focused and permits further thinking to be carried out in a larger range of medical facilities (Fan et al., 2025).

14. DISCUSSION

This chapter represents a complete and timely review of radiomics as a paradigm shift in cancer diagnostics and manages to bridge the gap between traditional medical imaging and quantitative precision medicine. The scientific detail of the radiomics workflows, starting with the image acquisition and ending with clinical use, provides a high level of methodological rigor and provides the readers with a logical comprehension of the complex area. The combination of various imaging techniques with CT, MRI, PET, ultrasound, and mammography is also worth noting since it stresses the versatility of radiomics in various cancers and situations. The fact that the chapter has real-world studies with their respective performance measures (AUC values between 0.724 and 0.997) helps to strengthen the empirical basis of the chapter and makes it a strong evidence of the clinical usefulness of radiomics in lung, breast, brain, liver, and pancreatic cancers.

The multidimensional nature of the chapter is a strong point because it covers not solely the technical side but also the economic, ethical implications, and the issue of fairness, which remains largely ignored in radiomics literature. The following discourse regarding the concept of algorithmic bias and the health equity issue reflects the realization of the more society-wide effects of AI-driven diagnostics, which will be necessary to conduct responsible clinical translation. In addition to this, the combined application of machine learning and deep learning approaches depicts how technological progress is bringing the sphere closer to automated, reproducible analyses that could be extended across healthcare systems.

Nevertheless, this chapter also has some weaknesses that should be noted. As much as some of the challenges including variability of imaging protocols and limited availability of datasets have been correctly made, the solution proposals are somewhat generic without specification on road maps of implementation. Regulatory landscape discussion is also very significant however not very specific when it comes to region specific approval pathways or actually an actionable approach to meet the explainability requirements imposed by regulatory agencies. Also, the chapter can use a stronger critique on the failure cases of radiomics or those situations, in which conventional imaging is still better than radiomics because such a balanced point of view would increase the credibility of the chapter and the corresponding application of radiomics in clinical work.

Although the economic analysis has been presented, it needs further discussion with actual cost-effectiveness evidence of actual or real-world practices. Although these are the limitations, the current chapter is a good addition to radiomics literature as it places it in a holistic perspective, which clinicians, researchers, and policy makers can use to embrace this promising technology in their oncological practice.

15. CONCLUSION

Radiomics is a game changer in oncology since it is able to transform routine medical images into quantitative data to discover tumor heterogeneity, biology, and treatment response, which cannot be detected using visual interpretation. Radiomics, with regard to CT, MRI, PET, ultrasound, and mammography extremes, provides non-invasive information to help in cancer detection, determine correct subtypes, risk assessments, and monitoring therapy. The results of the lung, breast, brain, liver, and pancreatic cancer biopsies all lead us to believe that the predictive accuracy is high, and most of the models have AUC values that surpass 0.90, indicating that radiomics is a useful complement to the conventional diagnostics test.

Radiomics can be improved by the integration of artificial intelligence - especially machine learning and deep learning - automating feature selection and predictive modeling, with further integration of multi-omics giving it the potential to achieve highly individualized precision oncology. Radiomics has a number of clinical benefits: it helps = reduce invasive biopsies to prospective identification of tumors via virtual tumor profiling, allow the use of the current amount of imaging facilities at a relatively low cost, and expand the opportunities of advanced diagnostics across various medical facilities.

Nevertheless, radiomics has obstacles, such as inconsistency of imaging protocols, reproducibility, dearth of annotated datasets and regulatory and ethical issues. Efforts like Image Biomarker Standardisation Initiative, federated learning of shared data privacy and explainable artificial intelligence tools are combating these challenges and bringing the field to clinical implementation.

REFERENCES

Abbas, E., Fanni, S. C., Bandini, C., Francischello, R., Febi, M., Aghakhanyan, G., Ambrosini, I., Faggioni, L., Cioni, D., Lencioni, R. A., & Neri, E. (2023). Delta-radiomics in cancer immunotherapy response prediction: A systematic review. *European Journal of Radiology Open, 11*, 100511. DOI: 10.1016/j.ejro.2023.100511 PMID: 37520768

Aerts, H. J. W. L., Velazquez, E. R., Leijenaar, R. T. H., Parmar, C., Grossmann, P., Carvalho, S., Bussink, J., Monshouwer, R., Haibe-Kains, B., Rietveld, D., Hoebers, F., Rietbergen, M. M., Leemans, C. R., Dekker, A., Quackenbush, J., Gillies, R. J., & Lambin, P. (2014). Decoding tumour phenotype by noninvasive imaging using a quantitative radiomics approach. *Nature Communications, 5*(1), 4006. DOI: 10.1038/ncomms5006 PMID: 24892406

Ahmed, H. S. (2025). Navigating ethical dimensions in algorithmic radiology: A call for action to ensure representation of low-resource contexts. *Indian Journal of Medical Ethics, 10*(2), 138–145. DOI: 10.20529/IJME.2025.001 PMID: 40036128

Ahrari, S., Zaragori, T., Zinsz, A., Oster, J., Imbert, L., & Verger, A. (2024). Application of PET imaging delta radiomics for predicting progression-free survival in rare high-grade glioma. *Scientific Reports, 14*(1), 3256. DOI: 10.1038/s41598-024-53693-x PMID: 38332004

Bordron, A., Rio, E., Badic, B., Miranda, O., Pradier, O., Hatt, M., Visvikis, D., Lucia, F., Schick, U., & Bourbonne, V. (2022). External Validation of a Radiomics Model for the Prediction of Complete Response to Neoadjuvant Chemoradiotherapy in Rectal Cancer. *Cancers (Basel), 14*(4), 1079. DOI: 10.3390/cancers14041079 PMID: 35205826

Boubnovski Martell, M., Linton-Reid, K., Chen, M., & Aboagye, E. O. (2025). Radiomics for lung cancer diagnosis, management, and future prospects. *Clinical Radiology, 86*, 106926. DOI: 10.1016/j.crad.2025.106926 PMID: 40344812

Camps, J., Jiménez-Franco, A., García-Pablo, R., Joven, J., & Arenas, M. (2025). Artificial intelligence-driven integration of multi-omics and radiomics: A new hope for precision cancer diagnosis and prognosis. *Biochimica et Biophysica Acta (BBA) -. Biochimica et Biophysica Acta. Molecular Basis of Disease, 1871*(6), 167841. DOI: 10.1016/j.bbadis.2025.167841 PMID: 40216368

El-Jammal, M., & Chung, C. (2025). Paving a Path to Clinical Impact with Radiomics: Enabling Reproducibility and Reach. *Cancer Research, 85*(13), 2353–2355. DOI: 10.1158/0008-5472.CAN-25-2083 PMID: 40598943

Fan, Y., Feigenberg, S. J., & Simone, C. B.II. (2025). Current and Future Applications of PET Radiomics in Radiation Oncology. *PET Clinics*, *20*(2), 185–193. DOI: 10.1016/j.cpet.2025.01.002 PMID: 39915189

Ferro, A., Bottosso, M., Dieci, M. V., Scagliori, E., Miglietta, F., Aldegheri, V., Bonanno, L., Caumo, F., Guarneri, V., Griguolo, G., & Pasello, G. (2024). Clinical applications of radiomics and deep learning in breast and lung cancer: A narrative literature review on current evidence and future perspectives. *Critical Reviews in Oncology/Hematology*, *203*, 104479. DOI: 10.1016/j.critrevonc.2024.104479 PMID: 39151838

Filippi, C. G., Stein, J. M., Wang, Z., Bakas, S., Liu, Y., Chang, P. D., Lui, Y., Hess, C., Barboriak, D. P., Flanders, A. E., Wintermark, M., Zaharchuk, G., & Wu, O. (2023). Ethical Considerations and Fairness in the Use of Artificial Intelligence for Neuroradiology. *AJNR. American Journal of Neuroradiology*, *44*(11), 1242–1248. DOI: 10.3174/ajnr.A7963 PMID: 37652578

Fournier, L., Costaridou, L., Bidaut, L., Michoux, N., Lecouvet, F. E., De Geus-Oei, L.-F., Boellaard, R., Oprea-Lager, D. E., Obuchowski, N. A., Caroli, A., Kunz, W. G., Oei, E. H., O'Connor, J. P. B., Mayerhoefer, M. E., Franca, M., Alberich-Bayarri, A., Deroose, C. M., Loewe, C., Manniesing, R., & deSouza, N. M.European Society of Radiology. (2021). Incorporating radiomics into clinical trials: Expert consensus endorsed by the European Society of Radiology on considerations for data-driven compared to biologically driven quantitative biomarkers. *European Radiology*, *31*(8), 6001–6012. DOI: 10.1007/s00330-020-07598-8 PMID: 33492473

. Froelich, M. F., Kunz, W. G., Tollens, F., Schnitzer, M. L., Schönberg, S. O., Kaiser, C. G., & Rübenthaler, J. (2022). Cost-effectiveness analysis in radiology: Methods, results and implications. *RöFo - Fortschritte auf dem Gebiet der Röntgenstrahlen und der bildgebenden Verfahren, 194*(1), 29–38. DOI: 10.1055/a-1502-7830

Garau, N., Paganelli, C., Summers, P., Choi, W., Alam, S., Lu, W., Fanciullo, C., Bellomi, M., Baroni, G., & Rampinelli, C. (2020). External validation of radiomics-based predictive models in low-dose CT screening for early lung cancer diagnosis. *Medical Physics*, *47*(9), 4125–4136. DOI: 10.1002/mp.14308 PMID: 32488865

Gillies, R. J., Kinahan, P. E., & Hricak, H. (2016). Radiomics: Images Are More than Pictures, They Are Data. *Radiology*, *278*(2), 563–577. DOI: 10.1148/radiol.2015151169 PMID: 26579733

Gillies, R. J., & Schabath, M. B. (2020). Radiomics Improves Cancer Screening and Early Detection. *Cancer Epidemiology, Biomarkers & Prevention*, *29*(12), 2556–2567. DOI: 10.1158/1055-9965.EPI-20-0075 PMID: 32917666

Guo, Y., Li, N., Song, C., Yang, J., Quan, Y., & Zhang, H. (2025). Artificial intelligence-based automated breast ultrasound radiomics for breast tumor diagnosis and treatment: A narrative review. *Frontiers in Oncology*, *15*, 1578991. DOI: 10.3389/fonc.2025.1578991 PMID: 40406239

Hanna, M. G., Pantanowitz, L., Jackson, B., Palmer, O., Visweswaran, S., Pantanowitz, J., Deebajah, M., & Rashidi, H. H. (2025). Ethical and Bias Considerations in Artificial Intelligence/Machine Learning. *Modern Pathology*, *38*(3), 100686. DOI: 10.1016/j.modpat.2024.100686 PMID: 39694331

Hertel, A., Kuru, M., Tollens, F., Tharmaseelan, H., Nörenberg, D., Rathmann, N., Schoenberg, S. O., & Froelich, M. F. (2024). Comparison of diagnostic accuracy of radiomics parameter maps and standard reconstruction for the detection of liver lesions in computed tomography. *Frontiers in Oncology*, *14*, 1444115. DOI: 10.3389/fonc.2024.1444115 PMID: 39435296

Hong, S., Hong, S., Oh, E., Lee, W. J., Jeong, W. K., & Kim, K. (2024). Development of a flexible feature selection framework in radiomics-based prediction modeling: Assessment with four real-world datasets. *Scientific Reports*, *14*(1), 29297. DOI: 10.1038/s41598-024-80863-8 PMID: 39592859

Horvat, N., Papanikolaou, N., & Koh, D.-M. (2024). Radiomics Beyond the Hype: A Critical Evaluation Toward Oncologic Clinical Use. *Radiology. Artificial Intelligence*, *6*(4), e230437. DOI: 10.1148/ryai.230437 PMID: 38717290

Ibrahim, A., Primakov, S., Beuque, M., Woodruff, H. C., Halilaj, I., Wu, G., Refaee, T., Granzier, R., Widaatalla, Y., Hustinx, R., Mottaghy, F. M., & Lambin, P. (2021). Radiomics for precision medicine: Current challenges, future prospects, and the proposal of a new framework. *Methods (San Diego, Calif.)*, *188*, 20–29. DOI: 10.1016/j.ymeth.2020.05.022 PMID: 32504782

Jha, A. K., Mithun, S., Sherkhane, U. B., Dwivedi, P., Puts, S., Osong, B., Traverso, A., Purandare, N., Wee, L., Rangarajan, V., & Dekker, A. (2023). Emerging role of quantitative imaging (radiomics) and artificial intelligence in precision oncology. *Exploration of Targeted Anti-tumor Therapy*, •••, 569–582. DOI: 10.37349/etat.2023.00153 PMID: 37720353

Li, S., Deng, Y.-Q., Zhu, Z.-L., Hua, H.-L., & Tao, Z.-Z. (2021). A Comprehensive Review on Radiomics and Deep Learning for Nasopharyngeal Carcinoma Imaging. *Diagnostics (Basel)*, *11*(9), 1523. DOI: 10.3390/diagnostics11091523 PMID: 34573865

Liu, X., Zhang, J., Zhou, J., He, Y., Xu, Y., Zhang, Z., Cao, G., Miao, H., Chen, Z., Zhao, Y., Jin, X., & Wang, M. (2022). Multi-modality radiomics nomogram based on DCE-MRI and ultrasound images for benign and malignant breast lesion classification. *Frontiers in Oncology*, *12*, 992509. DOI: 10.3389/fonc.2022.992509 PMID: 36531052

Magnin, C. Y., Lauer, D., Ammeter, M., & Gote-Schniering, J. (2025). From images to clinical insights: An educational review on radiomics in lung diseases. *Breathe (Sheffield, England)*, *21*(1), 230225. DOI: 10.1183/20734735.0225-2023 PMID: 40104259

Majumder, S., Katz, S., Kontos, D., & Roshkovan, L. (2023). State of the art: Radiomics and radiomics-related artificial intelligence on the road to clinical translation. *BJR|Open*, *6*(1), tzad004. DOI: 10.1093/bjro/tzad004

Maniaci, A., Lavalle, S., Gagliano, C., Lentini, M., Masiello, E., Parisi, F., Iannella, G., Cilia, N. D., Salerno, V., Cusumano, G., & La Via, L. (2024). The Integration of Radiomics and Artificial Intelligence in Modern Medicine. *Life (Chicago, Ill.)*, *14*(10), 1248. DOI: 10.3390/life14101248 PMID: 39459547

Martin, P., Holloway, L., Metcalfe, P., Koh, E.-S., & Brighi, C. (2022). Challenges in Glioblastoma Radiomics and the Path to Clinical Implementation. *Cancers (Basel)*, *14*(16), 3897. DOI: 10.3390/cancers14163897 PMID: 36010891

Mayerhoefer, M. E., Materka, A., Langs, G., Häggström, I., Szczypiński, P., Gibbs, P., & Cook, G. (2020). Introduction to Radiomics. *Journal of Nuclear Medicine*, *61*(4), 488–495. DOI: 10.2967/jnumed.118.222893 PMID: 32060219

Miles, K. (2020). Radiomics for personalised medicine: The long road ahead. *British Journal of Cancer*, *122*(7), 929–930. DOI: 10.1038/s41416-019-0699-8 PMID: 31937924

Nardone, V., Reginelli, A., Rubini, D., Gagliardi, F., Del Tufo, S., Belfiore, M. P., Boldrini, L., Desideri, I., & Cappabianca, S. (2024). Delta radiomics: An updated systematic review. *La Radiologia Medica*, *129*(8), 1197–1214. DOI: 10.1007/s11547-024-01853-4 PMID: 39017760

Osei-Afriyie, S., Addae, A. K., Oppong, S., Amu, H., Ampofo, E., & Osei, E. (2021). Breast cancer awareness, risk factors and screening practices among future health professionals in Ghana: A cross-sectional study. *PLoS One*, *16*(6), e0253373. DOI: 10.1371/journal.pone.0253373 PMID: 34166407

Parmar, C., Grossmann, P., Rietveld, D., Rietbergen, M. M., Lambin, P., & Aerts, H. J. W. L. (2015). Radiomic Machine-Learning Classifiers for Prognostic Biomarkers of Head and Neck Cancer. *Frontiers in Oncology, 5*. Advance online publication. DOI: 10.3389/fonc.2015.00272 PMID: 26697407

Quang, L. T., Baek, B. H., Yoon, W., Kim, S. K., & Park, I. (2024). Comparison of Normalization Techniques for Radiomics Features From Magnetic Resonance Imaging in Predicting Histologic Grade of Meningiomas. *Investigative Magnetic Resonance Imaging, 28*(2), 61. DOI: 10.13104/imri.2024.0010

Quraishi, M. I. (2022). Radiomics-Guided Precision Medicine Approaches for Colorectal Cancer. *Frontiers in Oncology, 12*, 872656. DOI: 10.3389/fonc.2022.872656 PMID: 35756680

Russo, L., Charles-Davies, D., Bottazzi, S., Sala, E., & Boldrini, L. (2024). Radiomics for clinical decision support in radiation oncology. *Clinical Oncology, 36*(8), e269–e281. DOI: 10.1016/j.clon.2024.03.003 PMID: 38548581

Spaanderman, D. J., Hakkesteegt, S. N., Hanff, D. F., Schut, A. R. W., Schiphouwer, L. M., Vos, M., Messiou, C., Doran, S. J., Jones, R. L., Hayes, A. J., Nardo, L., Abdelhafez, Y. G., Moawad, A. W., Elsayes, K. M., Lee, S., Link, T. M., Niessen, W. J., Van Leenders, G. J. L. H., Visser, J. J., & Starmans, M. P. A. (2024). Multicenter external validation of an automated method segmenting and differentiating atypical lipomatous tumors from lipomas using radiomics and deep-learning on MRI. *EClinicalMedicine, 76*, 102802. DOI: 10.1016/j.eclinm.2024.102802 PMID: 39351025

Stefano, A. (2024). Challenges and limitations in applying radiomics to PET imaging: Possible opportunities and avenues for research. *Computers in Biology and Medicine, 179*, 108827. DOI: 10.1016/j.compbiomed.2024.108827 PMID: 38964244

Van Timmeren, J. E., Cester, D., Tanadini-Lang, S., Alkadhi, H., & Baessler, B. (2020). Radiomics in medical imaging—"How-to" guide and critical reflection. *Insights Into Imaging, 11*(1), 91. DOI: 10.1186/s13244-020-00887-2 PMID: 32785796

Zhang, Y.-P., Zhang, X.-Y., Cheng, Y.-T., Li, B., Teng, X.-Z., Zhang, J., Lam, S., Zhou, T., Ma, Z.-R., Sheng, J.-B., Tam, V. C. W., Lee, S. W. Y., Ge, H., & Cai, J. (2023). Artificial intelligence-driven radiomics study in cancer: The role of feature engineering and modeling. *Military Medical Research, 10*(1), 22. DOI: 10.1186/s40779-023-00458-8 PMID: 37189155

Zhou, A., Yousem, D. M., & Alvin, M. D. (2018). Cost-Effectiveness Analysis in Radiology: A Systematic Review. *Journal of the American College of Radiology, 15*(11), 1536–1546. DOI: 10.1016/j.jacr.2018.06.018 PMID: 30057243

Chapter 3
Revolutionizing Early Cancer Diagnosis Using Artificial Intelligence: A Systematic Review

Tariq Saeed Mian
https://orcid.org/0000-0003-2666-9223
Taibah University, Saudi Arabia

Hisham Farooq Saeed
Fatima Medical and Saleem Surgical Hospital, Sheikhupura, Pakistan

Eman M. Alatawi
Taibah University, Saudi Arabia

ABSTRACT

Early cancer diagnosis significantly improves treatment outcomes and survival rates. While traditional diagnostic methods face challenges in accuracy, speed, and accessibility, artificial intelligence (AI) offers transformative solutions. AI models, particularly machine learning (ML) and deep learning (DL), excel at learning complex data patterns to predict early-stage cancer, enhancing existing diagnostics. This review examines the scope of AI in early cancer detection, analysing studies categorised by cancer type, diagnostic modality, AI methodology, and performance. AI consistently demonstrates superior sensitivity and specificity compared to conventional methods, especially in radiology, pathology, and genomics. Despite promising advancements, further exploration and collaborative efforts between clinicians, researchers, and technologists are crucial to address limitations and ensure effective clinical implementation.

DOI: 10.4018/979-8-3373-4312-9.ch003

1. INTRODUCTION

Early detection of cancer has acquired immense exposure among other researchers, clinicians and oncologists to enhance the survival rate and cure. Due to the development of oncology, along with the introduction of advanced methods, the procedure of cancer diagnosis has been dramatically changed. As stressed in many pieces of evidence, screening can be used to detect cancer at early stages and decrease mortality (Crosby et al., 2022). Nevertheless, despite successful screening, a doubt about the accuracy of diagnostics persists. Majority of the existing screening procedures use a single proven model which usually collides with the concepts of personalised medicine (Maroni et al., 2021). One of the challenges is the identification of the right patients to screen using relevant risk factors. The diagnosis process has also been automated under conditions of artificial intelligence (AI) techniques, which have led to the precise diagnosis of cancer tumours (Houssami et al., 2019) . Artificial intelligence (AI) approaches of ML and DL have been demonstrated to be effective to address complicated medical problems, such as cancer detection and diagnosis. These models can become a significant contribution to the enhancement of these processes in the near future (Dembrower et al., 2020; Tharwat et al., 2022; Hirsch et al., 2025) . Also, AI may enhance the diagnosis of cancer through automation of clinical practices founded on clinical data of individuals who undergo screening, especially in case of limited resources (Bi et al., 2019).

Previously, a number of studies have surveyed the role of AI in early detection of different types of cancer (Cheung and Rubin, 2021; Jones et al., 2022). AI models have better potential of classification of cancer into various types with the highest accuracy. The usefulness of these models was confirmed in a number of studies, and the utilization of AI should be properly studied to make it more useful in the healthcare systems. Given the eminence of AI, the current review paper discusses the role played by these models in enhancing the process of early cancer diagnosis.

1.1 Importance of Early Cancer Diagnosis and Challenges

Early cancer detection is of utmost importance in enhancing the outcome of patients by boosting their survival chances and facilitating its timely and less expensive treatment while minimizing the risks of the disease (Fitzgerald et al., 2022). Some studies have suggested that the early detection of cancer greatly enhances the prognosis of cancer. Irrespective of its importance, there are certain critical issues associated with early cancer diagnosis. Given the difficulty of detecting cancer in its initial stages, it is necessary to consider new methods, including AI in oncology, to address the problem and improve the efficiency of early diagnosis. To set the scene for this literature review, the following diagram (Figure 1) illustrates the key evolutionary milestones in the field.

1.2 Contributions of the Review Paper

This review paper emphasises the early diagnosis of cancer using advanced AI models. The primary contributions of the reviewed paper are as follows:

- Introduction to Early Cancer Diagnosis: The importance of early cancer diagnosis with different AI models is discussed in this review.
- Survey of AI models: The use of different AI models including ML and DL models was also thoroughly reviewed and discussed, including the role of AI and medical imaging instruments, including X-rays, MRI, CT scans, and histopathology and digital pathology developments.
- AI-Powered Multi-Omics in Early Cancer Detection: In this review, the authors highlight the implementation of AI-based multi-omics to detect cancer at an early diagnosis stage.
- Challenges and Future Recommendations: The paper outlines the challenges and problems that may arise and proposes possible directions in the future, to overcome the changing challenges in improving the diagnosis process to detect early cancer.

1.3 Organisation of the Paper

The structure of the paper is in the following way: Section 2 will discuss the methodology of how the review was conducted. Section 3 is the detailed analysis of the use of various AI models in early cancer diagnosis. The fourth section deals with the use of AI-enabled multi-omics to diagnose cancer at the early stage. Section 5 gives a short description of the datasets used in the diagnosis of cancer. Section 6 will address identified challenges and research gaps in available literature and will give future research directions, and Section 7 will provide a conclusion of the paper with the notable observations.

2. METHODOLOGY USED FOR CONDUCTING LITERATURE REVIEW

An organized approach was taken to undertake a thorough investigation of the application of AI in the early diagnosis of cancer. The review paper is organised into summarising the relevant research articles and knowing the research gaps and challenges of the study.

Table 1. PRISMA Flow Diagram – Literature Search and Screening Process

Stage	Resources
Identification	• **Records identified from databases (n = 2,480)** o Springer (620) o IEEE Xplore (410) o ResearchGate (350) o Google Scholar (1,100) • **Records after duplicates removed (n = 1,430)**
Screening	• **Records screened (title & abstract) (n = 1,430)** • **Records excluded (n = 1,080)**
Eligibility	• **Full-text articles assessed (n = 350)** • **Full-text articles excluded (n = 252)** • **Reasons:** o Not in English o Conference papers o Non-academic/grey literature o Older than 2019 o Insufficient methodology o Outside IEEE/Springer/ResearchGate • • **Not related to early cancer diagnosis with AI**
Included	• **Studies included in qualitative synthesis (n = 80)** • **These studies represent:** o AI in radiology o AI-enabled histopathology o Multi-omics & precision oncology o Biomarker discovery • **ML & DL models for early cancer detection**

2.1 Data Sources and Search Strategy

Their review is achieved through searching of the relevant articles on the search keywords and search strings. The keywords and strings are searched across four search engines: Springer, ResearchGate, IEEE Xplore, and Google Scholar. The selection of articles is mainly based on the finalised keywords such as 'Early Cancer Diagnosis', 'Artificial Intelligence', 'Machine Learning', 'Deep Learning', 'Systematic Review', 'Cancer Detection', and 'Medical Imaging'.

2.2 Inclusion and Exclusion Criteria

The shortlisted articles were investigated, and duplicates were removed. Papers analysing the concept of early cancer diagnosis using AI were reviewed. In addition, articles not written in English, duplicate articles, articles published in conference proceedings and journals other than IEEE, Springer, and ResearchGate, non-academic articles, and articles older than 2019 were excluded from the review.

3. AI TECHNIQUES IN EARLY CANCER DIAGNOSIS

This section provides a comprehensive analysis of the application of different AI models for early cancer diagnosis.

3.1 Machine Learning Classifiers

Conventional ML classifiers are used to identify and classify cancerous and non-cancerous tumours based on clinical information (Maurya et al., 2023; Painuli & Bhardwaj, 2022; Tembhurne et al., 2023). Traditional detection techniques rely on predefined rule sets and feature sets for cancer detection. Hence, these techniques are often limited to detecting cancer only after certain stages and are unable to detect it in its early stages. This section highlights the application of different ML classifiers for early cancer detection.

3.1.1 Support Vector Machines (SVM)

The authors Hage Chehade et al. (2022) examined the role of various ML classifiers including SVM for accurately classifying colon and lung cancer types. The classifiers were trained using histopathological images for the analysis which were obtained from the LC25000 dataset. Experimental outcomes suggest that the SVM model achieved an accuracy of 94.68% in comparison to ANN and KNN classifiers The SVM classifier was also used by Daghrir et al. (2020) for classifying skin cancer. A hybrid approach was designed wherein the SVM classifier was used with other two classifiers for improving the accuracy of prediction. The result was based on the prediction of all three classifiers which were trained using skin lesion images. The accuracy of SVM alone was found to be 71.8%. a SVM based approach is discussed in Al Mudawi & Alazeb (2022) for detecting cervical cancer. The SVM classifier along with other ML classifiers such as KNN, regression algorithms and tree-based algorithms. For predicting cervical cancer SVM achieved an excellent accuracy of 99%. A comprehensive examination of the use of ML models in cancer prediction along the lines of the expression of single genes in the paper by Khalsan et al. (2022) is provided.

3.1.2 Tree-Based and Ensemble Methods (RF, DT, Gradient Boosting, AdaBoost)

The work presented by Ali et al. (2021) investigated the role of ML in detecting early-stage cervical cancer. Clinical features were used to train three different ML classifiers, namely Random Tree, Random Forest (RF) and K-Nearest Neighbours (KNN) to achieve an accurate classification. Following transformations of features, the models had 98% to 99% accuracy. It was found that with fine-tuning ML models, cervical cancer at its early stages can be detected successfully. A novel boosting-based approach is proposed in Vo et al. (2019) for classifying breast cancer types. A Gradient boosting tree (GBDT) classifier is combined with a deep learning model for building a strong classifier. The proposed approach effectively classifies the cancer images as benign and malignant with an accuracy of 99.5%. The authors Gamil et al. (2024) employed an AdaBoost algorithm for detecting and classifying skin cancer. A feature extraction technique is used to reduce the dimensionality of the dataset and the accuracy was 93%. A similar AdaBoost algorithm is implemented in Li et al. (2025) for predicting lymph node metastasis in cervical cancer patients. Results show that the AdaBoost classifier exhibited excellent accuracy in comparison to SVM and RF.

3.1.3 k-Nearest Neighbours (KNN)

The KNN classifier was used by Fahami et al. (2021) for detecting effective genes in colon cancer. The KNN classifier along with DT was used to extract essential features related to effective genes in patients with colon cancer. This extraction of genes helped in the early cancer detection. A novel KNN classifier was implemented in Sachdeva et al. (2024) for diagnosing lung cancer. The conventional KNN classifier was modified using a Pearson correlation which was proved to be more resilient, adaptable and accurate for real-time cancer detection in comparison to KNN and other conventional ML classifiers. The authors Vemula et al. (2024) revolutionized detection of breast cancer using KNN classifier along with SVM. The study suggested that the KNN classifier has the potential to transform the way of cancer detection.

3.1.4 Logistic Regression (LR) and Other Classical Models

The investigation of applying LR for cancer detection is discussed in several research works. A comprehensive analysis of LR for diagnostic biomarker studies to aid cancer detection is discussed in Elkahwagy et al. (2024). The study emphasized the implementation of LR algorithms and enhance the potentiality of biomarkers by employing different statistical techniques for cancer detection. A comparison of

LR with other ML classifier for predicting metastasis in gastric cancer patients is discussed in Lu et al. (2024). The review indicates that ML models could be used to better the precision of early cancer detection and also to present meaningful information to radiologists, endoscopists, and pathologists to aid in diagnosis and treatment planning. However, ML models often suffer from issues such as limited labelled data, imbalanced datasets, and lack of generalization problems.

3.2 Deep Learning Models

This section highlights some of the DL models used for cancer detection.

3.2.1 Convolutional Neural Networks (CNN) for Imaging

The authors Yurttakal et al. (2020) employed a Deep CNN (DCNN) model for detecting breast cancer. The DCNN model used MRI images for classifying breast cancer in the early stage. A multi-layered CNN architecture was employed which yielded an accuracy of 98.33%.

The article structured by Hosseini et al. (2023) talks about a systematic review of ML models to detect oesophageal cancer at an early stage. The overall accuracy of the models to analyse endoscopy and CT images was above 89%. This indicates that the ML efficiency is high in the early detection of oesophageal cancer. The similar survey is available in Islam et al. (2022), where the researchers discuss the problem of the introduction of DL into the first cut of identifying the presence of oesophagus cancer. The authors Gouda et al. (2022) used CNN for classifying skin lesion images to detect skin cancer. The model was trained using ISIC2018 dataset which achieved an accuracy of 83.2%. The researchers conducted a meta-analysis to analyze the effectiveness of the ML in the diagnosis of early gastric cancer (EGC) Shi et al. (2024). As discussed, the application of ML models is ideal in the diagnosis of EGC, and the highest success is achieved. A comprehensive review of DL for diagnosing cancer is presented in (Tandon et al., 2024). The analysis revealed that CNNs were the most commonly used and consistently delivered high accuracy.

3.2.2 Deep Neural Networks (DNNs, MLPs, Autoencoders)

A DNN based architecture was designed in Maqsood et al. (2022) for detecting multimodal brain tumor. The DNN was combined with a multiclass SVM for enhancing the accuracy of detection. The maximum accuracy achieved by the DNN architecture was 98.92%. A deep MLP along with a feature-fused Autoencoder was proposed by Hameed Alsaedi et al. (2025) for classifying breast cancer. The Autoencoder model was found to be more effective in classifying cancerous images and improving the cancer diagnosis process. An autoencoder based stacked approach is presented in Ogundokun et al. (2025) for classifying cervical cancer. The model is accompanied by feature extraction and an ensemble learning approach. A summary of different ML and DL models used for early cancer detection is presented in Table 2.

Table 2. Summary of ML and DL models for early cancer detection

Reference	ML/DL Model	Type of Cancer Analysis	Accuracy	Observation
(Yurttakal et al., 2020)	Deep CNN (DCNN)	Breast Cancer	98.33%	The model is faster in classifying cancerous and noncancerous tumours. It also prevents unnecessary biopsies.
(Vo et al., 2019)	DCNN, Gradient boosting tree (GBDT) classifier	Breast Cancer	4-class = 96.4% 2-class = 99.5%	GBDT effectively handles imbalanced training data and avoids overfitting.
(Fahami et al., 2021)	Decision Tree (DT), KNN	Colon Cancer	97.49 ± 2.92%	More DL models need to be explored for colon cancer diagnosis. In addition, techniques such as normalisation and clustering can be applied to improve the performance.
(Hage Chehade et al., 2023)	SVM, ANN, KNN	Lung and Colon Cancer	KNN = 92.10% SVM = 94.68% ANN = 92.58%	Feature extraction techniques can be implemented to improve the performance of SVM and KNN models.
(Daghrir, et al., 2020)	KNN, SVM, CNN	Skin Cancer	KNN = 57.3% SVM = 71.8% CNN = 85.5%	CNN performs better compared to other ML models. However, the fusion of all three models yields better results; hence, adopting a hybrid model should be explored.
(Gouda et al., 2022)	CNN, Resnet50, InceptionV3, Inception Resnet	Skin Cancer	CNN = 83.2% Resnet50 = 83.7% InceptionV3 = 85.8% Inception Resnet = 84%	CNN, along with multiple transfer learning models, performs better than a single CNN architecture

continued on following page

Table 2. Continued

Reference	ML/DL Model	Type of Cancer Analysis	Accuracy	Observation
(Al Mudawi & Alazeb, 2022)	Logistic Regression, SVM, RF, DT, Adaptive Boosting, KNN	Cervical Cancer	Logistic Regression = 98%, SVM = 99%, RF = 100%, DT = 100%, Adaptive Boosting = 100%, KNN = 95%	The models need to be evaluated using diverse and large-scale datasets in order to validate their performance
(Maqsood et al., 2022)	Deep Neural Network with Multi-class SVM	Brain Tumor	98.92%	The proposed method overcomes issues such as low-contrast images and incorrect tumour-region segmentation, yielding superior results.

Whereas, DL models have been found to be more reliable than ML, they also have a problem of class imbalance and bias in the datasets. This highlights the need to test DL algorithms to predict and diagnose cancer early. Moreover, the lack of data to train models and the use of patient-sensitive information can also be considered as obstacles to the training of DL models.

3.3 AI and Medical Imaging

AI has revolutionized medical imaging, which has risen the level of early cancer diagnosis. A sample illustration of how CNN is used in the process of lung nodule detection is shown in figure 2.

In this section, the author explains the use of AI and medical imaging in the early diagnosis of cancer.

3.3.1 AI in Radiology

Radiomics, the segment of medical research that is rapidly developing, is being fueled by the integration of radiographic images with clinical outcome data with the help of AI tools (Bi et al., 2019; Jin et al., 2021) . Table 3 shows conventional imaging modalities that are applicable in the detection of early cancer.

Table 3. Conventional imaging modalities for early cancer diagnosis

Type of Cancer	Primary Screening Tools
Lung Cancer	LDCT / DxCT
Breast Cancer	Mammography Images or Digital Images
Pancreatic Cancer	Pancreatic Juice and Serum
Skin	Optical Images
Gastrointestinal Cancer	Optical (OCT)
Liver	CT or MRI Images
Cervical Cancer	Optical Images

AI systems can address these shortcomings of traditional imaging modalities by allowing algorithms to learn on their own strategies of which parts of an image are most strongly correlated with a particular outcome. Such models also acquire the distinguishing characteristics in those areas in multi-layered hierarchical levels, which minimizes the reliance on manual information (Gillies et al., 2020) . The discussion of the place of AI in changing the traditional radiology process is discussed in the below section using a flowchart.

Table 4.

Step	Process Description	Key Technologies/Methods	Output
1. Image Acquisition	Get raw medical images.	**Radiology:** CT, MRI, Ultrasound, X-ray, Mammography. **Pathology:** Whole Slide Images (WSI) from digitised glass slides.	Raw Digital Image Dataset
2. Pre-processing & Augmentation	Prepare the raw images (i.e. enhance image quality and standardise the data) for the model.	**Normalisation:** Adjusting contrast/ brightness. **Filtering:** Removing noise. **Augmentation:** Creating variations (rotation, scaling, cropping) to increase the dataset size.	Clean, Standardised Image Set
3. Segmentation & Localisation	Identify and isolate the region of interest (ROI) (a tumour, lesion, or specific tissue area).	**Deep Learning:** U-Net, Mask R-CNN. **Traditional:** Thresholding, Active Contours.	Identified and Labelled ROI
4. Feature Extraction (For Traditional ML/Radiomics)	Extract the relevant quantitative features (texture, shape, intensity) of the ROI.	**Radiomics:** Extraction of high-throughput features. **Deep Learning:** Features learned internally by CNN layers.	Quantified Feature Vector
5. AI Model Training & Classification	Train the machine to recognise patterns associated with cancer.	**Deep Learning:** CNNs like ResNet, VGG), Transformers. **Traditional ML:** Support Vector Machines (SVM), Random Forests.	Trained Model and Cancer Classification

continued on following page

Table 4. Continued

Step	Process Description	Key Technologies/Methods	Output
6. Post-processing & Visualisation	Refine the model output and present it in an interpretable format for the clinician.	**Heatmaps (e.g., Grad-CAM):** To show *why* the model made a prediction (Explainable AI - XAI). **Thresholding:** Converting probability scores into a binary Yes/No prediction.	Diagnostic Report with Prediction & Confidence Score
7. Clinical Decision Support	The final prediction is integrated into the clinical workflow to aid the physician in making the definitive diagnosis and treatment plan.	**Integration:** Electronic Health Records (EHR) systems. **Multi-Modal Fusion:** Combining AI imaging results with clinical/genomic data.	Final Diagnostic Prediction (e.g., Benign or otherwise)

(i) ***Improving workflow for disease diagnosis:*** AI technologies may help organize the schedule of imaging appointments and anticipate the availability of patients, allowing it to be managed more efficiently even prior to the arrival of the patients at the radiology department. Also, AI can transform the process of diagnostics. The article offered by Derevianko et al. (2023) applied the AI in the field of radiology to enhance the interaction between patients and doctors during the diagnosis of cancer. The other article reported in (Tran et al., 2021) addressed the use of AI in the field of computational radiology to diagnose breast cancer. In contrast to the current computer-based methods to aid diagnoses, AI demonstrated promising results, improving the accuracy of the diagnoses.

(ii) ***Early Detection:*** AI is currently used to analyze CT scans and CT angiograms to notify radiologists and clinicians to act prior to the critical situation which is beneficial to treatment. RAD can prioritise the process of diagnosis according to the urgency of the findings with the help of AI (O'Connor and Bhalla, 2021). As an illustration, a simulation study carried at a university hospital in Germany regarding historical chest radiographs showed that the time to report serious cases reduced to 80mins, (Baltruschat et al., 2021). Besides urgent diagnosis, AI can also assist in incidental diagnoses in the earlier stages, particularly cancer. Routine test or CT scan analyses using AI can be effectively used to identify possible early warning signs of various types of cancer.

(iii) ***Improved diagnostic accuracy:*** About half of the AI tools currently offered in radiology are mainly oriented at improving diagnostic precision in order to reduce cases of missed diagnosis and to avoid unnecessary procedures and follow-up examinations, which ultimately leads to the achievement of improved patient outcomes (van Leeuwen et al., 2022; Qin et al., 2019). Moreover, AI devices support radiologists in the process of image clarification by showing visual cues, e.g., bounding boxes, markers, and probability scores, in real-time or as a subsequent evaluation (van Leeuwen et al., 2024).

(iv) ***Personalised diagnostics:*** The AI algorithms allow precision medicine to predict risks and outcomes. Such a personalised solution can enhance clinical outcomes and better resource allocation. A prospective study showed that it was possible to avoid unnecessary biopsies when there was an assessment of the risk of malignancy through a commercially existing AI tool (Lu et al., 2019). Breast density classification is another form of personalisation in breast cancer screening. Females having thick breast tissue are considered to be more vulnerable to cancer (Bakker et al., 2019). A more personalized screening approach can be made by using an automated AI-based approach, and with this approach, women with dense breasts can have more frequent screenings or may adopt other imaging methods like MRI.

In spite of the fact that AI can greatly enhance clinical outcomes in radiology, the latter is usually associated with some issues, including variability of data, lack of annotated data, and decreased extrapolation to other populations. To achieve the full potential of AI in the field of medical imaging in detecting early cancer there is a need to ensure that these issues are addressed through sound validation, multicenter datasets, and regulatory oversight.

3.3.2 AI-Enabled Histopathology and Digital Pathology Advancements

The integration of AI into the field of digital pathology is altering the process of diagnosing cancer by allowing it to automatically analyze histological samples, enhance the prediction of prognostic outcomes and detection accuracy (Bera et al., 2019). Traditional pathology methods largely depend on manual inspection with a microscope of tissue samples (Acs et al., 2020). Conversely, AI-based computational pathology with ML or DL algorithms has shown impressive results in the analysis of the tumour microenvironment, detection of cancer and prediction of patient outcome based on the analysis of detailed histological data.

Whole-slide imaging (WSI) has transformed digital pathology by allowing the high-quality digitisation of histology slides. In contrast to the traditional microscopy that is based on manual analysis of the tissue samples, WSI allows analyzing the digital tissue samples, provides the possibility to conduct remote consultations, store a lot of data, and effectively integrate with AI technologies (Bera et al., 2020). One area that the innovation has significantly influenced is oncology, where the accurate diagnosis, staging, and prognosis of cancer depend on precise examination of tissues (Huang et al., 2021). Besides the efficiency of the workflow, the digitisation of the glass slides into the image also has a solid route to the achievement of artificial intelligence-driven pathology results (Shmatko et al., 2022). Among these learning methods, supervised learning-based models exhibit higher accuracy because they are trained on labelled datasets to categorise cancerous tissues from benign tissues and identify biomarkers (Musulin et al., 2021). These models address the drawbacks of conventional models that rely on manual annotation of histopathological slides, such as high time consumption and labour intensity. However, one of the most complex issues is the reliability of the outcome generated by supervised models (Rakha et al., 2022)

To mitigate the limitations of supervised models, other scholars have proposed semi-supervised learning models (Youseif et al., 2022) . Moreover, the unsupervised forms of learning are not dependent on labelled data, which is why they are one of the most popular to detect cancerous tissues as well. Unsupervised models give possibilities to AI tools to find peculiar morphological patterns related to disease development (Bizzego et al., 2019). Researchers are investigating more complex DL-based models for cancer diagnosis and prediction, for customised treatment (Wong et al., 2022). It is anticipated that integrating AI models into histopathology analysis would improve diagnostic consistency and, eventually, cancer patient care, as these models become more interpretable and resilient (Rathore et al., 2020). The effectiveness of oncology treatment can be enhanced by incorporating multimodal information in the traditional pathology information. Combining histopathological data with other data of imaging (clinical, molecular, and genomic) can be used to give a more comprehensive picture of tumour biology and permits better-informed treatment approaches in the end. Basic histopathology analysis lays emphasis on the morphological characteristics, thus not taking into consideration the heterogeneity of tumours Various concepts can be used to summarise the role of AI in histopathology and digital pathology as shown in Table 5.

Table 5. Summary of AI in histopathology for cancer diagnosis

AI in Pathology	Observations	Reference
Histopathological Features for Cancer Grading	AI models reduce inter-observer variability and enhance visibility. Therefore, the reliability and throughput of the analysis can be improved.	(Mantrala et al., 2022) (Rodriguez et al., 2022)
Automating Cancer Grading Systems	Models such as CNNs, Generative Adversarial Networks (GANs), and transformer models are widely used to automate the grading of histopathological images with high accuracy. Pre-trained AI models accurately distinguish between low-grade and high-grade cancer tumours, whereas ML models do not.	(Klein et al., 2021) (Großerueschkamp et al., 2021)
	AI-based grading yields excellent outcomes when applied to breast, lung, and prostate cancer. These systems achieved 94.6% accuracy in prostate cancer. While DL models were found to be highly accurate when handling histopathology images of breast cancer.	(Viswanathan et al., 2022) (Lagree et al., 2021)
Reducing Observer Variability and Improving Reliability	In cancer grading, interobserver variability has been reported as a very complex issue. Interobserver variability affects diagnosis and treatment outcomes. AI can successfully address this issue and significantly improve the reliability of assessing and grading histopathological images.	(Laury et al., 2021)
	The manual analysis suffers from high deviation, while the AI model minimises the deviation and makes the classification of the cancerous tumours accurate and precise. In prostate cancer, the AI models are found to be more consistent. It has also been observed that by using AI, interobserver variability reduces by approximately 35%.	(Musulin et al., 2021) (Rakha et al., 2022)

4. AI-POWERED MULTI-OMICS FOR EARLY CANCER DETECTION

Combined with multi-omics data, AI has revolutionized early cancer detection through offering a comprehensive view of tumour history. Nevertheless, this data is complex and has a high dimension and is difficult to analyse using conventional methods. This problem can be addressed using AI-based ML and DL models capable of working with complex data, detecting underlying patterns, and early biomarkers due to the predictive capabilities. In this section, the author talks about using AI-based multi-omics to diagnose early cancer.

4.1 Multi-Omics Analysis Using AI

The latest research has shown that fusing omics data with AI algorithms are much better than single-omics models in cancer detection. The machinery of multi-omics data analysis (pattern recognition, prediction, and data integration) has been automated by ML and DL (Chukwunweike et al., 2024). Sixty-six AI models are capable of an accurate analysis of nonlinear data and complex patterns across omics layers (Wen et al., 2023). One of the popular AI models in multi-omics analysis is DL. The neural network architecture of DL fits well in the extraction of exploitive features and data patterns of high dimensional data. The advantages of autoencoders (AEs) include effective unsupervised models that can reduce multi-omics data without including any valuable data on the disease (Debbadi and Boateng, 2025).

Both ML and DL models can remove any additional noise of data and find important and significant molecular features in relation to cancer (Alves et al., 2021). SVMs help to adopt a more detailed approach to medicine by categorizing cancer patients based on a combination of genomic and transcriptomic data (Debbadi and Boateng, 2025). On the other hand, RF model is applied to identify biomarkers and depict the most prevalent features and traits of multi-omics findings (Acharjee et al., 2020; Dhillon et al., 2023). Other than the selection of useful features, AI has been used in the refinement of multi-omics data analysis by generating biological interaction maps to determine basic molecular interactions. Another DL model that can identify unique therapeutic targets and can analyse complicated patterns and connections among genes, proteins and metabolites is Graph Neural Network (GNN) (Alharbi et al., 2024). Besides that, AI solutions, such as natural language processing (NLP) and knowledge graphs, are used to fuse multi-omics data with biomedical data. They learn and discover the biological features of cancer and patient data due to their internal structure (Karim et al., 2023). The other powerful and efficient AI model that can be utilized in the analysis of the multi-omics data is the use of reinforcement learning (RL) algorithms to enhance the omics data fruits strategies. The RL algorithms are leaner and better at improving the integration, which guarantees the protection of important features to be analyzed later (Mohammed et al., 2023). As AI continues to develop, its integration into multi-omics analysis is expected to lead to more accurate disease models, better biomarker discovery, and personalized treatment plans, and hopefully, precision medicine will become a more efficient and more universal process.

4.2 AI-Driven Biomarker Discovery Using Multi-Omics Data

Another notable use of AI in the analysis of multi-omics data is biomarker discovery. AI strategies facilitate the identification of multi-omics dataset patterns and as a result discover biomarkers to diagnose and prognose early cancer (Zhang et al., 2025). RF algorithm has been applied frequently in the context of finding biomarkers by picking Informative features among large data sets. RF models have been found to be quite useful in the identification of gene expression biomarkers in the classification of cancerous tissues versus benign tissues. With the help of

SVM techniques, the early detection of the signs of a disease is enhanced since the classification boundary is optimized between a healthy sample and a diseased sample (Ali and Mohammed, 2024). CNNs and AEs are examples of DL models that have transformed the process of biomarker detection in omics and imaging studies. CNNs are superior at processing radiomic data of MRI and CT scans and locating biomarkers to detect cancer at an early stage (Hassan, 2024). AEs are specialised DL architectures capable of greatly reducing the dimensionality of large-scale omics data without losing significant disease-related features and with a minimal amount of noise. Another potentially useful AI tool in biomarker discovery and in interaction mapping between genes, proteins, and metabolites is network-based analysis on the basis of GNNs (Alharbi et al., 2025). Such models are useful in revealing key regulatory nodes in disease pathways, and as a result, the highly interconnected biomarkers can be identified, and they have a mechanistic role. Several reinforcement learning (RL) methods optimise biomarker selection, which is done through an iterative process of picking the most informative molecular features to classify illnesses and predict prognosis (Mohammed et al., 2023). Such models increase the sensitivity and specificity of biomarkers to such serious diseases as cancer and autoimmune conditions (Pauly & Schwartz, 2019). The discovery process can be redefined with the introduction of AI as a biomarker analyzer and the processing time can be minimized and the precision medicine process can be more efficient to improve the outcome of the treatment (Ali, 2023). Table 6 demonstrates that the efficacy of AI-driven biomarker discovery is greater than the conventional models.

Table 6. Comparison of AI-based and conventional biomarker discovery methods

Parameters / Functionalities	AI-based Biomarker Discovery Methods	Traditional Biomarker Discovery Methods
Methodology	ML or DL-based data-driven analysis	Hypothesis-based analysis
Data Integration	Multi-omics	Single omics
Processing Speed	High and Automated	Manual and Slow Processing
Sensitivity	High	Low and Moderate
Scalability	High scalability even for larger datasets	Limited scalability for high-dimensional data

4.3 Application of AI in Precision Oncology

Precision oncology primarily involves prescribing therapies that target the molecular driver alterations of a cancer type in an individual (Azuaje, 2019). This paradigm has become increasingly popular as multi-omics data and molecular profiling techniques have been integrated into the core of clinical oncology. Besides, precision oncology has also led to the validation of various molecularly targeted agents, which have enhanced treatment outcomes for different cancer types. Although targeted treatments such as trastuzumab or vemurafenib have exhibited their proficiency in improving cancer treatment along with immune checkpoint inhibitors, the need for personalised cancer treatment has always been in demand. This aspect has increased the demand for personalised treatment, which is a part of precision oncology (Ballester & Carmona, 2021).

With tremendous advancements in DL, the application of these models in precision oncology has increased significantly (Wang et al., 2022). DL models are highly capable of classifying high-dimensional data across various domains and cancer patients, yielding accurate results. DL models have proven their ability to classify brain tumours and skin lesions, detect breast cancer, and classify lung tumours. ML models are used to analyse various datasets and multi-omics data and categorise tumours into their own category. RF, SVMs, DTs, and gradient boosting algorithms are among the widely used models in tumour and cancerous cells classification (Wu and Hicks, 2021; Mao et al., 2022; Vindhya et al., 2023).

The other impressive use of the DL model is whole-genome sequencing (WGS) and RNA sequencing (RNA-seq) analysis, which allows identifying driver mutations and actable genetic changes in lung, breast, and colorectal cancer (Alharbi and Rashid, 2022). The DL model was able to interpret every genomic, transcriptomic, and proteomic data of individuals and propose a personalized treatment plan that is determined by the needs of the patient. The experimental analysis shows that the suggested treatment plan was consistent with the one developed by the oncologists, which suggests the prospects of using AI-based models in clinical decision-making (Ali, 2023). Another outstanding development in precision oncology changing how cancer is treated is AI-based forecasting of immunotherapy response. GANs and variational autoencoders (VAEs) use of the DL models have helped scientists find new combinations of drugs to treat various cancer types, which in turn decreases the death rate.

5. CHALLENGES, RESEARCH GAPS, AND FUTURE DIRECTIONS

The introduction of AI in the diagnosis of cancer has resulted in a significant change of the traditional diagnostic procedure. There are a number of studies that confirm the effectiveness of AI models in changing the treatment process. Nevertheless, there are certain obstacles and problems that should be overcome. In this review, several challenges and research gaps that were identified in the existing literature are highlighted and the future research directions are presented.

5.1 Challenges in the AI-based Cancer Diagnosis Process

The challenges identified with respect to benchmarking AI models for cancer treatment are as follows:

(i) **Data Imbalance:** The lack of early-stage malignant samples relative to benign or advanced-stage cases is primarily the causative factor of the class imbalance problem. This makes the model more biased and it does not detect the cancers at early stages despite giving high accuracy.

(ii) **Data Availability:** A number of studies indicate that AI models primarily rely on patient information received through hospital, which in many cases has sensitive data and is not publicly available.

(iii) **Insufficient Explainability**: The majority of AI models are black box (in particular, DNNs), and the clarity of the result of their work is frequently restricted. The absence of explainability impedes the adoption of AI into the diagnostic processes and undermines the regulatory approval initiatives.

(iv) **Generalisation Problems:** It is possible that models that are trained on a single dataset will do badly on a different dataset. Demographic differences, patient data, population genetics and data quality can have a notable impact on the reliability and accuracy of AI models. Therefore, an alternative model that can be developed to tackle the problem of generalisation through training in various clinical settings is necessary.

(v) **AI Deployment in Real-World Healthcare:** Seamless integration of AI into analysing clinical processes and disease diagnosis processes is highly challenging due to differences in electronic health record (EHR) systems, resistance to workflow changes, and the need for real-time performance. Additionally, limited infrastructure availability in resource-constrained medical and healthcare centres can hinder the deployment of AI in real-time healthcare applications.

(vi) **Regulatory concerns and FDA approvals:** Regulatory entities such as the FDA require AI models to demonstrate safety, effectiveness, and consistency, particularly in adaptive (continuously learning) models. In addition, the lack of standardisation of AI models and performance evaluation metrics further slows regulatory acceptance.

(vii) **Ethics and patient privacy:** The use of confidential data of patients in the training of AI models is a major risk to the privacy of the data and raises the issue of the misuse of data. Violations of data protection or the illegal use of patient clinical information may interfere with the trust of the population.

5.2 Future Recommendations

In accordance with the overarching issues, this review provides potential future research directions based on the identified challenges.

(i) Creation of Balanced and Representative Datasets: To minimize the bias and enhance the model performance, it is important to create large, diversified, and well-annotated datasets with a balanced class distribution. The multi-ethnic multi-centre datasets that reflect more closely the real-life scenarios could be developed through collaboration across hospitals, research institutions, and countries.
(ii) Explainable and Interpretable AI: AI models to be used to diagnose cancer in particular should focus on explainability and interpretability, where attention maps, saliency visualisation, and decision trees are examples.
(iii) Robust Generalisation: AI models should be more generally validated on data sets of other populations and clinical setting to guarantee generalisation. With the domain adaptation and transfer learning techniques, it is possible to enhance cross-site performance without necessarily retraining.
(iv) Fitting into Clinical Workflows: Clinicians, radiologists, and pathologists should be consulted to find out how best the AI systems can integrate into the existing workflow. The use of real-time decision support systems and user friendly interfaces will be important in enhancing use in the day to day field.
(v) Enhancement of Regulatory and Standardisation Structures: Uniform guidelines and regulatory frameworks in the field of healthcare (specifically adaptive models) need to be developed on AI. Cooperation with the FDA and EMA is to be directed towards the formulation of effective model validation, safety and monitoring standards.
(vi) Ethical Use and Data Privacy: AI development should be guided by stringent ethical guidelines such as informed consent, anonymisation of data, as well as responsible data sharing. Training models would be possible with fair protection of patient confidentiality with the aid of federated learning and differential privacy methods.
(vii) Multimodal and Multi-Omics AI: Future studies are needed to integrate imaging, clinical records, genomic and proteomic information to enhance the accuracy of the diagnosis. Multimodal AI models can identify new biomarkers and offer risk personalisation.

Future suggestions may help researchers to extend the investigation of the application of AI to the problem of early diagnosing of cancer.

6. CONCLUSION

This review paper analysed the application of various AI-based ML and DL models for diagnosing cancer at its early stages. As inferred from the study, the cancer diagnosis process is a highly critical area that is subject to continuous changes driven by demographic shifts and patient diversity. Given the criticality, traditional diagnostic models, such as hypothesis-based imaging modalities, fail to achieve the desired performance in detecting cancer occurrences at early stages from clinical data. ML and DL models are generally trained to accurately detect and categorise cancerous tissues from noncancerous tissues by analysing patient data. This review discusses the application of AI across different aspects of cancer diagnosis, including AI in radiology, histopathology, and digital pathology; multi-omics analysis using AI; biomarker discovery using AI; and AI in precision oncology. This review is offered in a detailed analysis to assist researchers to achieve significant information with regard to the use of AI models in the early detection of cancer. The information presented in the review may be applied to analyze the implementation of different AI models and provide insights into AI-based cancer detection to detect various types of cancer. Even though AI-based ML and DL models can effectively detect cancer using clinical data, there are numerous issues that may be an obstacle to their implementation. Therefore, the need to delve further into this aspect exists even though various research works are available. These issues are those that require more research, which are presented in this review. The recommendations made in this review could be adopted to make early diagnosis of cancer much better. The AI models can be used to realise early detection, diagnosis, and treatment of cancer and support the transformation of the diagnostic process with the help of advanced technologies including explainable AI and Generative AI.

REFERENCES

Acharjee, A., Larkman, J., Xu, Y., Cardoso, V. R., & Gkoutos, G. V. (2020). A random forest-based biomarker discovery and power analysis framework for diagnostics research. *BMC Medical Genomics, 13*(1), 1–14. DOI: 10.1186/s12920-020-00826-6 PMID: 33228632

Acs, B., Rantalainen, M., & Hartman, J. (2020). Artificial intelligence is the next step towards precision pathology. *Journal of Internal Medicine, 288*(1), 62–81. DOI: 10.1111/joim.13030 PMID: 32128929

Al Mudawi, N., & Alazeb, A. (2022). A model for predicting cervical cancer using machine learning algorithms. *Sensors (Basel), 22*(11), 4132. DOI: 10.3390/s22114132 PMID: 35684753

Alharbi, F., Vakanski, A., Zhang, B., Elbashir, M. K., & Mohammed, M. (2024). Comparative Analysis of Multi-Omics Integration Using Advanced Graph Neural Networks for Cancer Classification. *arXiv preprint arXiv:2410.05325.*

Alharbi, F., Vakanski, A., Zhang, B., Elbashir, M. K., & Mohammed, M. (2025). Comparative Analysis of Multi-Omics Integration Using Graph Neural Networks for Cancer Classification. *IEEE Access : Practical Innovations, Open Solutions, 13*, 37724–37736. DOI: 10.1109/ACCESS.2025.3540769 PMID: 40123934

Alharbi, W. S., & Rashid, M. (2022). A review of deep learning applications in human genomics using next-generation sequencing data. *Human Genomics, 16*(1), 26. DOI: 10.1186/s40246-022-00396-x PMID: 35879805

Ali, A. M., & Mohammed, M. A. (2024). Optimized Cancer Subtype Classification and Clustering Using Cat Swarm Optimization and Support Vector Machine Approach for Multi-Omics Data. *Journal of Soft Computing and Data Mining, 5*(2), 223–244. DOI: 10.30880/jscdm.2024.05.02.017

Ali, H. (2023). Artificial intelligence in multi-omics data integration: Advancing precision medicine, biomarker discovery and genomic-driven disease interventions. *Int J Sci Res Arch, 8*(1), 1012–1030. DOI: 10.30574/ijsra.2023.8.1.0189

Ali, M. M., Ahmed, K., Bui, F. M., Paul, B. K., Ibrahim, S. M., Quinn, J. M., & Moni, M. A. (2021). Machine learning-based statistical analysis for early-stage detection of cervical cancer. *Computers in Biology and Medicine, 139*, 104985. DOI: 10.1016/j.compbiomed.2021.104985 PMID: 34735942

Alves, M. A., Lamichhane, S., Dickens, A., McGlinchey, A., Ribeiro, H. C., Sen, P., Wei, F., Hyötyläinen, T., & Orešič, M. (2021). Systems biology approaches to study lipidomes in health and disease. *Biochimica et Biophysica Acta (BBA)-. Biochimica et Biophysica Acta. Molecular and Cell Biology of Lipids*, *1866*(2), 158857. DOI: 10.1016/j.bbalip.2020.158857 PMID: 33278596

Azuaje, F. (2019). Artificial intelligence for precision oncology: Beyond patient stratification. *NPJ Precision Oncology*, *3*(1), 6. DOI: 10.1038/s41698-019-0078-1 PMID: 30820462

Bakker, M. F., de Lange, S. V., Pijnappel, R. M., Mann, R. M., Peeters, P. H., Monninkhof, E. M., Emaus, M. J., Loo, C. E., Bisschops, R. H. C., Lobbes, M. B. I., de Jong, M. D. F., Duvivier, K. M., Veltman, J., Karssemeijer, N., de Koning, H. J., van Diest, P. J., Mali, W. P. T. M., van den Bosch, M. A. A. J., Veldhuis, W. B., & van Gils, C. H. (2019). Supplemental MRI screening for women with extremely dense breast tissue. *The New England Journal of Medicine*, *381*(22), 2091–2102. DOI: 10.1056/NEJMoa1903986 PMID: 31774954

Ballester, P. J., & Carmona, J. (2021). Artificial intelligence for the next generation of precision oncology. *NPJ Precision Oncology*, *5*(1), 79. DOI: 10.1038/s41698-021-00216-w PMID: 34408248

Baltruschat, I., Steinmeister, L., Nickisch, H., Saalbach, A., Grass, M., Adam, G., Knopp, T., & Ittrich, H. (2021). Intelligent chest X-ray worklist prioritisation using artificial intelligence: A clinical workflow simulation. *European Radiology*, *31*(6), 3837–3845. DOI: 10.1007/s00330-020-07480-7 PMID: 33219850

Bera, K., Katz, I., & Madabhushi, A. (2020). Reimagining T staging through artificial intelligence and machine learning image processing approaches in digital pathology. *JCO Clinical Cancer Informatics*, *4*(4), 1039–1050. DOI: 10.1200/CCI.20.00110 PMID: 33166198

Bera, K., Schalper, K. A., Rimm, D. L., Velcheti, V., & Madabhushi, A. (2019). Artificial intelligence in digital pathology—New tools for diagnosis and precision oncology. *Nature Reviews. Clinical Oncology*, *16*(11), 703–715. DOI: 10.1038/s41571-019-0252-y PMID: 31399699

Bi, W. L., Hosny, A., Schabath, M. B., Giger, M. L., Birkbak, N. J., Mehrtash, A., Allison, T., Arnaout, O., Abbosh, C., Dunn, I. F., Mak, R. H., Tamimi, R. M., Tempany, C. M., Swanton, C., Hoffmann, U., Schwartz, L. H., Gillies, R. J., Huang, R. Y., & Aerts, H. J. (2019). Artificial intelligence in cancer imaging: Clinical challenges and applications. *CA: a Cancer Journal for Clinicians*, *69*(2), 127–157. DOI: 10.3322/caac.21552 PMID: 30720861

Bi, W. L., Hosny, A., Schabath, M. B., Giger, M. L., Birkbak, N. J., Mehrtash, A., Allison, T., Arnaout, O., Abbosh, C., Dunn, I. F., Mak, R. H., Tamimi, R. M., Tempany, C. M., Swanton, C., Hoffmann, U., Schwartz, L. H., Gillies, R. J., Huang, R. Y., & Aerts, H. J. (2019). Artificial intelligence in cancer imaging: Clinical challenges and applications. *CA: a Cancer Journal for Clinicians*, *69*(2), 127–157. DOI: 10.3322/caac.21552 PMID: 30720861

Bizzego, A., Bussola, N., Chierici, M., Maggio, V., Francescatto, M., Cima, L., Cristoforetti, M., Jurman, G., & Furlanello, C. (2019). Evaluating reproducibility of AI algorithms in digital pathology with DAPPER. *PLoS Computational Biology*, *15*(3), e1006269. DOI: 10.1371/journal.pcbi.1006269 PMID: 30917113

Cheung, H. M. C., & Rubin, D. (2021). Challenges and opportunities for artificial intelligence in oncological imaging. *Clinical Radiology*, *76*(10), 728–736. DOI: 10.1016/j.crad.2021.03.009 PMID: 33902889

Chukwunweike, J. N., Praise, A., & Bashirat, B. A. (2024). Harnessing Machine Learning for Cybersecurity: How Convolutional Neural Networks are Revolutionising Threat Detection and Data Privacy. *International Journal of Research Publication and Reviews*, *5*(8), 3608–3617. DOI: 10.55248/gengpi.5.0824.2402

Crosby, D., Bhatia, S., Brindle, K. M., Coussens, L. M., Dive, C., Emberton, M., Esener, S., Fitzgerald, R. C., Gambhir, S. S., Kuhn, P., Rebbeck, T. R., & Balasubramanian, S. (2022). Early detection of cancer. *Science*, *375*(6586), eaay9040. DOI: 10.1126/science.aay9040 PMID: 35298272

Daghrir, J., Tlig, L., Bouchouicha, M., & Sayadi, M. (2020, September). Melanoma skin cancer detection using deep learning and classical machine learning techniques: A hybrid approach. In *the 5th International Conference on Advanced Technologies for Signal and Image Processing (ATSIP)* (pp. 1-5). IEEE. DOI: 10.1109/ATSIP49331.2020.9231544

Debbadi, R. K., & Boateng, O. (2025). Developing intelligent automation workflows in Microsoft Power Automate by embedding deep learning algorithms for real-time process adaptation. *Int J Sci Res Arch*, *14*(2), 802–820. DOI: 10.30574/ijsra.2025.14.2.0449

Debbadi, R. K., & Boateng, O. (2025). Optimising end-to-end business processes by integrating machine learning models with UiPath for predictive analytics and decision automation. *Int J Sci Res Arch*, *14*(2), 778–796. DOI: 10.30574/ijsra.2025.14.2.0448

Dembrower, K., Wåhlin, E., Liu, Y., Salim, M., Smith, K., Lindholm, P., Eklund, M., & Strand, F. (2020). Effect of artificial intelligence-based triaging of breast cancer screening mammograms on cancer detection and radiologist workload: A retrospective simulation study. *The Lancet. Digital Health*, *2*(9), e468–e474. DOI: 10.1016/S2589-7500(20)30185-0 PMID: 33328114

Derevianko, A., Pizzoli, S. F. M., Pesapane, F., Rotili, A., Monzani, D., Grasso, R., Cassano, E., & Pravettoni, G. (2023). The use of artificial intelligence (AI) in the radiology field: What is the state of doctor–patient communication in cancer diagnosis? *Cancers (Basel)*, *15*(2), 470. DOI: 10.3390/cancers15020470 PMID: 36672417

Dhillon, A., Singh, A., & Bhalla, V. K. (2023). A systematic review on biomarker identification for cancer diagnosis and prognosis in multi-omics: From computational needs to machine learning and deep learning. *Archives of Computational Methods in Engineering*, *30*(2), 917–949. DOI: 10.1007/s11831-022-09821-9

Elkahwagy, D. M. A. S., Kiriacos, C. J., & Mansour, M. (2024). Logistic regression and other statistical tools in diagnostic biomarker studies. *Clinical & Translational Oncology*, *26*(9), 2172–2180. DOI: 10.1007/s12094-024-03413-8 PMID: 38530558

Fahami, M. A., Roshanzamir, M., Izadi, N. H., Keyvani, V., & Alizadehsani, R. (2021). Detection of effective genes in colon cancer: A machine learning approach. *Informatics in Medicine Unlocked*, *24*, 100605. DOI: 10.1016/j.imu.2021.100605

Fitzgerald, R. C., Antoniou, A. C., Fruk, L., & Rosenfeld, N. (2022). The future of early cancer detection. *Nature Medicine*, *28*(4), 666–677. DOI: 10.1038/s41591-022-01746-x PMID: 35440720

Gamil, S., Zeng, F., Alrifaey, M., Asim, M., & Ahmad, N. (2024). An efficient AdaBoost algorithm for enhancing skin cancer detection and classification. *Algorithms*, *17*(8), 353. DOI: 10.3390/a17080353

Gillies, R. J., & Schabath, M. B. (2020). Radiomics improves cancer screening and early detection. *Cancer Epidemiology, Biomarkers & Prevention*, *29*(12), 2556–2567. DOI: 10.1158/1055-9965.EPI-20-0075 PMID: 32917666

Gouda, W., Sama, N. U., Al-Waakid, G., Humayun, M., & Jhanjhi, N. Z. (2022, June). Detection of skin cancer based on skin lesion images using deep learning. [). MDPI.]. *Health Care*, *10*(7), 1183. PMID: 35885710

Großerueschkamp, F., Jütte, H., Gerwert, K., & Tannapfel, A. (2021). Advances in digital pathology: From artificial intelligence to label-free imaging. *Visceral Medicine*, *37*(6), 482–490. DOI: 10.1159/000518494 PMID: 35087898

Hage Chehade, A., Abdallah, N., Marion, J. M., Oueidat, M., & Chauvet, P. (2022). Lung and colon cancer classification using medical imaging: A feature engineering approach. *Physical and Engineering Sciences in Medicine*, *45*(3), 729–746. DOI: 10.1007/s13246-022-01139-x PMID: 35670909

Hameed Alsaedi, N. R., & Akay, M. F. (2025). Effective Breast Cancer Classification Using Deep MLP, Feature-Fused Autoencoder and Weight-Tuned Decision Tree. *Applied Sciences (Basel, Switzerland)*, *15*(13), 7213. DOI: 10.3390/app15137213

Hassan, Z. (2024). Application of Deep Learning in Cancer Prognosis: Predicting Tumour Progression, Recurrence, and Patient Outcomes Using Multi-Omics Data. *Journal of Biosciences and Innovations*, *1*(01), 44–53.

Hirsch, L., Huang, Y., Makse, H. A., Martinez, D. F., Hughes, M., Eskreis-Winkler, S., Pinker, K., Morris, E. A., Parra, L. C., & Sutton, E. J. (2025). Early detection of breast cancer in MRI using AI. *Academic Radiology*, *32*(3), 1218–1225. DOI: 10.1016/j.acra.2024.10.014 PMID: 39482209

Hosseini, F., Asadi, F., Emami, H., & Harari, R. E. (2023). Machine learning applications for early detection of oesophageal cancer: A systematic review. *BMC Medical Informatics and Decision Making*, *23*(1), 124. DOI: 10.1186/s12911-023-02235-y PMID: 37460991

Houssami, N., Kirkpatrick-Jones, G., Noguchi, N., & Lee, C. I. (2019). Artificial Intelligence (AI) for the early detection of breast cancer: A scoping review to assess AI's potential in breast screening practice. *Expert Review of Medical Devices*, *16*(5), 351–362. DOI: 10.1080/17434440.2019.1610387 PMID: 30999781

Huang, B., Tian, S., Zhan, N., Ma, J., Huang, Z., Zhang, C., Zhang, H., Ming, F., Liao, F., Ji, M., Zhang, J., Liu, Y., He, P., Deng, B., Hu, J., & Dong, W. (2021). Accurate diagnosis and prognosis prediction of gastric cancer using deep learning on digital pathological images: A retrospective multicentre study. *EBioMedicine*, *73*, 73. DOI: 10.1016/j.ebiom.2021.103631 PMID: 34678610

Islam, M. M., Poly, T. N., Walther, B. A., Yeh, C. Y., Seyed-Abdul, S., Li, Y. C., & Lin, M. C. (2022). Deep learning for the diagnosis of oesophageal cancer in endoscopic images: A systematic review and meta-analysis. *Cancers (Basel)*, *14*(23), 5996. DOI: 10.3390/cancers14235996 PMID: 36497480

Jin, D., Harrison, A. P., Zhang, L., Yan, K., Wang, Y., Cai, J., & Lu, L. (2021). Artificial intelligence in radiology. In *Artificial Intelligence in Medicine* (pp. 265–289). Academic Press. DOI: 10.1016/B978-0-12-821259-2.00014-4

Jones, M. A., Islam, W., Faiz, R., Chen, X., & Zheng, B. (2022). Applying artificial intelligence technology to assist with breast cancer diagnosis and prognosis prediction. *Frontiers in Oncology, 12*, 980793. DOI: 10.3389/fonc.2022.980793 PMID: 36119479

Karim, M. R., Comet, L. M., Shajalal, M., Beyan, O. D., Rebholz-Schuhmann, D., & Decker, S. (2023). From large language models to knowledge graphs for biomarker discovery in cancer. *arXiv preprint arXiv:2310.08365.*

Khalsan, M., Machado, L. R., Al-Shamery, E. S., Ajit, S., Anthony, K., Mu, M., & Agyeman, M. O. (2022). A survey of machine learning approaches applied to gene expression analysis for cancer prediction. *IEEE Access : Practical Innovations, Open Solutions, 10*, 27522–27534. DOI: 10.1109/ACCESS.2022.3146312

Klein, C., Zeng, Q., Arbaretaz, F., Devêvre, E., Calderaro, J., Lomenie, N., & Maiuri, M. C. (2021). Artificial intelligence for solid tumour diagnosis in digital pathology. *British Journal of Pharmacology, 178*(21), 4291–4315. DOI: 10.1111/bph.15633 PMID: 34302297

Lagree, A., Shiner, A., Alera, M. A., Fleshner, L., Law, E., Law, B., Lu, F.-I., Dodington, D., Gandhi, S., Slodkowska, E. A., Shenfield, A., Jerzak, K. J., Sadeghi-Naini, A., & Tran, W. T. (2021). Assessment of digital pathology imaging biomarkers associated with breast cancer histologic grade. *Current Oncology (Toronto, Ont.), 28*(6), 4298–4316. DOI: 10.3390/curroncol28060366 PMID: 34898544

Laury, A. R., Blom, S., Ropponen, T., Virtanen, A., & Carpén, O. M. (2021). Artificial intelligence-based image analysis can predict outcome in high-grade serous carcinoma via histology alone. *Scientific Reports, 11*(1), 19165. DOI: 10.1038/s41598-021-98480-0 PMID: 34580357

Li, N., Peng, E., & Liu, F. (2025). Prediction of lymph node metastasis in cervical cancer patients using AdaBoost machine learning model: Analysis of risk factors. *American Journal of Cancer Research, 15*(3), 1158–1173. DOI: 10.62347/UMKG8609 PMID: 40226481

Lu, T., Fang, Y., Liu, H., Chen, C., Li, T., Lu, M., & Song, D. (2024). Comparison of machine learning and logic regression algorithms for predicting lymph node metastasis in patients with Gastric Cancer: A two-Center Study. *Technology in Cancer Research & Treatment, 23*. DOI: 10.1177/15330338231222331 PMID: 38190617

Lu, Y., Shi, X. Q., Zhao, X., Song, D., & Li, J. (2019). Value of computer software for assisting sonographers in the diagnosis of Thyroid Imaging Reporting and Data System grade 3 and 4 thyroid space-occupying lesions. *Journal of Ultrasound in Medicine, 38*(12), 3291–3300. DOI: 10.1002/jum.15065 PMID: 31237716

Mantrala, S., Ginter, P. S., Mitkari, A., Joshi, S., Prabhala, H., Ramachandra, V., Kini, L., Idress, R., D'Alfonso, T. M., Fineberg, S., Jaffer, S., Sattar, A. K., Chagpar, A. B., Wilson, P., Singh, K., Harigopal, M., & Koka, D. (2022). Concordance in breast cancer grading by artificial intelligence on whole slide images compares with a multi-institutional cohort of breast pathologists. *Archives of Pathology & Laboratory Medicine, 146*(11), 1369–1377. DOI: 10.5858/arpa.2021-0299-OA PMID: 35271701

Mao, Y. J., Lim, H. J., Ni, M., Yan, W. H., Wong, D. W. C., & Cheung, J. C. W. (2022). Breast tumour classification using ultrasound elastography with machine learning: A systematic scoping review. *Cancers (Basel), 14*(2), 367. DOI: 10.3390/cancers14020367 PMID: 35053531

Maqsood, S., Damaševičius, R., & Maskeliūnas, R. (2022). Multimodal brain tumour detection using deep neural networks and multiclass SVM. *Medicina, 58*(8), 1090. DOI: 10.3390/medicina58081090 PMID: 36013557

Maroni, R., Massat, N. J., Parmar, D., Dibden, A., Cuzick, J., Sasieni, P. D., & Duffy, S. W. (2021). A case-control study to evaluate the impact of the breast screening programme on mortality in England. *British Journal of Cancer, 124*(4), 736–743. DOI: 10.1038/s41416-020-01163-2 PMID: 33223536

Maurya, S., Tiwari, S., Mothukuri, M. C., Tangeda, C. M., Nandigam, R. N. S., & Addagiri, D. C. (2023). A review on recent developments in cancer detection using machine learning and deep learning models. *Biomedical Signal Processing and Control, 80*, 104398. DOI: 10.1016/j.bspc.2022.104398

Mohammed, M. A., Lakhan, A., Abdulkareem, K. H., & Garcia-Zapirain, B. (2023). A hybrid cancer prediction based on multi-omics data and reinforcement learning, state action reward state action (SARSA). *Computers in Biology and Medicine, 154*, 106617. DOI: 10.1016/j.compbiomed.2023.106617 PMID: 36753981

Musulin, J., Štifanić, D., Zulijani, A., Ćabov, T., Dekanić, A., & Car, Z. (2021). An enhanced histopathology analysis: An AI-based system for multiclass grading of oral squamous cell carcinoma and segmenting of epithelial and stromal tissue. *Cancers (Basel), 13*(8), 1784. DOI: 10.3390/cancers13081784 PMID: 33917952

O'Connor, S. D., & Bhalla, M. (2021). Should artificial intelligence tell radiologists which study to read next? *Radiology. Artificial Intelligence, 3*(2), e210009. DOI: 10.1148/ryai.2021210009 PMID: 33939773

Ogundokun, R. O., Owolawi, P. A., Tu, C., & van Wyk, E. (2025). Autoencoder-Assisted Stacked Ensemble Learning for Lymphoma Subtype Classification: A Hybrid Deep Learning and Machine Learning Approach. *Tomography : a Journal for Imaging Research, 11*(8), 91. DOI: 10.3390/tomography11080091 PMID: 40863882

Painuli, D., Bhardwaj, S., & köse, U. (2022). Recent advancement in cancer diagnosis using machine learning and deep learning techniques: A comprehensive review. *Computers in Biology and Medicine, 146*, 105580. DOI: 10.1016/j.compbiomed.2022.105580 PMID: 35551012

Pauly, R., & Schwartz, C. E. (2019). The future of clinical diagnosis: Moving functional genomics approaches to the bedside. *Advances in Molecular Pathology, 2*(1), 13–19. DOI: 10.1016/j.yamp.2019.08.001

Qin, Z. Z., Sander, M. S., Rai, B., Titahong, C. N., Sudrungrot, S., Laah, S. N., Adhikari, L. M., Carter, E. J., Puri, L., Codlin, A. J., & Creswell, J. (2019). Using artificial intelligence to read chest radiographs for tuberculosis detection: A multi-site evaluation of the diagnostic accuracy of three deep learning systems. *Scientific Reports, 9*(1), 15000. DOI: 10.1038/s41598-019-51503-3 PMID: 31628424

Rakha, E. A., Vougas, K., & Tan, P. H. (2022). Digital technology in diagnostic breast pathology and immunohistochemistry. *Pathobiology, 89*(5), 334–342. DOI: 10.1159/000521149 PMID: 34969036

Rathore, S., Niazi, T., Iftikhar, M. A., & Chaddad, A. (2020). Glioma grading via machine learning analysis of digital pathology images. *Cancers (Basel), 12*(3), 578. DOI: 10.3390/cancers12030578 PMID: 32131409

Rodriguez, J. P. M., Rodriguez, R., Silva, V. W. K., Kitamura, F. C., Corradi, G. C. A., de Marchi, A. C. B., & Rieder, R. (2022). Artificial intelligence as a tool for diagnosis in digital pathology whole slide images: A systematic review. *Journal of Pathology Informatics, 13*, 100138. DOI: 10.1016/j.jpi.2022.100138 PMID: 36268059

Sachdeva, R. K., Bathla, P., Rani, P., Lamba, R., Ghantasala, G. P., & Nassar, I. F. (2024). A novel K-nearest neighbor classifier for lung cancer disease diagnosis. *Neural Computing & Applications, 36*(35), 22403–22416. DOI: 10.1007/s00521-024-10235-w

Shi, Y., Fan, H., Li, L., Hou, Y., Qian, F., Zhuang, M., & Fei, S. (2024). The value of machine learning approaches in the diagnosis of early gastric cancer: A systematic review and meta-analysis—World. *Journal of Surgical Oncology, 22*(1), 40. PMID: 38297303

Shmatko, A., Ghaffari Laleh, N., Gerstung, M., & Kather, J. N. (2022). Artificial intelligence in histopathology: Enhancing cancer research and clinical oncology. *Nature Cancer, 3*(9), 1026–1038. DOI: 10.1038/s43018-022-00436-4 PMID: 36138135

Tandon, R., Agrawal, S., Rathore, N. P. S., Mishra, A. K., & Jain, S. K. (2024). A systematic review of deep learning-based automated cancer diagnosis models. *Journal of Cellular and Molecular Medicine, 28*(6), e18144. DOI: 10.1111/jcmm.18144 PMID: 38426930

Tembhurne, J. V., Hebbar, N., Patil, H. Y., & Diwan, T. (2023). Skin cancer detection using an ensemble of machine learning and deep learning techniques. *Multimedia Tools and Applications, 82*(18), 27501–27524. DOI: 10.1007/s11042-023-14697-3

Tharwat, M., Sakr, N. A., El-Sappagh, S., Soliman, H., Kwak, K. S., & Elmogy, M. (2022). Colon cancer diagnosis based on machine learning and deep learning: Modalities and analysis techniques. *Sensors (Basel), 22*(23), 9250. DOI: 10.3390/s22239250 PMID: 36501951

Tran, W. T., Sadeghi-Naini, A., Lu, F. I., Gandhi, S., Meti, N., Brackstone, M., Rakovitch, E., & Curpen, B. (2021). Computational radiology in breast cancer screening and diagnosis using artificial intelligence. *Canadian Association of Radiologists Journal, 72*(1), 98–108. DOI: 10.1177/0846537120949974 PMID: 32865001

Van Leeuwen, K. G., de Rooij, M., Schalekamp, S., van Ginneken, B., & Rutten, M. J. (2022). How does artificial intelligence in radiology improve efficiency and health outcomes? *Pediatric Radiology, 52*(11), 1–7. DOI: 10.1007/s00247-021-05114-8 PMID: 34117522

van Leeuwen, K. G., de Rooij, M., Schalekamp, S., van Ginneken, B., & Rutten, M. J. (2024). Clinical use of artificial intelligence products for radiology in the Netherlands between 2020 and 2022. *European Radiology, 34*(1), 348–354. DOI: 10.1007/s00330-023-09991-5 PMID: 37515632

Vemula, C., Chavva, P., Battu, U., Vemulapalli, S., Prasad, K. V., & Kannaiah, S. K. (2024, May). Revolutionizing Breast Cancer Diagnosis: Insights from KNN and SVM Models in Machine Learning. In *2024 5th International Conference for Emerging Technology (INCET)* (pp. 1-9). IEEE.

Vindhya, J., Pooja, C., Dongre, M. H., Gowrishankar, S., Srinivasa, A. H., & Veena, A. (2023). Skin Lesion Classification Using Machine Learning. In *Inventive Computation and Information Technologies Proceedings of ICICIT, 2022*, 385–397.

Viswanathan, V. S., Toro, P., Corredor, G., Mukhopadhyay, S., & Madabhushi, A. (2022). The state of the art for artificial intelligence in lung digital pathology. *The Journal of Pathology*, *257*(4), 413–429. DOI: 10.1002/path.5966 PMID: 35579955

Vo, D. M., Nguyen, N. Q., & Lee, S. W. (2019). Classification of breast cancer histology images using incremental boosting convolution networks. *Information Sciences*, *482*, 123–138. DOI: 10.1016/j.ins.2018.12.089

Wang, C. W., Khalil, M. A., & Firdi, N. P. (2022). A survey on deep learning for precision oncology. *Diagnostics (Basel)*, *12*(6), 1489. DOI: 10.3390/diagnostics12061489 PMID: 35741298

Wen, Y., Ma, L., & Ju, C. (2023). Recent insights into the pathogenesis and therapeutic targets of chronic liver diseases. *eGastroenterology*, *1*(2), e100020. DOI: 10.1136/egastro-2023-100020 PMID: 38074919

Wong, A. N. N., He, Z., Leung, K. L., To, C. C. K., Wong, C. Y., Wong, S. C. C., Yoo, J. S., Chan, C. K. R., Chan, A. Z., Lacambra, M. D., & Yeung, M. H. Y. (2022). Current developments of artificial intelligence in digital pathology and its future clinical applications in gastrointestinal cancers. *Cancers (Basel)*, *14*(15), 3780. DOI: 10.3390/cancers14153780 PMID: 35954443

Wu, J., & Hicks, C. (2021). Breast cancer type classification using machine learning. *Journal of Personalized Medicine*, *11*(2), 61. DOI: 10.3390/jpm11020061 PMID: 33498339

Yousif, M., van Diest, P. J., Laurinavicius, A., Rimm, D., van der Laak, J., Madabhushi, A., & Pantanowitz, L. (2022). Artificial intelligence applied to breast pathology. *Virchows Archiv*, •••, 1–19. PMID: 34791536

Yurttakal, A. H., Erbay, H., İkizceli, T., & Karaçavuş, S. (2020). Detection of breast cancer via deep convolutional neural networks using MRI images. *Multimedia Tools and Applications*, *79*(21), 15555–15573. DOI: 10.1007/s11042-019-7479-6

Zhang, W., Huang, H., Wang, L., Lehmann, B. D., & Chen, S. X. (2025). An Integrative Multi-Omics Random Forest Framework for Robust Biomarker Discovery. bioRxiv, 2025-03.

Chapter 4
Breast Cancer Detection Using Machine Learning: A New Frontier in Early Diagnosis

Priyanka Pradhan
https://orcid.org/0000-0001-5892-9312
Regional College of Professional Studies and Research, India

Afshan Zameer
Rakshpal Bahadur Management Institute, India

Manvi Mishra
http://orcid.org/0000-0001-6764-3789
SRMS College of Engineering Technology and Research, Bareilly, India

Kirti Seth
https://orcid.org/0009-0003-6582-9549
School of Computer Science and Engineering, INHA University, Tashkent, Uzbekistan

ABSTRACT

Breast cancer remains one of the most widespread and life-threatening diseases affecting women worldwide. The early detection and accurate diagnosis of breast cancer are crucial for reducing death rates and improving patient outcomes. Machine learning (ML), a subset of artificial intelligence, has recently emerged as a powerful tool in the healthcare sector, offering promising solutions to the challenges posed by traditional diagnostic methods. This chapter aims to present a comprehensive exploration of how machine learning techniques can revolutionize the process of breast cancer detection and classification. It delves into a wide array of ML algorithms, data acquisition techniques, feature extraction, model evaluation

DOI: 10.4018/979-8-3373-4312-9.ch004

metrics, and real-world implementation challenges, providing a solid theoretical and practical foundation for researchers, practitioners, and students. The vision is to create a holistic and accessible resource that not only informs but also inspires further innovation in the use of ML for breast cancer detection.

1. INTRODUCTION

Breast cancer continues to be one of the deadliest cancers impacting women across the globe. It is marked by abnormal cell proliferation within the breast, which often results in a tumor that can be visualized on imaging studies or palpated as a lump. The etiology of breast cancer is complex and includes genetic factors (like mutations in BRCA1 and BRCA2), hormonal changes, lifestyle choices, and specific genes. Some of the common symptoms are lumps in the breast, change/s in its shape,skindimpling,pain, and nipple discharge. Global statistics indicate it is the most diagnosed cancerous tumor among women, maintaining a prominent position as one of the highest contributors to oncological mortality. There is no question that early detection significantly improves prognosis. Early stage diagnosis directly correlates with successful treatment outcomes. Enhanced awareness coupled with screening services has proven to improve both early diagnosis and survival rates. Modern diagnostic techniques such as mammograms, ultrasound scans,and biopsies continue to play a pivotal role in breast cancer detection.

Nevertheless, these methods face challenges such as high expenses, false positives/negatives, invasive procedures, and difficulty accessing remote areas. Much recently, there have been advancements in technology with healthcare Machine Learning (ML) emerging as a new promising approach on cancer detection and prognosis. With the ability to assess and analyze large datasets, ML algorithms capture intricate correlations and can make precise predictions far surpassing traditional diagnostic techniques. The aim of integrating ML systems into breast cancer detection is to improve accuracy and promptness of diagnosis while aiding in clinically informed decisions.

This chapter outlines crucial matters relating to breast cancer including the need for timely interventions alongside an assessment of the fundamental issues within standard diagnostic practice followed by the application of machine learning aimed at improving detection and prevention methodologies. The following sections will focus on ML models and associated datasets, performance benchmarks, as well as prospects for future work in this area.

2. BACKGROUND

2.1 Examination of Medical Imaging Techniques in Breast Cancer Detection

Medical imaging is essential for breast cancer diagnosis, treatment planning, and on-going disease progression monitoring (He et al., 2025). Mammography, which uses low-dose X-rays to view breast tissue and spot suspicious abnormalities, is still the gold standard for early-stage detection among the widely used imaging modalities. Despite its benefits, mammography has drawbacks, especially when it comes to identifying tumors concealed in dense breast tissue, which can result in false negative results. Ultrasound is commonly used in conjunction with mammography because it can distinguish between solid tumors and fluid-filled cystic lesions. Because it is non-invasive and radiation-free, it is especially appropriate for younger patients or for elucidating unclear mammography results.

Magnetic resonance imaging (MRI) offers superior soft tissue contrast and highly detailed visualization, making it possible to detect lesions that might otherwise go undetected in situations where conventional imaging is inconclusive or when patients present with high genetic or familial risk factors. These modalities play a vital role in clinical practice, but they are not without drawbacks. The need for more sophisticated imaging techniques is highlighted by problems like decreased sensitivity in specific patient populations, high expenses, restricted accessibility in low-resource settings, and difficulties with computational efficiency. These issues could be addressed by integrating cutting-edge technologies like artificial intelligence, machine learning, and multimodal imaging, which would increase diagnostic precision, improve patient outcomes, and make the detection of breast cancer more efficient and equitable.

2.2 Available Techniques for Breast Cancer Detection

Two primary approaches were used in the past to detect breast cancer: rule-based computer systems and manual interpretation by medical professionals. When radiologists or other experts closely inspect breast images, like mammograms, to search for indications of cancer, this is known as manual interpretation. This method heavily depends on the expertise and judgment of the physician. Although knowledgeable professionals are crucial, this approach can occasionally result in mistakes because it solely relies on human observation. The same image may be interpreted differently by different doctors, and even the same doctor may produce different results at different times. Accuracy may also be impacted by fatigue, workload, or minor variations in training. This can lead to missed cancers as well as false alarms (Elmore et al., 1994).

Rule-based systems were created to increase consistency. To aid in decision-making, these systems employ set rules or clinical guidelines (for instance, based on the size, shape, or type of a lump). They lack flexibility but are more structured than manual interpretation. They find it difficult to deal with uncommon situations or novel patterns that were not taken into account when creating the rules because they can only operate with the rules that are programmed into them.The primary drawback of both rule-based and manual approaches is their incomplete independence. They always need to be operated and the results interpreted by qualified human professionals. In areas with limited medical resources or a shortage of qualified physicians, this renders them less useful. Due to these difficulties, scientists and medical professionals have been gravitating toward more sophisticated technologies, like artificial intelligence (AI) and machine learning, which can decrease human error, increase precision, and contribute to the expansion of access to breast cancer detection (Doi, 2007; Litjens et al., 2017).

2.3 Review of Related Work Using ML/DL

The diagnosis and prevention of breast cancer are now supported by intelligent systems thanks to the quick development of machine learning (ML) and deep learning (DL). These tools enable doctors to make more accurate decisions by rapidly and reliably analyzing medical data. One important use is image classification, where sophisticated models like Convolutional Neural Networks (CNNs) can analyze breast images and determine whether they are benign or malignant by spotting even the smallest, most intricate patterns. Risk prediction, which uses predictive models to estimate a person's chance of getting breast cancer by combining genetic information, medical history, and lifestyle factors, is another significant application. This facilitates the scheduling of more frequent screenings and individualized examinations.

Furthermore, by suggesting lifestyle modifications or genetic testing for individuals who are more susceptible, ML can support preventative measures. According to research, ML-based systems can serve as a useful second opinion for medical professionals, increasing diagnostic precision, decreasing errors, and expediting the entire procedure—all of which contribute to the increased efficacy and dependability of breast cancer detection.

3. COMPILING AND GETTING READY FOR DATA

The quality and quantity of data available in a particular field have a significant impact on how well machine learning algorithms detect and categorize breast cancer. In this instance, we address some dataset-related concerns, data cleaning practices, ways to methodically extract relevant features, and augmentation strategies meant to improve model output outcomes using feature-rich synthetic data.

3.1 Datasets Used (e.g., UCI, Kaggle)

Several publicly available datasets have become industry standards for research on breast cancer. These datasets differ in terms of size, data type (tabular vs. image), and annotation quality.

a) Wisconsin Breast Cancer Dataset (WBCD): The UCI Machine Learning Repository provides access to one of the most widely used datasets for breast cancer classification tasks. It includes features like smoothness, area, perimeter, texture, and radius that are derived from digital images of breast masses obtained through fine needle aspiration (FNA) The target labels classify tumors as either benign or malignant.
b) Regular Images of IDC Breast Histopathology: This dataset is available on Kaggle and contains images of breast tissue from histopathology. The images are labeled according to whether invasive ductal carcinoma (IDC) is present or not. The dataset, which contains over 277,000 image patches, offers a plethora of data for deep learning methods.

CNN model training uses mammogram images from the Mammographic Image Analysis Society (MIAS) and the Digital Database for Screening Mammography (DDSM). These datasets are useful for tasks like tumor detection, segmentation, and classification. By using these datasets, researchers can train and validate machine learning models to precisely identify early indicators of breast cancer (Heat et al., 2000).

3.2 Normalization and Data Cleaning

To preserve accuracy and dependability, raw datasets must be cleaned before beginning the preprocessing phase. Since incomplete records or incorrect data entry frequently result in gaps in breast cancer datasets, handling missing values is one of the crucial steps. In these situations, statistical measures like the mean, median, or mode may be used to replace missing values; however, samples with an excessive number of missing values are frequently eliminated to prevent bias. Since undesired disturbances in medical images can lower classification accuracy, noise removal is another crucial step. Methods like median filtering and Gaussian blurring are frequently used to remove these superfluous variations while keeping crucial information.

Furthermore, feature engineering is essential for getting data ready for machine learning models. Algorithms like SVM and KNN, which otherwise assign equal weight to every input variable regardless of scale, treat all features equally thanks to techniques like normalization and scaling. Common methods include Z-score normalization, which centers data around the mean with unit variance, and Min-Max scaling, which modifies values to a fixed range (typically 0–1). Lastly, encoding techniques (such as label encoding or one-hot encoding) are used to translate text-based categories into numerical formats that machine learning algorithms can comprehend for categorical information like diagnostic labels (Han et al., 2012; Kuhn & Johnson, 2013).

3.3 Methods for Feature Extraction

Effective feature extraction is essential for machine learning algorithms to accurately distinguish between benign and malignant cases. Some of such types of features are as follows.

a) Statistical Features: The mean, standard error, and worst texture are statistical features that provide information about the statistics of tumor features in the WBCD dataset.
b) Texture and Morphological Features: The Gray-Level Co-occurrence Matrix, or GLCM, defines contour-based textural features that quantify the visual patterns of tumors in imaging datasets.
c) Deep Feature Extraction (CNN): In deep learning models, convolutional layers automate the process of recognizing complex, well-known patterns by performing hierarchical feature extraction over input images (Khalid et al., 2023).

Dimensionality Reduction: The following methods can be used to reduce high-dimensional feature sets:

- To preserve as much variance as possible, use Principal Component Analysis (PCA).
- t-SNE for 2D/3D visualization of complex datasets
- Deep learning autoencoders for feature compression without supervision

3.4 Techniques for Data Augmentation

For image-based models, where overfitting as a result of insufficient training samples is a significant concern, data augmentation is particularly crucial. Random rotations, flipping, cropping, and scaling of images are examples of geometric transformations that are used to artificially expand dataset sizes and model generalizability. Some of the commonly used data augmentation techniques are:

a) **Color and Contrast Adjustments:** Models can be made to be invariant to imaging conditions by adjusting brightness, contrast, or applying filters.
b) **Noise Injection:** By simulating imaging variability, Gaussian noise increases the robustness of the model.
c) **Synthetic Data Generation:** To balance class distribution, synthetic yet realistic samples are created using methods such as SMOTE (Synthetic Minority Over-sampling Technique) for tabular data and GANs (Generative Adversarial Networks) for image data (Alawee et al., 2024).

Together, these data preparation techniques serve as the foundation of a successful pipeline for the detection of breast cancer. In addition to increasing model accuracy, proper preprocessing guarantees that the predictions are applicable to various patient demographics and imaging scenarios.

4. DETECTION MACHINE LEARNING MODELS

Breast cancer can be identified from both structured and unstructured datasets using a variety of algorithms provided by machine learning (ML). Every algorithm has distinct advantages and disadvantages. Following an overview of popular machine learning models for classifying breast cancer, this section includes concepts, implementation code and visual outputs.

4.1 The Logistic Regression Model

A supervised learning technique for binary classification is called logistic regression (Khandezamin et al., 2020). It uses the sigmoid function to determine the likelihood that a sample belongs to a specific class. It works especially well with the Wisconsin Breast Cancer Dataset, where determining whether a tumor is benign or malignant is the aim. This model is easy to understand and comprehend as well as Quick and effective on data that is linearly separable. Below is the code snippet of logistic regression model.

Figure 1. Code snippet of breast cancer dataset

```
import numpy as np
import pandas as pd
import sklearn.datasets
from sklearn.model_selection import train_test_split
from sklearn.linear_model import LogisticRegression
from sklearn.metrics import accuracy_score
```

```
[ ] import seaborn as sns
    import matplotlib.pyplot as plt
```

```
[ ] # loading the data from sklearn
    breast_cancer_dataset = sklearn.datasets.load_breast_cancer()
```

```
[ ] print(breast_cancer_dataset)
```

```
{'data': array([[1.799e+01, 1.038e+01, 1.228e+02, ..., 2.654e-01, 4.601e-01,
        1.189e-01],
       [2.057e+01, 1.777e+01, 1.329e+02, ..., 1.860e-01, 2.750e-01,
        8.902e-02],
       [1.969e+01, 2.125e+01, 1.300e+02, ..., 2.430e-01, 3.613e-01,
        8.758e-02],
       ...,
       [1.660e+01, 2.808e+01, 1.083e+02, ..., 1.418e-01, 2.218e-01,
        7.820e-02],
       [2.060e+01, 2.933e+01, 1.401e+02, ..., 2.650e-01, 4.087e-01,
        1.240e-01],
       [7.760e+00, 2.454e+01, 4.792e+01, ..., 0.000e+00, 2.871e-01,
```

As shown in fig.1, it is clear that to make data handling, model building, and performance evaluation for breast cancer detection easier,the code makes use of a number of crucial Python libraries. While pandas facilitates structured data manipulation and analysis, the numpy library is utilized for effective numerical computations. The breast cancer dataset used in this study is one of the built-in datasets accessible through the sklearn.datasets module. Train_test_split from sklearn. model_selection is used to divide the dataset into training and testing subsets for model development. Because it works well for binary classification problems like cancer detection, a logistic regression model is used, implemented using sklearn. linear_model.LogisticRegression. Lastly, accuracy_score from sklearn.metrics, which measures the model's prediction accuracy on unseen data, is used to evaluate the model's performance.

Figure 2. Attribute values of breast cancer dataset

```
[ ] # loading the data to a data frame
    data_frame = pd.DataFrame(breast_cancer_dataset.data, columns = breast_cancer_dataset.feature_names)
```

```
[ ] # print the first 5 rows of the dataframe
    data_frame.head()
```

	mean radius	mean texture	mean perimeter	mean area	mean smoothness	mean compactness	mean concavity	mean concave points	mean symmetry	mean fractal dimension	...
0	17.99	10.38	122.80	1001.0	0.11840	0.27760	0.3001	0.14710	0.2419	0.07871	...
1	20.57	17.77	132.90	1326.0	0.08474	0.07864	0.0869	0.07017	0.1812	0.05667	...
2	19.69	21.25	130.00	1203.0	0.10960	0.15990	0.1974	0.12790	0.2069	0.05999	...
3	11.42	20.38	77.58	386.1	0.14250	0.28390	0.2414	0.10520	0.2597	0.09744	...
4	20.29	14.34	135.10	1297.0	0.10030	0.13280	0.1980	0.10430	0.1809	0.05883	...

5 rows × 30 columns

```
[ ] # adding the 'target' column to the data frame
    data_frame['label'] = breast_cancer_dataset.target
```

To make data manipulation and investigation simple, the breast cancer dataset is put into a Pandas DataFrame. The feature data and associated column names from the breast_cancer_dataset object are arranged in a tabular manner using the pd.DataFrame constructor. As shown in Fig. 2. The head() function is used to display the dataset's first five rows, giving a quick overview of its properties, including mean radius, texture, area, perimeter, and other pertinent metrics. The target labels that indicate whether breast cancer is present or not are added to the DataFrame under a new column called "label" in order to get the data ready for modeling. Effective preprocessing, visualization, and machine learning model construction are made possible by this standardized format. Once this standardized format of dataset is achieved we can analyse the dataset by doing data visualization by using matplot and seaborn libraries in python.

Figure 3. Data visualization of breast cancer dataset using pairplot method of seaborn library

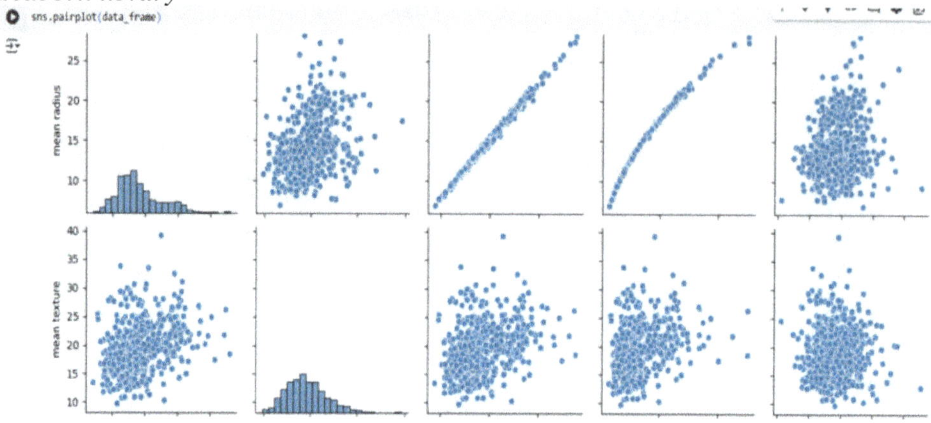

The pairplot created with the Seaborn library as shown in Fig.3. which shows the correlations between several features in a breast cancer dataset, is depicted in the image above. This pairplot specifically looks at the variables mean texture and mean radius, among others. While the diagonal plots illustrate the distribution of individual features, each scatter plot in the matrix displays the correlation between two different features. Some traits, for example, show a significant positive linear association, meaning that when one feature rises, the other likely to rise as well. These connections are essential for machine learning algorithms because they aid in determining the most important factors influencing the classification of cancer. This kind of data visualization helps us choose the best characteristics and models for precise breast cancer prediction by providing a better understanding of the structure, patterns, and possible separability of benign and malignant tumors.

Figure 4. Data visualization of breast cancer dataset using distplot method of seaborn library

```
sns.distplot(data_frame['mean radius'],bins=30)
<Axes: xlabel='mean radius', ylabel='Density'>
```

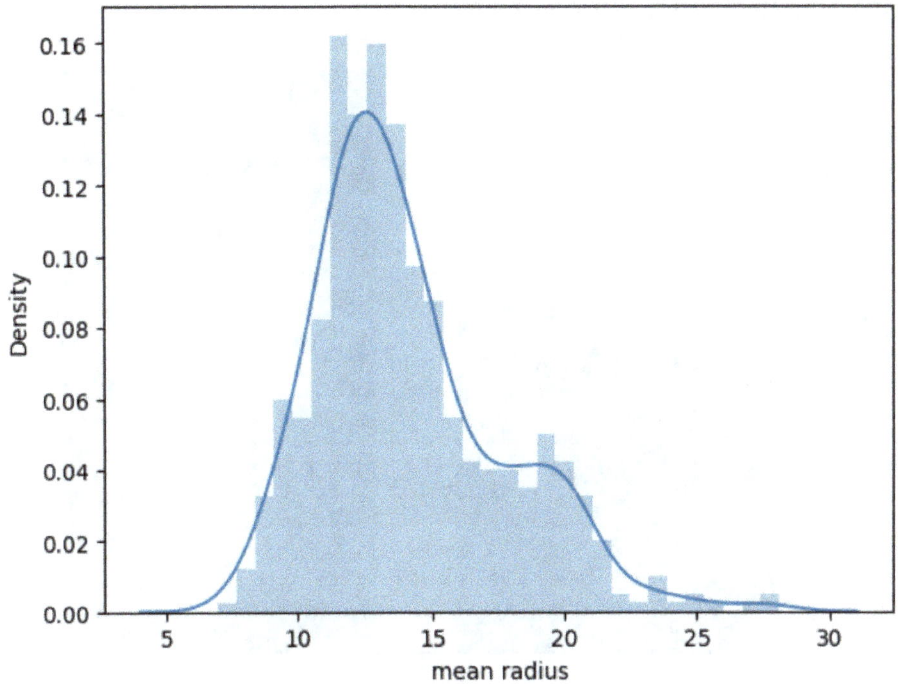

The distribution of the mean radius feature in the breast cancer dataset can be seen in depth in the histogram and density plot displayed in the above Fig.4. The sns.distplot() method from the Seaborn package with 30 bins is used to create this plot. The superimposed kernel density estimate (KDE) curve offers a smoothed approximation of the underlying probability density function, while the histogram (bar plot) shows the frequency of data points within designated intervals.

It can be seen from the plot that certain tumors have much bigger radii, even if the mean radius values are roughly normally distributed with a minor right skew. Around a mean radius of roughly 12 to 14 units, the majority of data points cluster. This information is useful for understanding the normal size range of cell nuclei in the dataset, as well as for preprocessing and feature scaling in machine learning workflows. Understanding the distribution facilitates the identification of outliers, the choice of transformation methods, and the enhancement of model performance in tasks involving the detection of breast cancer.

Figure 5. Data visualization of breast cancer dataset using countplot method of seaborn library

```
sns.countplot(x='label',data=data_frame)
```

```
<Axes: xlabel='label', ylabel='count'>
```

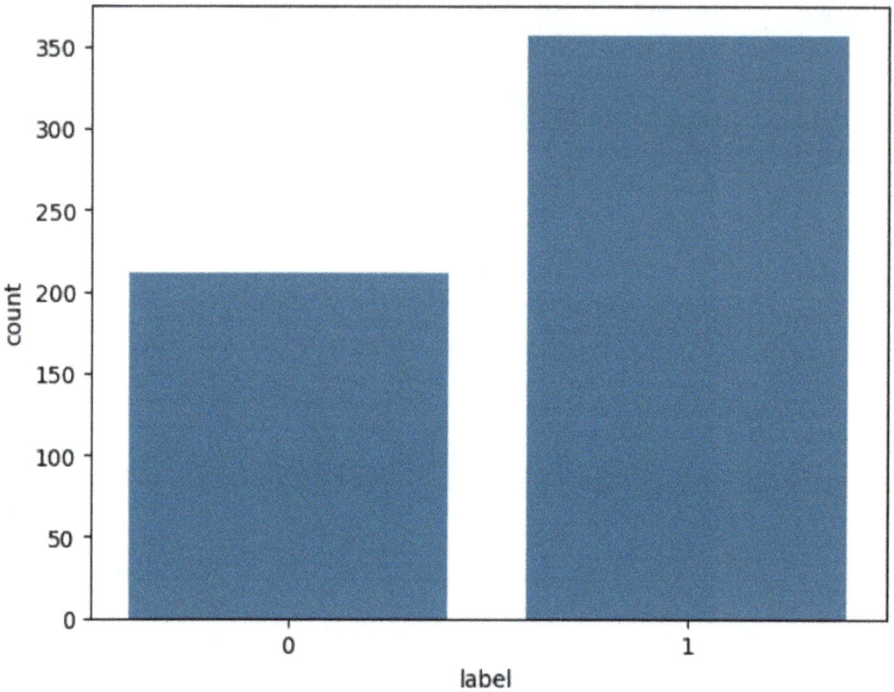

Using the Seaborn library's sns.countplot() method, the bar chart above shown in Fig.5 illustrates the distribution of the label column in the breast cancer dataset. According to the dataset documentation, this column usually represents the tumor classification, with 0 and 1 denoting malignant and benign cases, respectively.

The plot clearly shows a class imbalance in the dataset, with benign instances (label 1) substantially outnumbering malignant ones (label 0). Because it might result in biased predictions that favor the majority class, this imbalance is a typical problem in medical datasets and must be taken into account when training machine learning models. To guarantee that the model performs well across both classes—especially the minority class, which is frequently of higher clinical interest in cancer detection—it is imperative to properly handle such imbalance using techniques like resampling, weighted loss functions, or synthetic data generation (e.g., SMOTE).

Figure 6. Data visualization of breast cancer dataset using boxplot method of seaborn library

```
sns.boxplot(x='label',y='mean radius',data=data_frame)
```

```
<Axes: xlabel='label', ylabel='mean radius'>
```

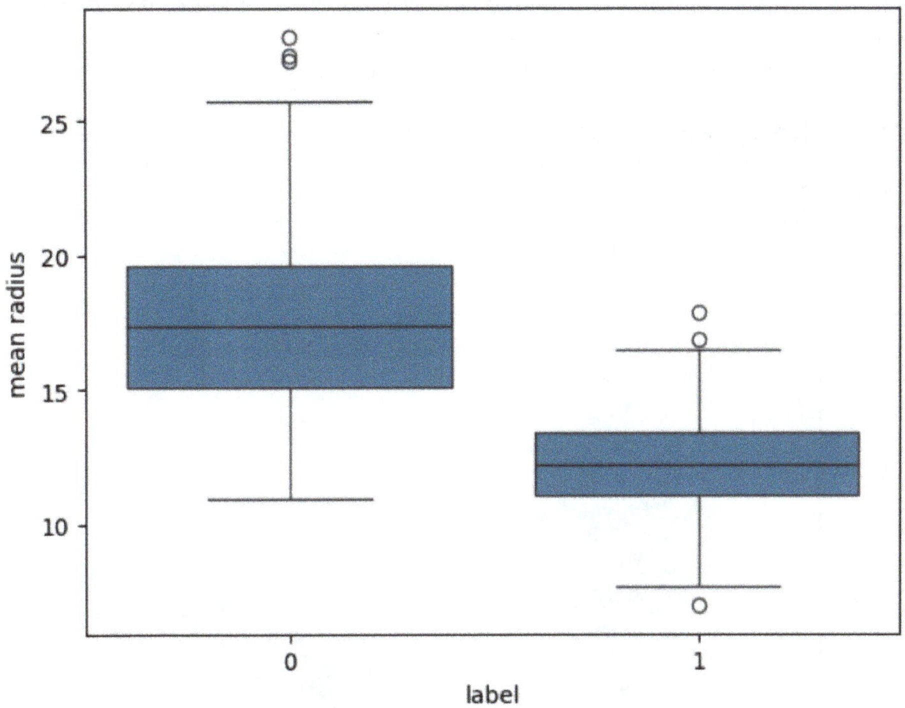

The distribution of the mean radius feature across the two tumor classes denoted by the label column is depicted in the boxplot in the above Fig.6, which was made with Seaborn'ssns.boxplot() tool. Malignant tumors are usually represented by label 0 in this plot, whereas benign tumors are represented by label 1 (or vice versa, depending on dataset encoding). An essential characteristic that characterizes the typical size of cell nuclei and is frequently a crucial marker in differentiating between benign and malignant growths is the mean radius.

The graphic shows that, in contrast to benign tumors (label 1), malignant tumors (label 0) typically have a substantially larger mean radius.There is more variation in size for malignant tumors, as evidenced by the bigger median value and wider interquartile range (IQR). Additionally, both groups contain outliers, which are represented as solitary points that are not included in the whiskers.

In the context of machine learning-based breast cancer detection, this visual distinction is crucial since it validates the discriminative nature of mean radius. By using these insights for feature selection and model training, algorithms can more effectively distinguish between benign and malignant cases based on their physical attributes.

Figure 7. Data visualization of breast cancer dataset using swarmplot method of seaborn library

```
sns.swarmplot(x='label',y='mean radius',data=data_frame)

<Axes: xlabel='label', ylabel='mean radius'>
/usr/local/lib/python3.11/dist-packages/seaborn/categorical.py:3399: User
  warnings.warn(msg, UserWarning)
```

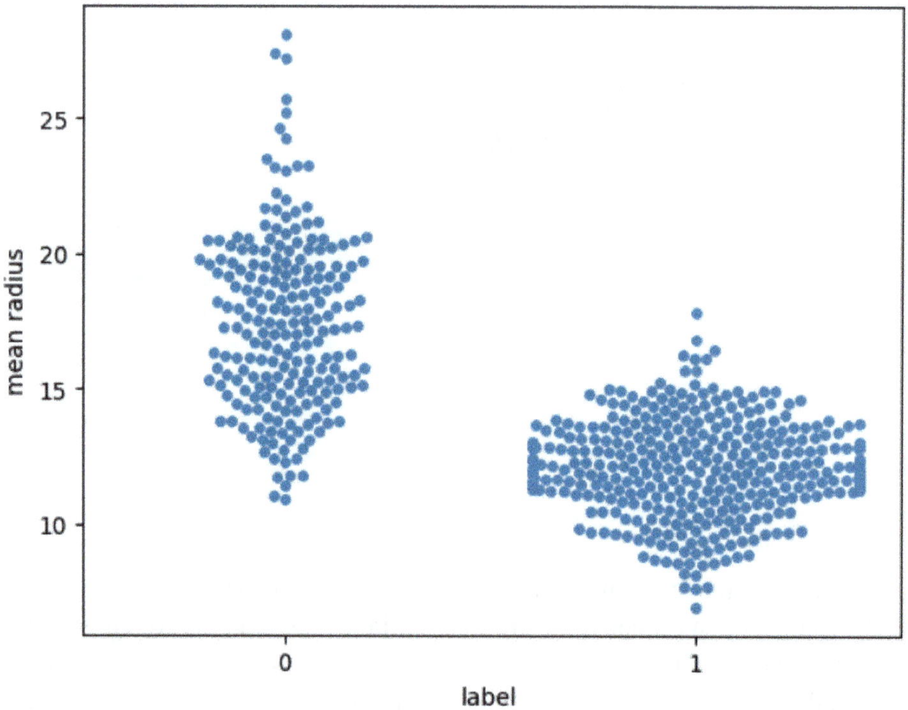

The distribution of the mean radius feature for each class in the label column of the breast cancer dataset is displayed in detail in the swarmplotin the above Fig.7, which was produced using Seaborn'ssns.swarmplot() method. The tumor kinds are usually represented by the labels in this plot: 0 for malignant and 1 for benign (or vice versa, depending on dataset encoding). The plot is perfect for illustrating the density and distribution of values in small to medium-sized datasets since each dot represents a single data point and is arranged to prevent overlap.

It is clear from the plot that benign tumors (label 1) have a more compact distribution centered on lower values, whereas malignant tumors (label 0) often have a higher and wider range of mean radius values. This visual distinction shows that mean radius is a useful characteristic for differentiating between benign and malignant tumors. Since the swarmplot does not aggregate the data like boxplots or histograms do, it is easier to see the true distribution and clustering patterns.

Exploratory data analysis (EDA) for machine learning tasks requires these kinds of visualizations in order to identify patterns, validate hypotheses, and choose useful features for the development of models for breast cancer diagnosis.

Figure 8. Data visualization of breast cancer dataset using stripplot method of seaborn library

```
sns.stripplot(x='label',y='mean radius',data=data_frame)
```

```
<Axes: xlabel='label', ylabel='mean radius'>
```

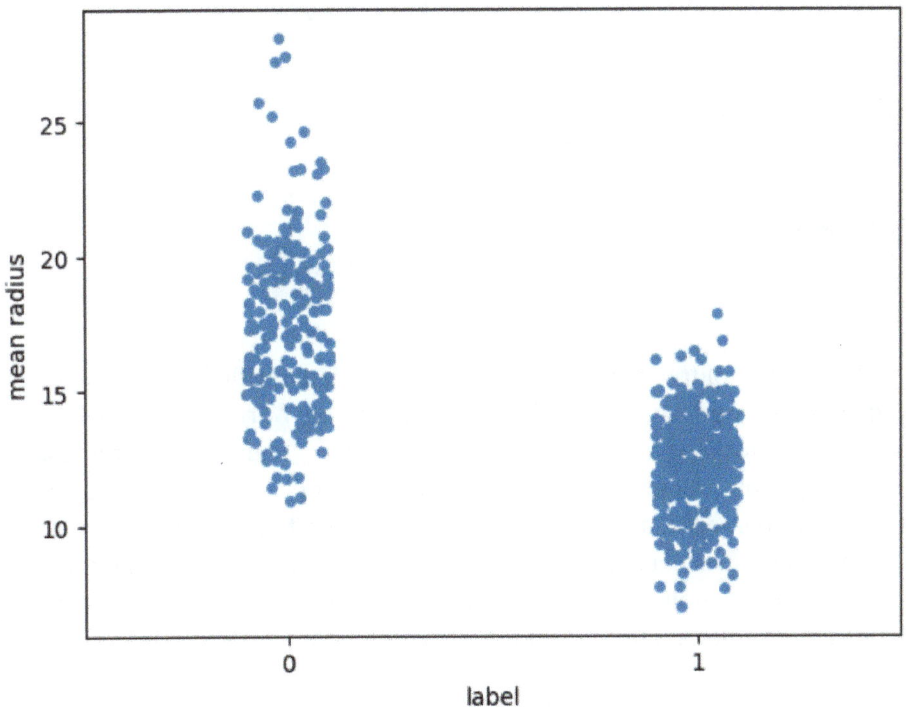

The distribution of the mean radius feature in relation to the label variable in a breast cancer dataset is clearly displayed in the above Fig.8 strip plot, which was produced using Seaborn'ssns.stripplot() tool. In this case, the label usually denotes the type of tumor, with 0 denoting malignant tumors and 1 denoting benign tumors (or vice versa, depending on the details of the dataset). A single observation is represented by each dot in the graphic.

It is clear from the plot that benign tumors (label 1) typically have lower mean radius values than malignant tumors (label 0). Malignant tumors exhibit a greater range and higher values overall, indicating a clear difference between the two groups. This implies that a significant characteristic that differentiates benign from malignant instances is mean radius.

Without aggregating the data, the strip plot is particularly helpful for determining the distribution, clustering, and any overlapping values between groups. Such visualizations are essential for identifying pertinent features that can improve model accuracy and facilitate accurate classification during the exploratory data analysis (EDA) stage of machine learning-based breast cancer diagnosis.

Figure 9. Training a Logistic Regression model with Python's scikit-learn module

```
model = LogisticRegression()

# training the Logistic Regression model using Training data

model.fit(X_train, Y_train)

/usr/local/lib/python3.11/dist-packages/sklearn/linear_model/_logistic.py:465: ConvergenceWarning: lbfgs failed to converge (status=1):
STOP: TOTAL NO. OF ITERATIONS REACHED LIMIT.

Increase the number of iterations (max_iter) or scale the data as shown in:
    https://scikit-learn.org/stable/modules/preprocessing.html
Please also refer to the documentation for alternative solver options:
    https://scikit-learn.org/stable/modules/linear_model.html#logistic-regression
  n_iter_i = _check_optimize_result(
▸ LogisticRegression
LogisticRegression()
```

The outcome of training a Logistic Regression model with Python's scikit-learn module is displayed in the Fig.9 above. A ConvergenceWarning is raised when the model is fitted to the training data (model.fit(X_train, Y_train)). This warning shows that the algorithm achieved the maximum number of permitted iterations without achieving a solution, indicating that the default solver lbfgs failed to converge.

When the data is not appropriately scaled or the problem is so complicated that it takes more iterations for the solver to resolve, this scenario frequently occurs. Two main remedies are recommended by the solution:

- Use the max_iter argument to increase the number of iterations, such as in LogisticRegression(max_iter=1000).
- Use standardization techniques to scale the data, such StandardScaler from sklearn.preprocessing, which normalizes feature values and frequently enhances convergence.

This warning is significant because it draws attention to a frequent problem that can arise during model training in the context of machine learning-based breast cancer diagnosis. By addressing it, the logistic regression model is guaranteed to learn the best weights for tumor classification, increasing prediction accuracy and dependability.

Figure 10. Logistic Regression-Based Breast Cancer Detection User Interface

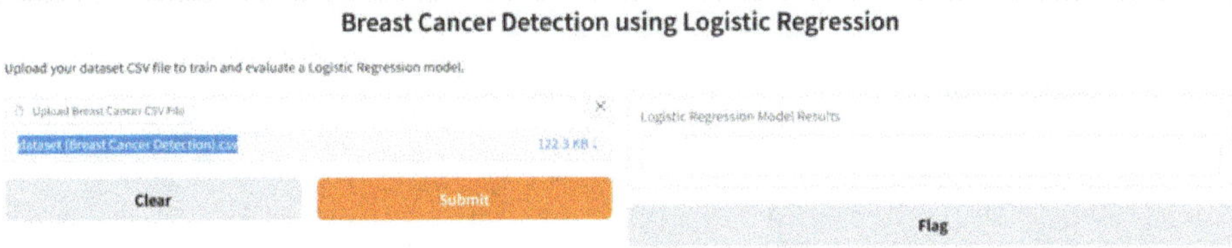

As shown in the above Fig.10, Users can upload a CSV dataset, submit it, and examine the model results on the image's online interface for Breast Cancer Detection using Logistic Regression. It offers a quick and interactive method for assessing how well the model performs with unique data.

Figure 11. The initial graphical user interface for detecting breast cancer.

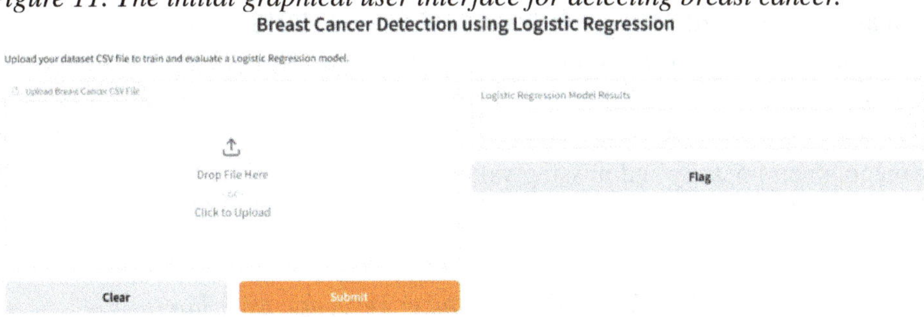

With the ability to publish, clear, or flag results, this interface enables users to train and assess a Logistic Regression model using a CSV file containing a breast cancer dataset as Shown in Fig.11.

Figure 12. Following dataset upload, the results of the logistic regression model

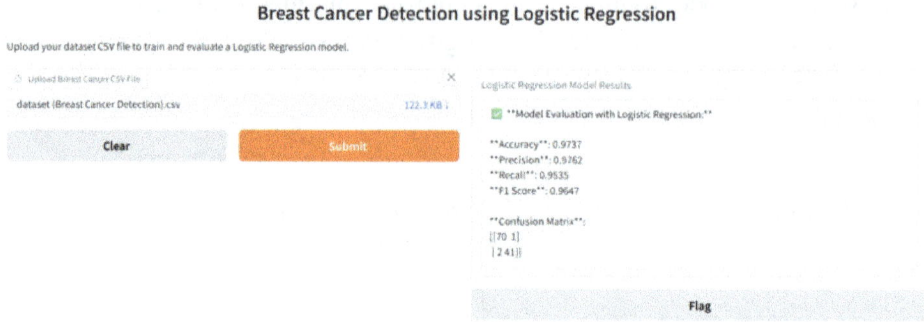

After a dataset is uploaded, this interface as shown in Fig.12, shows the results of the Logistic Regression model. It shows important metrics including accuracy (0.9737), precision (0.9762), recall (0.9535), F1 score (0.9647), and the confusion matrix, all of which show good model performance.

4.2 Random Forests and Decision Trees

Overview: To create a structure resembling a tree, decision trees divide the data according to feature values. Multiple decision tree ensembles called Random Forests increase accuracy and decrease over fitting (Dai et al., 2018).

Use in Breast Cancer: These models are frequently employed in medical decision-making systems and are capable of capturing intricate feature interactions.Decision trees are simple to understand and visualize. Random Forest algorithm help in managing non-linearity and missing values.

Code and Results:

Figure 13. Decision Tree-Based Breast Cancer Detection User Interface.

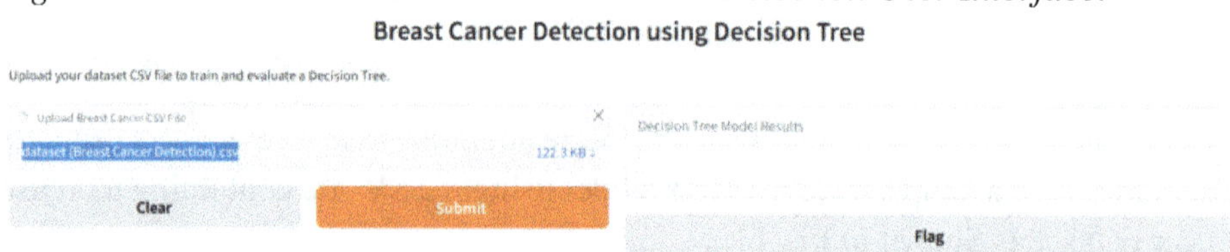

A graphical user interface (GUI) that uses a decision tree classifier to aid in breast cancer detectionis depicted in the above Fig.13. The interface makes it possible for users—especially those who are not programmers—to engage with the machine learning model in an intuitive way.

1. Important Elements:
   - **Section for Uploading Files:**Users can upload a dataset in.csv format by clicking the "Upload Breast Cancer CSV File" button.The dataset (Breast Cancer Detection.csv), which has a size of 122.3 KB, has been used for this example. Features including mean radius, texture, area, perimeter, and diagnosis labels (malignant or benign) are commonly included in this dataset.
2. Action Buttons:
   - Clear: Clears the data or allows a new file upload by resetting the interface.
   - Submit: After the dataset is uploaded, the Decision Tree algorithm starts the training and assessment process.
   - Flag: This can be used to indicate problems or unusualities in the dataset or findings.
3. Output Display: The output will be shown in a text box titled "Decision Tree Model Results" on the right-hand side. Following training and testing, this comprises accuracy, precision, recall, confusion matrix, and other evaluation measures.

The goal of this GUI is to provide a streamlined method of using machine learning in healthcare, specifically for the diagnosis of cancer. Such interfaces make machine learning accessible to researchers, physicians, and students who may not be comfortable with programming but are interested in predictive analytics for medical diagnosis by automating the data loading and model execution process.

Figure 14. the initial graphical user interface for detecting breast cancer.

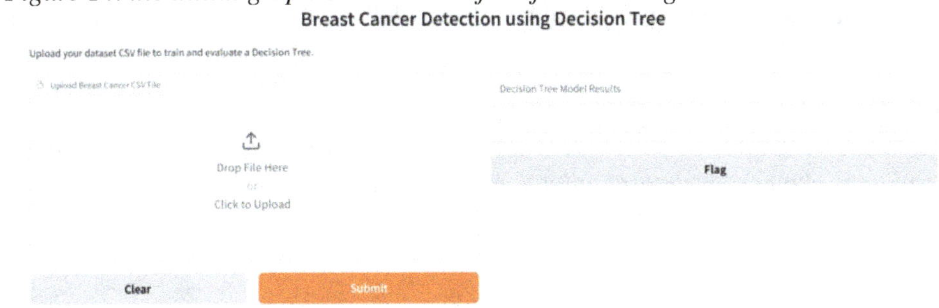

The first glimpse of a graphical user interface designed for the categorization of breast cancer using a Decision Tree algorithm is shown in the Fig.14. Users can either click to choose a file or drag & drop to upload a CSV dataset. The "Submit" button allows the user to start training the model after it has been uploaded, while the

"Clear" button resets the interface and the "Flag" button permits reporting problems. Following model evaluation, the output metrics will be shown in the "Decision Tree Model Results" panel on the right. Easy use in medical and research settings is made possible by this user-friendly design, which guarantees accessibility for individuals without programming experience.

Figure 15. Evaluation Results of a Decision Tree Model for the Detection of Breast Cancer.

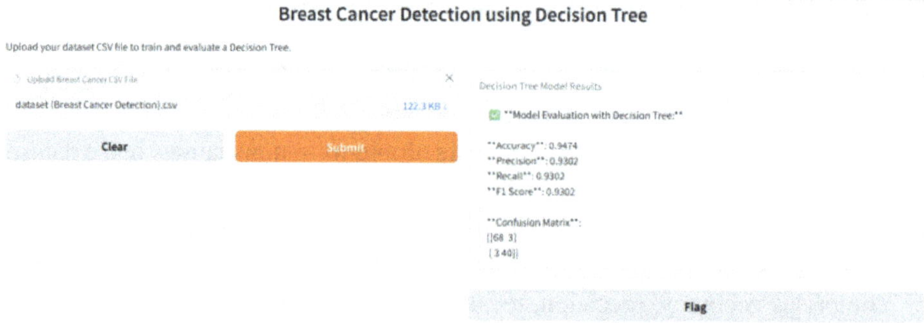

Following the upload of a dataset and the execution of the Decision Tree model, the Fig.15displays the final output of the breast cancer detection GUI. The model performed well, as evidenced by the results panel on the right, which shows important evaluation measures such as an accuracy of 94.74%, precision of 93.02%, recall of 93.02%, and an F1 score of 93.02%. The number of accurate and inaccurate classifications for benign and malignant cases is indicated by the confusion matrix [[68, 3], [3, 40]]. Without having to manually execute scripts or decipher code, this output enables users to rapidly evaluate the model's performance on the uploaded breast cancer dataset.

Figure 16. User interface for Random Forest classifier-based breast cancer detection, displaying choices for dataset upload, model execution, and result presentation.

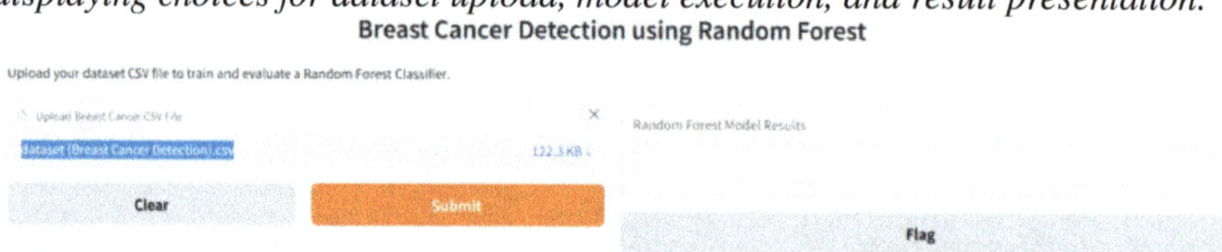

The user interface of a Random Forest classifier-based breast cancer detection system is depicted in the Fig.16. It offers a straightforward and interactive platform that allows users to train and assess the model by uploading a breast cancer dataset in CSV format, such as "dataset (Breast Cancer Detection).csv". Users can start the process by clicking the "Submit" button after uploading the file. This will cause the Random Forest algorithm to examine the data and generate findings. The "Random Forest Model Results" section then shows these findings. Additional buttons such as "Clear" enable the interface to be reset, while "Flag" can be used to report problems or issues. This configuration exemplifies the efficient use of machine learning, specifically Random Forest classification, in real-time applications for breast cancer diagnosis, supporting prompt and precise medical evaluations.

Figure 17. The first interface of a Random Forest-based breast cancer detection system, displaying the model result display part and the file upload area.

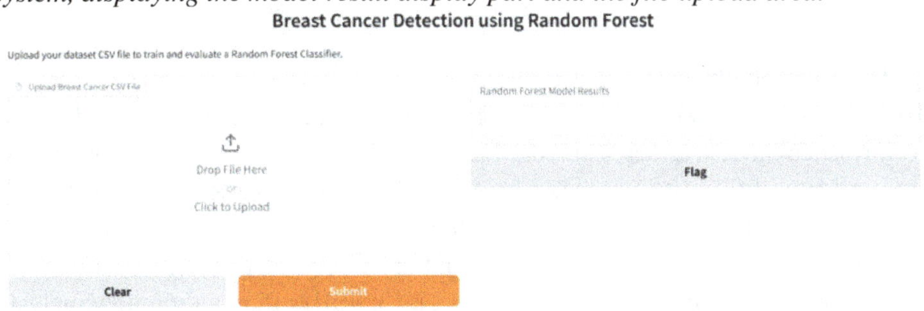

The first glimpse of a web application that uses a Random Forest algorithm to identify breast cancer is shown in the Fig.17. To upload a breast cancer dataset in CSV format, users can either click or drag the file into the "Drop File Here" upload section on the site. By selecting the "Submit" button after uploading the dataset, users can start the detection process, which will use the supplied data to train and assess the Random Forest model. The "Random Forest Model Results" section on the right will then show the evaluation metrics or prediction results. A "Clear" button to reset the interface and a "Flag" button to report problems or defects are two more features. The user-friendly design intended to make machine learning-based breast cancer diagnosis easier for non-technical users is depicted in this figure.

Figure 18. Following successful model execution, the Random Forest-based breast cancer detection system's result display displays assessment metrics and a confusion matrix.

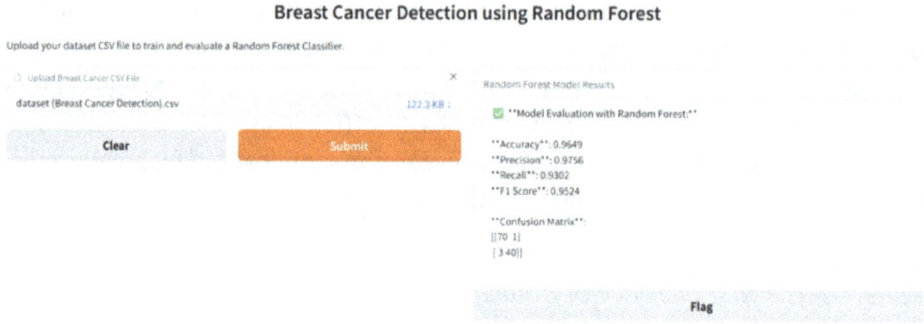

The final output stage of a Random Forest classifier-powered breast cancer detection system is depicted in the Fig.18. The system analyses the data and shows performance metrics under "Random Forest Model Results" on the right when the dataset "dataset (Breast Cancer Detection).csv" has been uploaded and submitted. These include F1 Score (0.9524), Accuracy (0.9649), Precision (0.9756), and Recall (0.9302), all of which demonstrate how well the model detects malignant instances. Furthermore, the Confusion Matrix ([[70, 1], [3, 40]]) offers a thorough analysis of true/false positives and negatives, assisting users in assessing the classifier's dependability. The "Clear" and "Flag" buttons on the user-friendly interface enable users to report problems or clear the input, respectively. This phase verifies that the model was executed successfully and demonstrates how machine learning can provide valuable insights for medical diagnosis.

4.3 SVMs (support vector machines)

SVM seeks to identify the best hyperplane with the greatest margin between classes. In high-dimensional spaces, it works incredibly well. This is used on tabular data with distinct class boundaries, like FNA-derived features from WBCD, SVM performs admirably (Wang et al., 2018). SVM algorithm is effective with small datasets and sturdy against overfitting in high-dimensional environments.

Code and Results:

Figure 19. Support Vector Machine user interface for breast cancer diagnosis, showing model results after running and allowing CSV file upload.

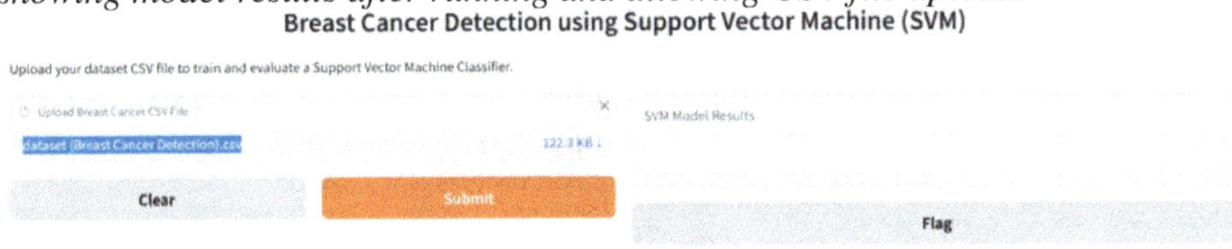

The interface of a breast cancer detection system using a Support Vector Machine (SVM) classifier is depicted in the Fig.19. Users may submit a breast cancer dataset in CSV format, like "dataset (Breast Cancer Detection).csv"—for analysis thanks to the user-friendly design. The SVM algorithm is activated to train on the provided data and produce classification results when the Submit button is clicked. These results are shown in the SVM Model Results section on the right. In order to reset the input and report any problems, respectively, this interface also has Clear and Flag buttons. By examining trends in clinical data, the system demonstrates how SVM, a potent supervised learning algorithm, can be used to support early and precise breast cancer diagnosis.

Figure 20. the initial interface of an SVM-based breast cancer detection system with a display area for results and the ability to add datasets.

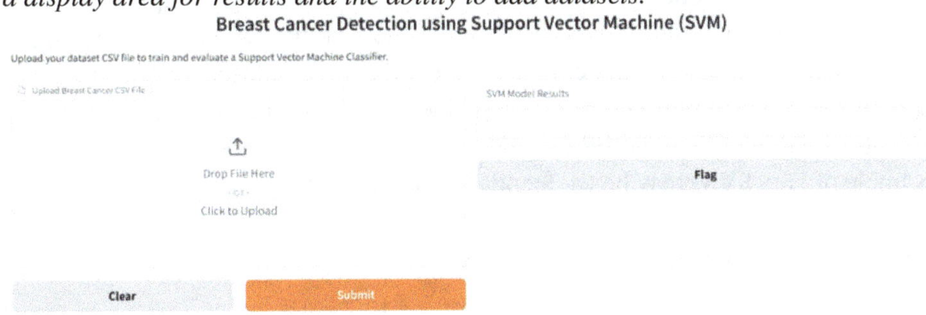

The first user interface of a breast cancer detection system using a Support Vector Machine (SVM) classifier is shown in the Fig.20. Users can submit a breast cancer dataset in CSV format by clicking to pick the file or by dragging and dropping the file. The Submit button starts the SVM algorithm-based model training and evaluation procedure as soon as the data is uploaded. The SVM Model Results section on the right side then shows the model's output.To reset the inputs or report any problems, the interface also has Clear and Flag buttons. Through effective data analysis and classification, this configuration highlights the incorporation of machine learning in an approachable manner to support early breast cancer detection.

Figure 21. After dataset processing, the output interface of an SVM-based breast cancer detection system displays the confusion matrix and model evaluation metrics.

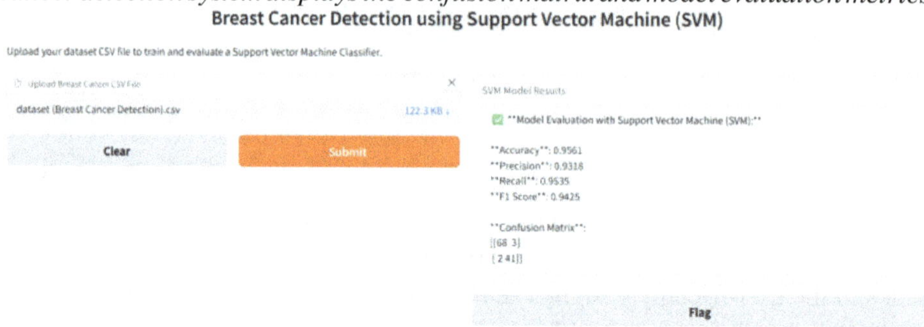

The final output screen of a breast cancer detection system using a Support Vector Machine (SVM) classifier is shown in the Fig.21. The system evaluates the data and displays the assessment results under the SVM Model Results section once the user uploads the dataset file named "dataset (Breast Cancer Detection).csv" and hits the Submit button. Accuracy (0.9561), Precision (0.9318), Recall (0.9535), and F1 Score (0.9425) are among the key performance measures displayed, which demonstrate how well the SVM model classifies cancer cases. The number of samples that were properly or wrongly identified is displayed in the Confusion Matrix ([[68, 3], [2, 41]]), which sheds light on the classification outcomes. Additionally, the interface has Clear and Flag buttons for reporting problems and resetting inputs, respectively. With its strong classification abilities and high accuracy, this output screen is a perfect example of how SVM may be a dependable tool in the diagnosis of breast cancer.

4.4 k-NN, or k-Nearest Neighbors

A data point is classified using the majority class of its "k" nearest neighbors in the feature space by the straightforward k-NN algorithm. KNN is Excellent in situations where clusters of benign and malignant samples can be easily distinguished from one another (Verma et al., 2010). In K-NN algorithm, no time is needed for training also it is non-parametric and simple to use.

Code and Results:

Figure 22. K-Nearest Neighbors (KNN) model user interface for breast cancer detection, displaying sections for uploading datasets and displaying results before the model runs.

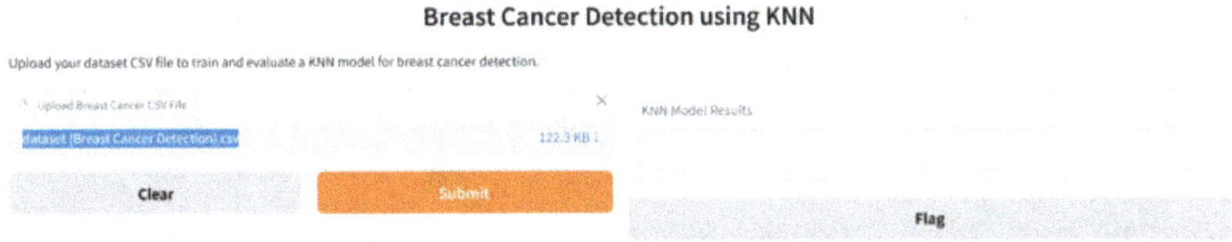

The K-Nearest Neighbors (KNN) algorithm-based breast cancer detection system's user interface is depicted in the Fig.22. At this point, the user has started the training and assessment procedure by uploading a dataset file called "dataset (Breast Cancer Detection).csv". The KNN model processes the uploaded data and presents the findings in the KNN Model findings section on the right after being triggered by the Submit button on the interface. The layout is intended to display important performance measures including accuracy, precision, recall, and F1 score, even if the assessment result has not yet been produced.Other options include Flag to report any problems and Clear to reset the input. This configuration provides a simplified procedure for clinical data analysis by showcasing the incorporation of the KNN algorithm into a useful, user-friendly web application for breast cancer categorization.

Figure 23. The KNN-based breast cancer detection system's initial interface, which displays the results display section and dataset upload option before the model is run.

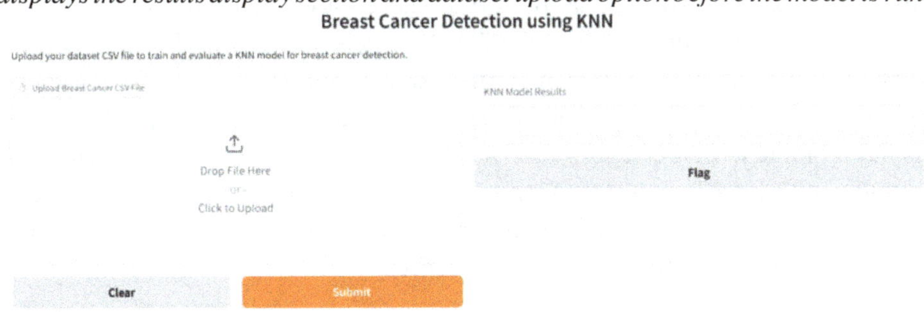

The K-Nearest Neighbors (KNN) algorithm-based breast cancer detection system's initial user interface is shown in the Fig.23. Users can submit a breast cancer dataset in CSV format using this web-based interface by either clicking to pick the file or dragging and dropping it into the appropriate location. After uploading the data, users can click the Submit button to start training and evaluating the model.

The KNN Model Results area on the right will show the KNN model's output, along with performance indicators like accuracy, precision, recall, and F1 score. The interface also has buttons labeledClear and Flag that allow you to reset inputs and report issues or errors. By enabling people to investigate the KNN algorithm for breast cancer classification, this visual interface highlights the simplicity and accessibility of machine learning technologies in medical diagnostics.

Figure 24. Following a successful model run, the output screen of the KNN-based breast cancer detection system shows the confusion matrix and assessment metrics.

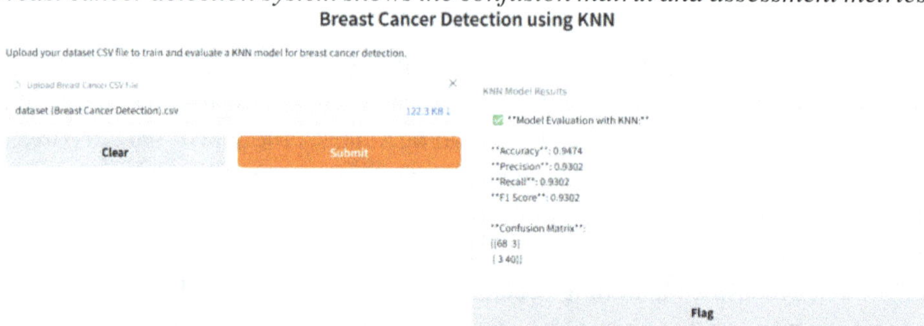

The K-Nearest Neighbors (KNN) algorithm-based breast cancer detection system's final output screen is depicted in the Fig.24 . The user runs the KNN model by clicking the Submit button after downloading the dataset file called "dataset (Breast Cancer Detection).csv". The system shows evaluation metrics in the KNN Model Results section once it has been run. These show good and balanced model performance and comprise Accuracy (0.9474), Precision (0.9302), Recall (0.9302), and F1 Score (0.9302). The amount of true positives, false positives, true negatives, and false negatives is displayed in the Confusion Matrix ([[68, 3], [3, 40]]), which displays comprehensive categorization results. Additionally, there are Clear and Flag buttons on this intuitive interface for resetting and reporting problems, respectively. All things considered, the graphic demonstrates how well the KNN algorithm is applied to reliably identify data on breast cancer.

4.5 Deep Learning (CNN) Convolutional Neural Networks

CNNs are specialized neural networks made for image data. Convolutional layers are used to automatically learn the spatial hierarchies of features.CNNs are especially well-suited for imaging-based diagnosis tasks such as mammograms and histopathology images (Rajkumari & Kalaivani, 2022). CNN shows excellent image classification performance as in this manual feature extraction is not required.

Code and Results:

Figure 25. The CNN-based breast cancer detection system's interface, displaying the uploading of datasets and the area for displaying results before the model runs.

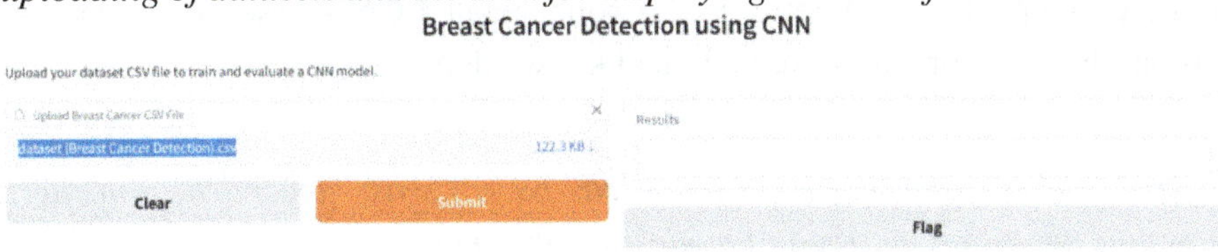

The interface of a Convolutional Neural Network (CNN) model-based breast cancer detection system is shown in the Fig.25 . The "dataset (Breast Cancer Detection). csv" file that the user submitted is meant to be used for CNN model evaluation and training. The CNN analyzes the dataset after clicking the Submit button, producing prediction results that show up in the Results area on the right. Additionally, the interface has a Flag button to report problems and a Clear button to reset the file input. This configuration exemplifies the application of deep learning methods, particularly CNNs, for the identification of breast cancer and shows how these models can be included into an intuitive user interface for practical diagnostic assistance.

Figure 26. CNN-based breast cancer detection user interface that allows CSV upload, model training, and result visualization.

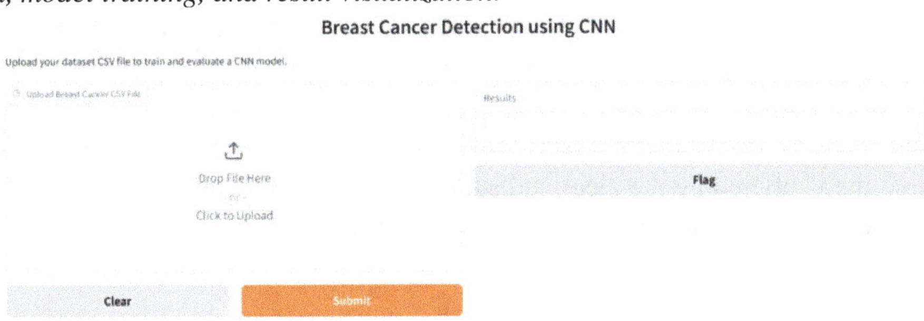

A user interface for Convolutional Neural Networks (CNNs)-based breast cancer detection is shown in Fig.26. Users can upload a CSV file with data pertaining to breast cancer for model training and assessment. Users can drag and drop the CSV file or click to upload it manually thanks to the interface's straightforward, user-friendly style. The "Submit" button allows users to start the model training process after the file has been uploaded, while the "Clear" button resets the input. The "Results" field is used to represent the prediction or evaluation's outcomes, such as model accuracy or categorization outcome (e.g., benign or malignant). There is also a "Flag" button available, which may be used to report problems or identify particular outputs. This interface shows how machine learning may be used practically in the healthcare industry by enabling people to access sophisticated CNN-based diagnostic tools without the need for extensive technical knowledge.

Figure 27. After submitting a dataset, a CNN-based breast cancer detection interface shows the confusion matrix and model performance metrics.

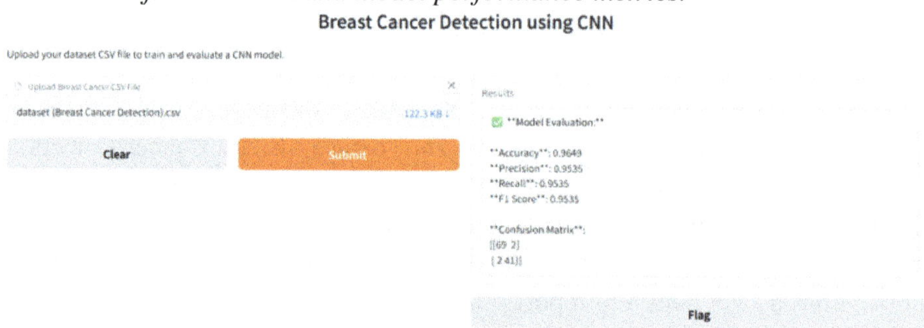

After uploading a dataset called dataset (Breast Cancer Detection.csv), the above Fig.27 displays the assessment results of a Convolutional Neural Network (CNN) model used for breast cancer detection. When the dataset is submitted, the system shows the following important performance metrics: 96.49% accuracy, 95.35% precision, 95.35% recall, and 95.35% F1 score. These metrics show how reliable the model is at accurately detecting cases of breast cancer. The model's classification efficacy is further assessed by presenting a confusion matrix that displays the distribution of true positives, true negatives, false positives, and false negatives. Control over file handling is offered by the clear and submit buttons, while any problems with the procedure or outcomes are probably reported using the flag button.

5. VALIDATION AND ASSESSMENT OF THE MODEL

5.1 Measures of Performance

When assessing how well machine learning models detect breast cancer, performance metrics are crucial. These metrics capture the whole picture of a model's predictive ability in healthcare, especially in diagnostic tasks, and go beyond simple accuracy (Vaka et al., 2020). Both false positives and false negatives should be kept to a minimum because these applications are life-critical.

The following are the primary performance indicators frequently employed in medical classification issues, like the detection of breast cancer:

1. **Accuracy:** Accuracy is the percentage of true results (both true positives and true negatives) among all cases analyzed, which indicates the model's overall correctness.

The formula is: Accuracy=Accuracy = (TP + TN)/(TP + TN + FP + FN)

Use Case: When classes are balanced, accuracy is helpful. In datasets that are unbalanced, such as when there are substantially more benign cases than malignant ones, it could be misleading.

2. **Precision:** Precision is the percentage of positive identifications that were in fact accurate. It assesses how well the model prevents false positives.

The formula is: Precision=Precision =TP/(TP + FP)

Use Case: Reducing false alarms requires high precision. This results in fewer patients being misdiagnosed with breast cancer.

3. Sensitivity / True Positive Rate Recall

Definition: Recall is the percentage of true positives that the model correctly identified.

The formula is: Recall=Recall =TP/(TP + FN)

Use Case: In medical applications, high recall is essential because it guarantees that the majority of cancer cases are detected and not overlooked.

4. **F1-Score:** The F1-score is the harmonic mean of recall and precision. It offers a single metric that strikes a balance between recall and precision.

F1-score = 2×Precision×Recall is the formula.

Use Case: Beneficial in situations where it's crucial to take into account both false positives and false negatives, as is common in medical diagnosis.

5. Receiver Operating Characteristic – Area Under Curve, or ROC-AUC

Plotting the True Positive Rate (Recall) against the False Positive Rate is known as the ROC curve. The model's capacity to differentiate between positive and negative classes is summed up by the Area Under the Curve (AUC).

AUC = 1 = Perfect Classifier

AUC = 0.5 → No ability to discriminate (random guess)

Use Case: When assessing diagnostic models across a range of threshold settings, AUC-ROC is especially helpful.

6. MACHINE LEARNING EXPLAINABILITY AND INTERPRETABILITY

Explainability and interpretability have become crucial requirements as machine learning (ML) models get more complex, particularly in the healthcare industry. Accurate predictions alone are insufficient in clinical settings such as breast cancer detection; in order to gain the confidence of physicians, patients, and regulatory agencies, a model must also provide clear and convincing reasoning for its predictions.In order to improve interpretability in medical machine learning applications, this section addresses the significance of model transparency, presents popular explainable AI (XAI) techniques, and talks about visualization tools.

6.1 Significance in Medical Environments

Model choices have a direct impact on patient outcomes, diagnosis, and treatment in high-stakes settings like healthcare. Therefore, interpretability is not only desirable but also required for practical, ethical, and legal reasons.

- Important Advantages in Clinical Settings: Adoption and Trust: Physicians who comprehend the reasoning behind a decision are more likely to embrace ML-based diagnostic systems.
- Error Identification: Clinicians can identify possible model biases or poor judgments thanks to interpretability.
- Regulatory Compliance: To guarantee accountability, laws like the GDPR and medical device regulations demand explainability.
- Communication with Patients: Transparent models assist physicians in providing patients with straightforward explanations of complicated findings.

Example: In breast cancer detection, an interpretable model can show which specific features (e.g., tumor radius or cell texture) led to a classification of "malignant."

6.2 Explainable AI Techniques (like SHAP and LIME)

Explainable AI (XAI) techniques aid in comprehending the inner workings of intricate models such as ensemble algorithms or neural networks. LIME and SHAP (Arravalli et al., 2025) are two of the most widely used model-agnostic tools.

Local Interpretable Model-Agnostic Explanations or LIME

By locally approximating the model with an interpretable one (such as a decision tree or linear model), LIME clarifies individual predictions. This is helpful in determining which characteristics led to a particular conclusion (e.g., classifying a tumor as malignant).

Use Case in Breast Cancer: By emphasizing the areas of the mammogram that most influenced the decision, LIME can clarify why an image-based model identified malignancy.

SHAP (Shapley Additive explanations)

SHAP gives each feature an importance value for a specific prediction based on cooperative game theory. It provides interpretability on a local and global level. This makes it a more theoretically sound approach by guaranteeing additivity and consistency.

Use Case: SHAP can indicate the degree to which a tumor's texture, area, or radius influenced a prediction and whether that influence was positive or negative.

6.3 Techniques and Tools for Visualization

- Interpretability depends on visualization, particularly in clinical machine learning where stakeholders might not understand technical jargon. There are numerous tools available for visualizing model decisions and feature contributions:

  1. Graphs of Feature Importance utilized in tree-based models, such as XGBoost and Random Forest. This shows each input feature's proportional contribution.
  2. Force Plots and SHAP Summary

- Overall feature impact is displayed in summary plots.
- By illustrating how each feature influenced the prediction, force plots provide a visual representation of individual predictions.

7. DIFFICULTIES AND MORAL ISSUES

There are a number of significant obstacles and moral dilemmas associated with the use of machine learning (ML) models in breast cancer detection. If these problems are not adequately resolved, they may jeopardize the legitimacy, security, and uptake of these technologies in medical settings. The reliability and generalizability of machine learning systems, data privacy and legal compliance, and bias in models and datasets are the three main areas of concern highlighted in this section.

7.1 Prejudice in Datasets and Models

The Meaning and Source of Bias:

In machine learning models, bias refers to systematic errors that produce unfair or incorrect predictions; these errors are frequently caused by skewed data distributions or poor model design. Bias in medical AI can have major repercussions, including incorrect diagnoses, particularly for patient groups that are underrepresented.

- Bias sources include class imbalance, which occurs in most breast cancer datasets where there are significantly more benign cases than malignant ones. As a result, models may perform poorly in minority (critical) cases and favor the majority class.
- Demographic Bias: Some populations (such as younger women and ethnic minorities) may be underrepresented in datasets, which reduces the model's accuracy for these groups.
- Sampling bias: Information gathered from a single hospital or area might not accurately represent the diversity of patients worldwide.
- Use of balanced datasets or the application of oversampling methods like SMOTE are routine fairness testing and bias audits.
- Models are trained using representative and varied data from various sources.

Real-World Concern: Health disparities could result from a model that was trained solely on the mammograms of Caucasian women showing lower accuracy for Asian or African women.

7.2 Legal Frameworks and Data Privacy (HIPAA, GDPR)

The significance of data privacy

- ○ As medical data is so sensitive, improper use of it can result in discrimination, identity theft, or a decline in public confidence in healthcare organizations. ML systems must be developed and deployed under strict privacy regulations.

For instance, an ML model utilized in the EU must permit patients to obtain justifications for automated decisions, including those made by diagnostic tools, in accordance with GDPR (Sangaraju, 2025).

7.3 Generalizability and Model Reliability

- Model Reliability: The stability and consistency of a model over several runs or environments is referred to as reliability. Unreliable forecasts can be harmful, undermine trust, and prevent clinical adoption in medical settings.
- Model Generalizability: A model that can be applied to unseen data from various hospitals, devices, or patient populations does well in addition to the training data.

8. FUTURE RESEARCH DIRECTIONS

Machine learning models must be smoothly incorporated into the clinical workflow in order to have a significant impact on breast cancer detection. Integration entails making the system usable, reliable, and functional in actual healthcare settings; it goes beyond creating a highly accurate model. This section looks at the obstacles that currently stand in the way of the practical implementation of AI systems in clinical settings, how human-AI collaboration can be organized, and what usability and trust issues need to be addressed.

8.1 AI-Human Cooperation

Machine learning is meant to support human decision-making, not to take the place of clinicians. The use of collaborative systems in radiology and pathology, where AI aids in the doctor's diagnosis and treatment choices, is growing (Diaz et al., 2024).

Crucial Components of AI-Human Collaboration:

- Second Opinion Systems: Machine learning models can offer second opinions by spotting potential cancers that might be missed during manual review.
- Decision Support Tools: By highlighting regions of interest on histopathological slides or mammograms, AI can assist radiologists in focusing.

- Efficiency Gain: AI reduces workload and frees up doctors to concentrate on more complex cases by automating repetitive tasks (such as triaging routine cases).

For example, a CNN-based breast cancer detection system can spot suspicious areas on mammograms, which a radiologist can then confirm or refute. This ensures safety while boosting speed and accuracy.

8.2 Problems with Usability and Trust

In clinical practice, even the most accurate machine learning models may not work if they are difficult to use or do not gain the trust of clinicians. Adoption of AI depends heavily on usability and trust.

- Difficulties: Complicated Interfaces: Without clear dashboards or visualizations, clinicians may find it challenging to understand ML tools.
- Black-Box Models: Users find it challenging to comprehend or defend model predictions due to their lack of interpretability.
- Mistrust of Automation: Even when AI tools perform well, they may be rejected due to mistakes or a lack of transparency.

Solutions: Create user interfaces (UIs) that are friendly to clinicians (e.g., heatmaps, annotated images, confidence scores).

- Make outputs comprehensible by using explainable AI techniques like SHAP or LIME.
- To show dependability and get input, conduct clinical trials.

Real-World Perspective: Particularly in high-risk settings like oncology, many medical professionals favor "less accurate but more explainable" models.

8.3 Obstacles to Deployment in Practical Environments

Despite tremendous advancements in academia, organizational, legal, and technical obstacles still prevent the widespread use of ML systems in hospitals. Some more common deployment obstacles include interoperability of data because clinical data comes in a variety of formats (DICOM, HL7, FHIR) from various systems and institutions that becomes a challenging task. Another challenge is interoperability of data in deploying models. One of the obstacles is lack of standardization as generalizability of models is impacted by variations in imaging equipment, scanning protocols, and reporting styles. Some more obstacles can be regulatory obstacles that include extensive testing and documentation to obtain approval from regulatory agencies such as the FDA or CE. An infrastructure requirement for deep learning models that require GPUs or cloud based deployment, which may not be practical in the environment is the hurdle. And, the last obstacle is hospital information system integration that requires strong APIs and adherence to healthcare IT standard regulations which are necessary for integration of ML tools with Electronic Health Records system.

9. CONCLUSION

According to this study, machine learning (ML) approaches have a lot of promise for improving breast cancer early detection and precise diagnosis. We have observed notable gains in classification accuracy, sensitivity, and specificity by employing a variety of algorithms, including decision trees, random forests, and support vector machines (SVM). Model performance was found to be significantly influenced by feature selection, data preprocessing, and algorithm selection. Because of their capacity to identify intricate patterns in medical data, ensemble approaches and deep learning techniques frequently produced better results than the other models that were evaluated. Summarized Table 1 of all the algorithms is shown below.

Table 1: Performance table of all the algorithms

Algorithm	Accuracy	Precision	Recall	F1 Score	Confusion Matrix
Logistic Regression	0.9737	0.9762	0.9535	0.9647	[70 1] [2 41]
Decision Tree	0.9474	0.9302	0.9302	0.9302	[68 3][3 40]
Random Forest	0.9649	0.9756	0.9812	0.9574	[70 1] [3 40]
SVM	0.9561	0.9318	0.9535	0.9425	[68 3] [24 1]
KNN	0.9474	0.9302	0.9302	0.9302	[89 3] [3 40]
CNN	0.9649	0.9535	0.9535	0.9535	[69 2] [2 41]

With all methods attaining accuracy above 94%, the comparative analysis of machine learning algorithms for breast cancer detection demonstrates the powerful predictive powers of these models. With a 97.37% accuracy rate, Logistic Regression was the most successful model among them. Its consistency in striking a balance between sensitivity and specificity was demonstrated by its high precision, recall, and F1 score. With an accuracy of 96.49% and a high recall, Random Forest also showed competitive performance, making it especially useful for accurately identifying true positive cases.

Although interpretable and simple to use, the Decision Tree classifier performed relatively poorly, while SVM and KNN produced good but marginally worse results. These results align with broader research trends: Deep learning models like CNNs achieve excellent classification performance but require large amounts of labelled data and high processing power; Random Forests often deliver higher accuracy but demand more computational resources; and Decision Trees and SVMs are interpretable and simple but struggle with large or complex datasets.

Notwithstanding these developments, a number of issues still exist, such as uneven class distributions, sparse and irregular datasets, and the "black box" character of deep learning models, which raises questions regarding explainability, ethics, and legal responsibility in misdiagnosis situations. Overall, the findings imply that although Random Forest and Logistic Regression provide dependable and useful performance for the detection of breast cancer, further development of ML/DL methods is necessary to close current gaps and advance toward more precise, understandable, and morally sound diagnostic systems.

REFERENCES

Alawee, W. H., Al-Haddad, L. A., Basem, A., & Al-Haddad, A. A. (2024). A data augmentation approach to enhance breast cancer detection using generative adversarial and artificial neural networks. *Open Engineering, 14*(1), 20240052.

Arravalli, T., Chadaga, K., Muralikrishna, H., Sampathila, N., Cenitta, D., Chadaga, R., & Swathi, K. S. (2025). Detection of breast cancer using machine learning and explainable artificial intelligence. *Scientific Reports, 15*(1), 26931.

Dai, B., Chen, R. C., Zhu, S. Z., & Zhang, W. W. (2018, December). Using random forest algorithm for breast cancer diagnosis. In *2018 International symposium on computer, consumer and control (IS3C)* (pp. 449-452). IEEE.

Díaz, O., Rodríguez-Ruíz, A., & Sechopoulos, I. (2024). Artificial Intelligence for breast cancer detection: Technology, challenges, and prospects. *European Journal of Radiology, 175*, 111457.

Doi, K. (2007). Computer-aided diagnosis in medical imaging: Historical review, current status and future potential. *Computerized Medical Imaging and Graphics, 31*(4-5), 198–211.

Elmore, J. G., Wells, C. K., Lee, C. H., Howard, D. H., & Feinstein, A. R. (1994). Variability in radiologists' interpretations of mammograms. *The New England Journal of Medicine, 331*(22), 1493–1499.

Han, J., Kamber, M., & Pei, J. (2012). *Data mining: Concepts and. Techniques.* Morgan Kaufmann Publishers.

He, J., Liu, N., & Zhao, L. (2025). New progress in imaging diagnosis and immunotherapy of breast cancer. *Frontiers in Immunology, 16*, 1560257.

Heat, M., Bowyer, K., Kopans, D., Moore, R., & Kegelmeyer, P. (2000). The digital database for screening mammography. In *Digital Mammography–Proceedings of the 5th International Workshop on Digital Mammography (IWDM2000)* (pp. 212-218). Toronto.

Khalid, A., Mehmood, A., Alabrah, A., Alkhamees, B. F., Amin, F., AlSalman, H., & Choi, G. S. (2023). Breast cancer detection and prevention using machine learning. *Diagnostics (Basel), 13*(19), 3113.

Khandezamin, Z., Naderan, M., & Rashti, M. J. (2020). Detection and classification of breast cancer using logistic regression feature selection and GMDH classifier. *Journal of Biomedical Informatics, 111*, 103591.

Kuhn, M., & Johnson, K. (2013). *Applied predictive modeling*. Springer.

Litjens, G., Kooi, T., Bejnordi, B. E., Setio, A. A. A., Ciompi, F., Ghafoorian, M., & Sánchez, C. I. (2017). A survey on deep learning in medical image analysis. *Medical Image Analysis*, *42*, 60–88.

Rajakumari, R., & Kalaivani, L. (2022). Breast Cancer Detection and Classification Using Deep CNN Techniques. *Intelligent Automation & Soft Computing*, *32*(2).

Sangaraju, V. V. (2025). AI and Data Privacy in Healthcare: Compliance with HIPAA, GDPR, and emerging regulations. *International Journal of Emerging Trends in Computer Science and Information Technology*, 67-74.

Vaka, A. R., Soni, B., & Reddy, S. (2020). Breast cancer detection by leveraging Machine Learning. *ICT Express*, *6*(4), 320–324.

Verma, B., McLeod, P., & Klevansky, A. (2010). Classification of benign and malignant patterns in digital mammograms for the diagnosis of breast cancer. *Expert Systems with Applications*, *37*(4), 3344–3351.

Wang, H., Zheng, B., Yoon, S. W., & Ko, H. S. (2018). A support vector machine-based ensemble algorithm for breast cancer diagnosis. *European Journal of Operational Research*, *267*(2), 687–699.

Chapter 5
Advances in Brain Tumor Diagnosis Through Multimodal Imaging and Deep Learning Techniques

Liyakathunisa Syed
https://orcid.org/0000-0003-4513-1795
Taibah University, Saudi Arabia

Roba Alhashmiy Alamir
https://orcid.org/0009-0008-2343-2734
Taibah University, Saudi Arabia

Ghada Alharbi
Taibah University, Saudi Arabia

Abdullah Alsaeedi
Taibah University, Saudi Arabia

Ayman Noor
https://orcid.org/0000-0002-3344-2847
Taibah University, Saudi Arabia

Talal Noor
Taibah University, Saudi Arabia

ABSTRACT

Brain tumors represent abnormal growths of cells—either benign or malignant—within the confined space of the human skull. These growths can lead to severe health complications and long-term psychological and physical consequences, greatly diminishing a patient's quality of life. The survival rate for individuals diagnosed with malignant brain tumors decreases significantly over time if early interventions are not implemented. This study investigates advanced hybrid architectures, namely CNN-UNet, ResNet-UNet, EfficientNet-UNet, and EfficientNet integrated with Vision Transformers. A comprehensive comparative analysis of these hybrid architectures is conducted to recognize the most efficient model. The results

DOI: 10.4018/979-8-3373-4312-9.ch005

indicate that EfficientNet-UNet architecture achieved superior performance on the BraTS dataset with an accuracy of 99.47%, while EfficientNet-Vision Transformer on the Nickparvar dataset from Kaggle reached an accuracy of 97%. These findings highlight the efficiency of advanced hybrid deep learning models in detecting brain tumors from multimodal MRI images.

I. INTRODUCTION

Brain tumors are the leading cause of cancers deaths worldwide; in adults they arise due to the uncontrolled division of cells. The brain is an essential organ composed of neuronal cells, along with supporting tissues such as cells known as glial cells and meninges that surround them (Azzarelli et al., 2018). Damage to these brain regions is permanent and may lead to severe illnesses, including possibly fatal brain tumors. Abnormal growth of cells in the human brain leads to the formation of certain cancers. The National Brain Tumor Society (NBTS) predicts that by 2025, around 18,330 fatalities will occur due to malignant brain tumors, and over 93,000 Americans will have been diagnosed of serious brain tumors. Several obstacles arise during patient treatment, since the survival rate for malignant brain tumors is 35.7%, according to a survey done over the last five years (National Brain Tumor Society, 2023). It is furthermore predicted that the death rate for males is 2.8 per 100,000 and for females it is 2.0 per 100,000, according to global age-standardized for primary malignant brain tumors (National Brain Tumor Society, 2023). Accurate and early detection and diagnosis play a significant role in preventing mortalities related to brain tumors (Grant et al., 2020). There exist several imaging modalities to capture the tumors such as magnetic resonance imaging (MRI), computed tomography (CT), X-rays, and Ultrasound and are used in medical diagnostics. MRI is considered a powerful and significant tool for screening brain cancers, as it offers enhanced visibility of surrounding soft tissue features (Hussain et al., 2022). Traditional clinical based diagnosis potentially causes inaccuracies and delays and sometimes falls short of revealing the complete complexity of tumor features. Physicians are often dependent on multiple magnetic resonance imaging (MRI) images to assess tumor growth, but this procedure can be extremely intensive laborious and vulnerable to human inaccuracies, still MRI is widely used for brain tumor categorization and detection (Martucci et al., 2023). Automated techniques with the use of Artificial Intelligence tools could accelerate tumor diagnosis, reduce the occurrence of false positives rates, and minimize waiting times. For improving the health of patients, timely and precise diagnosis has become essential, and it alleviates adverse long-term effects.

Technological advancements have significantly enhanced the field of medical diagnostics, particularly in neuro-oncology. The integration of Artificial Intelligence (AI) into medical imaging is a transformative step toward improving diagnostic precision. Artificial intelligence possesses the potential to serve as a transformative tool in neuro-oncology, currently addressing challenges across several phases of therapeutic treatment (Jeong et al., 2025). Through the utilization of AI tools and techniques large amounts of MRI image data can be easily managed, it also has the capacity for accurate measurement, abnormality detection, tumor pattern recognition, early diagnosis, optimization of workflow and treatment planning. Individualized therapy can be provided to enhance patient outcomes with the integration of AI tools into clinical trials. Hence AI is significantly essential in clinical neuroimaging for tumor detection, segmentation and classifications, to evaluate post treatment responses and increase pre-treatment planning (Huang et al., 2025).

Machine learning techniques provide sophisticated methods for medical experts that enhance accuracy of diagnosis and expedite treatment planning. These deep neural networks architectures provide strong capabilities which substantially increase the performance of model by precise feature extraction. Recently advanced deep learning algorithms are utilized for tumor detection, segmentation, and classification (Satushe et al., 2025). For early detection of tumor lesions, DL algorithms provide precise, persistent and quantitative measures which are crucial for monitoring the tumor progression and timely intervention. Furthermore, DL algorithms can predict the tumor grade, kind, and genetic alterations to facilitate personalized medicine (Thaha et al., 2019). The high-resolution imaging offered by MRI scans makes it suitable for detecting abnormalities in the brain cells using artificial intelligence techniques such as deep learning to enhance the patient's survival rates by timely interventions.

This chapter emphasizes the development of complex deep learning frameworks, including CNN, ResNet50, U-Net, EfficientNetB0, and ViTs models, to analyze BraTS (Bra, 2025) and Nickparvar (Nickparvar, 2020) datasets. Five hybrid deep learning models (CNN-U-Net, ResNet50-UNet, EfficientNetB0-U-Net, and EfficientNetB0- ViTs) have been developed for tumor analysis, precise detection and classification. Furthermore, it demonstrates superior feature extraction capabilities of U-Net and EfficientNet's architectures which capture long-range relationships. This chapter further discusses several challenges such as data scarcity, class imbalance, computational complexity, and model generalization encountered during the implementation and mitigation to overcome the challenges. The proposed hybrid approaches, especially EfficientNetB0-U-Net, and EfficientNetB0- ViTs provide superior performance compared to traditional approaches it delineates the challenges and provides accurate diagnosis and can be deployed and adopted for clinical diagnosis.

This chapter is structured into seven sections. Section 1 provides a concise overview of brain tumors and the use of artificial intelligence technologies, particularly machine learning and deep learning, in their automated detection and classification. Section 2 reviews relevant research on brain tumor diagnosis using deep learning and machine learning methods. Section 3 describes various deep learning architectures employed for tumor identification. Section 4 introduces the proposed deep learning methodology for brain tumor detection. Section 5 summarizes the findings along with a comparative analysis. Section 6 addresses the key challenges and future research directions, and conclusion is provided in Section 7.

2. RELATED STUDIES

This section provides a succinct overview of current progress in brain tumor diagnosis by multimodal imaging and artificial intelligence (AI) methodologies. These studies utilize several data sources, including computed tomography (CT), and magnetic resonance imaging (MRI) scans, in conjunction with deep learning and machine learning techniques for tumor lesions localization, segmentation, classification, and prognosis.

Rahman et al. (Rahman et al., 2025) systematically analyzed and assessed several feature extraction techniques—Gabor filters, LBP, FFT, DWT, GLRLM, and CNN—alongside machine learning methods which includes k-NN, SVC, Random Forest, CNN, and PNN for the identification of brain tumors using MRI. The Brain Tumor MRI Dataset was utilized from Kaggle (Nickparvar, 2020). Results indicate that LBP combined with CNN and SVC obtains good accuracy, as it was validated by statistical tests and SHAP analysis for feature significance. In both short and big datasets, CNN surpassed other models, achieving an accuracy of up to 98.9%, indicating robust generalization. The study emphasizes CNN's capacity to utilize high-resolution MRI characteristics for rapid, consistent, and accurate tumor identification, hence enhancing therapeutic results.

Similarly, Dorfner et al. (Dorfner et al., 2025) presented a review to examine the transformational influence of deep learning on brain tumor analysis, emphasizing its applications in two primary domains: segmentation and classification. Their discussion was focused on how deep learning models provide a transformative impact on brain tumor analysis and precise tumor segmentation from medical images, thus providing objective and reproducible measures significant for disease monitoring, diagnosis, and treatment planning.

Razzaghi et al. (Razzaghi et al., 2022) suggested a multimodal deep transfer learning approach for the analysis of MRI brain images. They highlighted two primary contributions which includes a novel multimodal feature encoder and adaptation technique to alleviate distribution variations among test and training datasets. They assumed that not all modalities are available for every sample. This approach aims to improve segmentation effectiveness by using additional information provided by several imaging modalities. Figshare brain tumor datasets and IBSR were used for evaluating their techniques. Their proposed M-SVM classifier obtained an accuracy of 98.92% on the Figshare dataset for classification of the tumors form the MRI images.

Transfer learning-based approaches using pre-trained CNNs was suggested by Filatov et al. (Filatov & Yar, 2022) They applied EfficientNetB1, EfficientNetV2B1, ResNet50, and EfficientNetB7 models to Kaggle dataset on MRI scans which include pituitary, meningioma, glioma, and non-tumor cases. Their preprocessing techniques involved normalization and image augmentation. They achieved best accuracy of 89.55% for EfficientNetB1 when compared to their other models. Regardless of the results obtained being underscored, they illustrate the ability of EfficientNet's flexible design towards enhancing classification accuracy and future highlight the need for hybrid frameworks.

A comparative study on hybrid transformer-based models and CNNs was performed on the BRISC dataset by Thahiruddin et al. (Thahiruddin, 2025). This is a benchmark balanced dataset of 6,000 MRI scans. A comprehensive analysis was conducted on four architectures which includes MobileViTV2,ResNet18, MobileNetV3-Small, and EfficientNet-B0. The models were fine-tuned advanced regularization techniques with a rigorous 5-fold cross-validation scheme. They demonstrated that their models (MobileViTV2, ResNet18, and EfficientNet-B0) obtained an accuracy of 98.9%, while with MobileNetV3-Small an accuracy of 96.9% was obtained. Their study also addressed that performance of ResNet8 achieved the fastest inference latency despite being the largest model. Hence, the obtained results show the efficacy of EfficientNet-B0 and its ability to extract features for brain tumor classification. Furthermore, this study also addresses that the hybrid CNN–Transformer designs can handle complex neuroimaging tasks. The authors in (Deepak & Ameer, 2021) suggested SVM for classification and CNN for its feature extraction from MRI images. FigShare brain tumor dataset was utilized for model training and testing. They obtained an accuracy of 95.82% with SVM and CNN feature extraction technique. The limitations of this study are that it was constrained on model robustness, and low-resolution or noisy images.

Park et.al (Park & Kim, 2024) deploy deep neural networks and explainable artificial intelligence (XAI) to classify brain cancers from MRI scans. Four models (ResNet-50, VGG-16, Vision Transformer, and EfficientNetV2L) are compared. All models were fine-tuned using transfer learning and trained over 100 epochs using SGD and 0.001 learning rate. The researchers tuned hyperparameters for optimizers (SGD vs. Adam), learning rates, and training epochs. The study employed 3,164 brain MRI pictures from Kaggle. VGG-16 had the greatest classification accuracy at 97.62%, followed by ResNet-50 at 96.51%. EfficientNetV2L and the Vision Transformer (ViT-Base-16) scored poorly, scoring 89.68% and 88.89%, respectively. When data is scarce, classic CNNs outperform transformer-based models for tumor identification. Grad-CAM, LIME, and SHAP visualizations demonstrated that VGG-16 and ResNet-50 performed better and created more focused and interpretable heat maps that accurately highlighted tumor areas that impacted categorization. Larger and more diversified data sets are needed because data augmentation has little effect on accuracy. The study's limitation was the use of homogenous dataset which limits model generalizability to other clinical contexts. The underperformance of ViT-Base-16 shows that transformer systems need much bigger datasets. While the study established explainability tools, it did not systematically assess explanation consistency or reliability across patient instances or models. Finally, the study lacks real-world clinical validation, which is essential for assessing these models' diagnostic process applicability.

A hybrid EFFResNet-ViT model was introduced by Hussain et.al (Hussain et al., 2025). This model integrates features from a convolutional neural network (CNN) via ResNet with representations from a ViT model, to utilize both low-level feature extraction and high-level contextual information for medical images categorization. The design combines the advantages of residual CNN blocks for collecting detailed spatial characteristics with the self-attention technique of ViT for modeling long-range interdependence. The fusion occurs at the feature level before the final classification layer. A cross-entropy loss function is applied to train the model is trained in an end-to-end manner, along with conventional data augmentation methods employed to enhance generalization. The model was assessed using a Kaggle MRI dataset for brain cancers, encompassing images from several tumor types, such as pituitary, meningioma, and glioma tumors. The dataset comprises thousands of T1-weight MRI images with contrast enhancement. Images underwent preprocessing include data augmentation, normalization, and scaling to improve robustness. EFFResNet-ViT attained an overall classification accuracy of roughly 95.3%, surpassing the performance of standalone CNN or ViT models in baseline evaluations. The fusion method exhibited enhanced feature representation capabilities, resulting in superior differentiation across tumor types. Furthermore, explainability evaluations with Grad-CAM and attention visualization validated that the model concentrated on pertinent tumor locations during prediction, hence enhancing the clinical interpretability of the results. The primary weakness of the study is its dependence on a very small and homogeneous dataset, potentially constraining the model's applicability to varied clinical populations. The computational difficulty of integrating ResNet and ViT layers escalates training duration and resource demands.

The integration of MRI imaging and sophisticated AI methodologies has produced encouraging outcomes in enhancing the precision and efficacy of brain tumor detection. Nonetheless, obstacles persist, such as the necessity for extensive annotated datasets, standardization of imaging methods, data scarcity, and the need to create scalable models, which can generalize on cross platforms and with varying image settings. To overcome the mentioned drawbacks, we have suggested hybrid deep learning models such as CNN-U-Net, EfficientNetB0-U-Net, ResNet50-UNet, and EfficientNetB0-Vision Transformers (ViTs) for accurate detection, segmentation, and classification of brain tumors from MRI multimodal images.

3. DEEP LEARNING ARCHITECTURES FOR BRAIN TUMOR Detection

Recently, researchers have created sophisticated deep learning architectures applicable for the identification and classification of brain tumors. These encompass Convolutional Neural Networks (CNNs), ResNet, U-Net, EfficientNet, and Transformers. This section will explore diverse deep learning architectures utilized for the classification of different categories of aberrant brain tumors, which will be implemented in our proposed study.

3.1. Convolutional Neural Networks (CNN)

When dealing with MRI images, a traditional Deep Neural Network (DNN) tends to encounter the computational complexity associated with the parameters to process the data. For example, if a small square image containing 28 pixels (28 ×28) is forwarded through a single neuron, it will produce 784 parameters, which is manageable with traditional DNNs. Nonetheless, if the image has many more pixels, it will produce a much larger number of parameters that cannot be managed with standard DNNs. Convolutional neural networks (CNNs) were developed to solve this issue (Febrianto et al., 2020). Usually, CNN consists of three significant layers (convolutional layers, pooling layers, and fully connected layers) as shown in Figure 1. When an input image that has a height n_h and width n_w and color channels $d(n_h \times n_w \times d)$ is passed through these layers, it will be dimensionally transformed to become denser in depth and the spatial dimension $(n_h \times n_w)$ tends to get smaller. In the convolutional layer, the image will be convolved with a given set of filters across the spatial dimension, producing a 2D matrix. This matrix is fed into the pooling layer to reduce its dimensions. As the number of parameters are reduced, the model decreases its computational complexity. These two processes are repeated until the features are learned to the desired degree of complexity. Finally, the FC layers will connect each neuron, hence producing many parameters that will help predict the class of the input image. CNN performance can be optimized by setting appropriate values of padding and stride. In addition, some sophisticated operations such as dropouts and regularization can help increase performance (Sarvamangala & Kulkarni, 2022). This is how the CNNs were shown to perform better than usual DNNs. Thereby, they were widely adopted by computer vision researchers.

Figure 1. General Convolutional Neural Network (CNN) Architecture

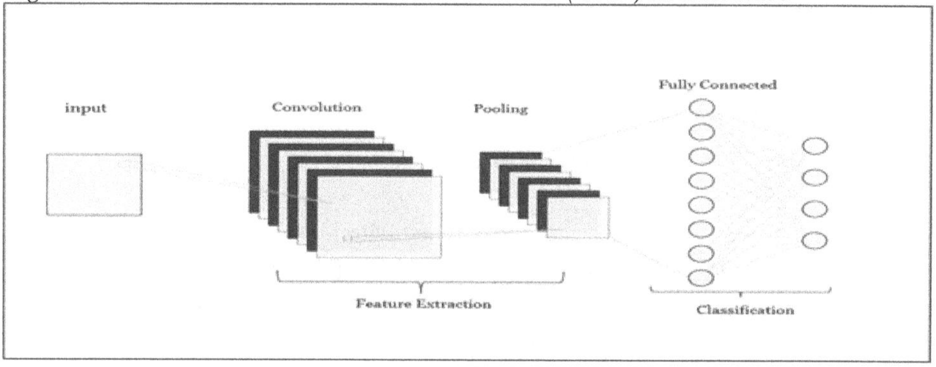

3.2 U-Net

In 2015, Ronneberger et. al (Ronneberger et al., 2015) presented a sophisticated CNN architecture able to sufficiently perform biomedical image segmentation called U-Net. U-Net can be trained on a significantly small image dataset yet delivers outstanding performance in segmentation. Figure 2 illustrates the U-Net framework which consists of two symmetric parts (a contracting path and an expansive path). The contracting path consists of the convolutional procedure as in CNN. The expansive path consists of the transposed 2D convolutional layers to execute the up-sampling operation. Every process employs two convolution steps. U-Net delivers fast image classification and segmentation that can be used individually and can be embedded within several types of DNNs for other purposes.

Figure 2. U-Net architecture (Ronneberger et al., 2015)

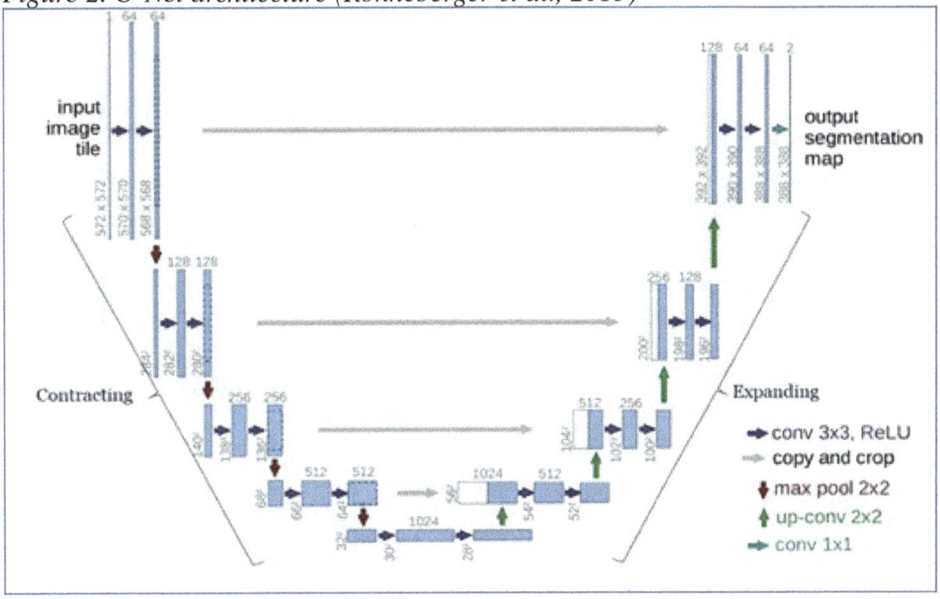

U-Net is extremely adept in brain tumor identification because of its U-shaped design, which facilitates accurate tumor segmentation by integrating high-resolution and contextual data. It operates effectively with constrained MRI datasets, captures multi-scale tumor characteristics, and facilitates rapid, precise inference for clinical applications.

3.3 ResNets

In 2015, Residual Network (ResNet) was first introduced as the winner of the ImageNet contest (He et al., 2016). The main issue ResNet solved was the vanishing gradient effect. This model can be up to 152 layers deep and still manages to achieve an outstanding performance of a 3.57% error rate. ResNet has the standard components of a classic CNN, yet it introduces a new module called the skip connection, illustrated in Figure 3. A skip connection creates a shortcut within layers by transferring the output of a layer, skipping several layers, and sending it into the next layers via addition. To avoid the input-output dimension variations, zero-padding is performed. As ResNets tolerate having large numbers of layers, many versions can be produced. Such as (ResNet-34, ResNet-50, ResNet-101, ResNet-1202, ResNet-152) and more depending on the number of layers (He et al., 2016).

Figure 3. Skip connection block in ResNets

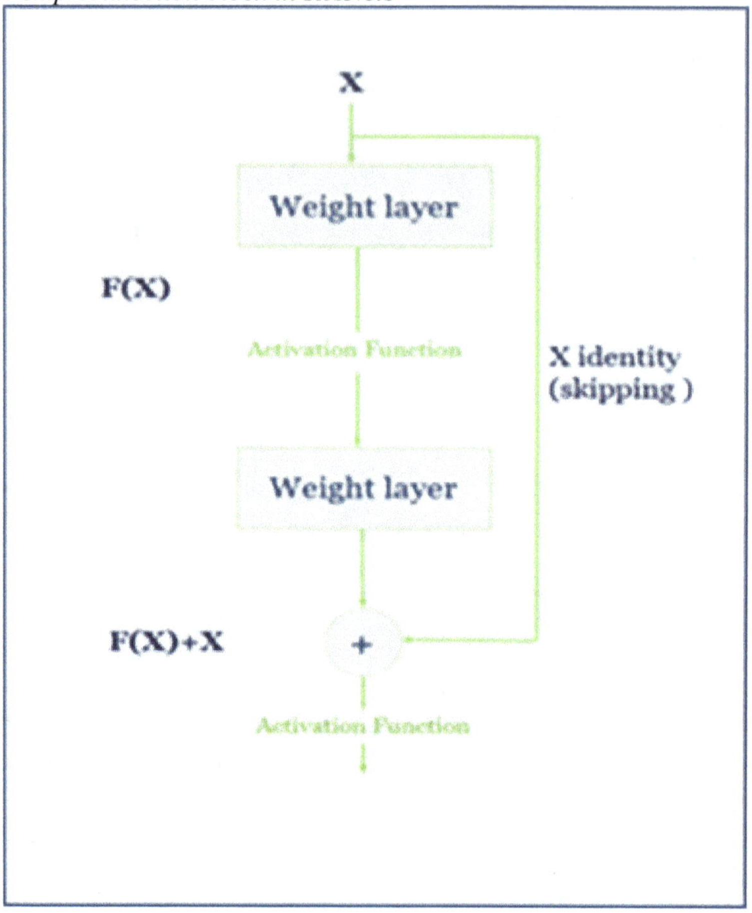

ResNet is exceptionally proficient in brain tumor identification due to its residual connections, which overcomes the problem of the vanishing gradient, enabling extremely deep networks to discern intricate details in MRI data. This results in enhanced accuracy and resilience in differentiating between tumor categories. Utilizing transfer learning techniques with pre-trained ResNet models diminishes the requirement for extensive medical datasets, rendering it feasible for clinical use. ResNet enhances feature extraction, patient generalization, and diagnostic reliability in brain tumor classification.

3.4 EfficientNet

EfficientNet is a variation of CNN model that improves performance by using a composite scaling method to consistently adjust all dimensions such as resolution, depth, and breadth. Unlike many traditional CNNs, which tend to scale layers in an inconsistent way, EfficientNet adopts a more systematic strategy. By scaling depth, width, and resolution in a balanced manner, the model can reach higher accuracy while keeping parameter counts and computational cost under control (Tan & Le, 2019). The EfficientNet family (B0–B7) is pre-trained on large datasets such as ImageNet, it provides multiple variants that can be chosen depending on the available hardware resources. In the context of brain tumor segmentation, EfficientNet has delivered promising results. It can detect subtle variations in MRI scans such as shifts in intensity and texture that conventional CNNs often struggle to capture. At the same time, it manages to keep the architecture lightweight and reduce training time, which is particularly useful in medical environments where both computing resources and time are often constrained (Iqbal et al., 2024). Its effectiveness likely comes from the way it balances accuracy and efficiency, offering both strong predictive power and practical usability. Figure 4 below shows the general architecture of EfficientNet.

Figure 4. EfficientNet's Architecture (Zhou et al., 2023)

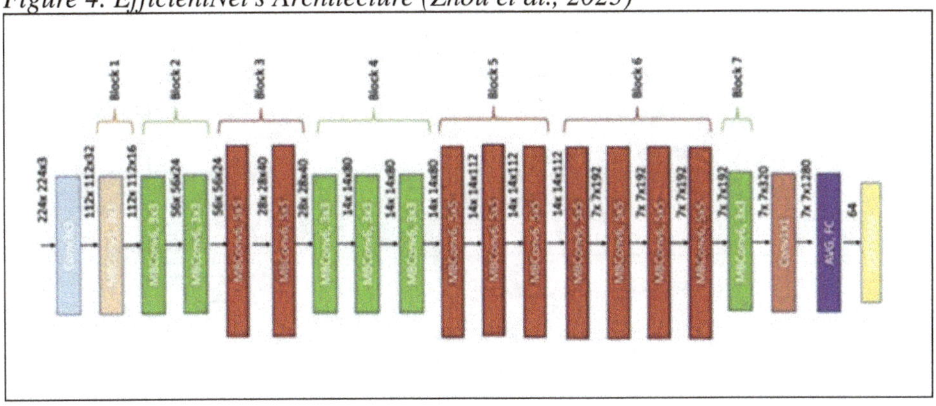

3.5 Vision Transformers (ViTs)

The Vision Transformer (ViT) represents a deep learning architecture specifically tailored for image classification tasks. Instead of processing the entire image directly, ViT partitions the input into fixed-size, non-overlapping patches (Dosovitskiy et al., 2020). Each patch is subsequently transformed into a one-dimensional embedding vector, which is then passed through a transformer encoder to capture global contextual relationships across the image. To enable classification, a special class token is appended to the sequence and passed through a multilayer perceptron

(MLP) for final prediction (Manzari et al., 2023). The key strength of ViT lies in its use of self-attention mechanism, which allows the model to selectively focus on relevant features, thereby capturing both local and global dependencies. This capability enhances the accuracy of image classification tasks.

$$Attention(Q,K,V) = softmax\left(\frac{QK^T}{\sqrt{d_k}}\right)V \quad (1)$$

Here, Q denotes the query matrix representing the current elements under consideration, K is the key matrix representing all elements, and V is the value matrix containing the associated information to be aggregated (Byeon et al., 2025). The dot product QK^T measures similarity between query and key vectors, scaled by $\frac{1}{\sqrt{d_k}}$ to ensure numerical stability. The SoftMax function normalizes these similarity scores into probabilities, and the final weighted sum of V refines the representation based on these attention weights. Figure 5 illustrates the overall architecture of the Vision Transformer.

Figure 5. General Architecture of The Vision Transformer (Dosovitskiy et al., 2020)

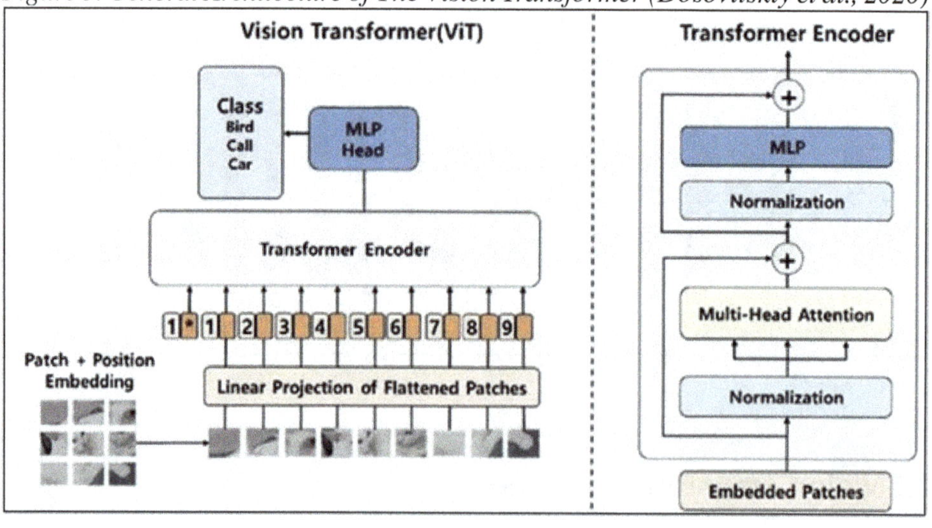

Vision Transformers offer a robust methodology for medical imaging tasks by integrating global context, comprehensive feature representation, and adaptability across imaging modalities, rendering them very useful for illness and tumor identification.

3.6 Hybrid Architecture EfficientNet-ViTs

Recent progress in medical image analysis has encouraged the integration of EfficientNet and ViTs into a unified framework that leverages the strengths of both approaches for brain tumor classification. EfficientNet, a CNN-based architecture, demonstrates strong capability in feature extraction, particularly in capturing spatial and local dependencies within MRI scans, such as tissue textures and tumor boundaries. By employing compound scaling, EfficientNet balances network depth, width, and resolution, enabling efficient learning with fewer parameters while maintaining high accuracy. In CNN architectures by applying adaptive filters(kernels) essential features from the input image are automatically learnt and extracted form convolutional layer. They observe morphological structures, such as edges and intensities fluctuations of the tumor, while retaining the general anatomical structure of the brain (Alzubaidi et al., 2021). The issue of model overfitting and computational cost can be reduced by pooling operations in CNN, which extract only the important and significant features. This phase is particularly critical in medical imaging, as the goal is to compress data while capturing vital tumor information (Rajatha & Ashoka, 2025). The resulting feature maps, which carry localized tumor information, are then passed to the Vision Transformer (ViT) module for further refinement and contextual analysis.

Unlike CNNs, which are usually limited to capturing local spatial features, the Vision Transformer (ViT) introduces global self-attention. This is an important step because it allows the model to relate information from different and sometimes distant regions of the image something that CNNs often fail to do effectively. In practical terms, MRI scans are first divided into non-overlapping patches, with each patch converted into a low-dimensional embedding and then passed through the transformer encoder (Han et al., 2022). By doing so, ViT can capture subtle but clinically relevant differences in tumor morphology, texture, and intensity. These details often require a broader view of the image in order to achieve reliable classification.

When EfficientNet is combined with ViT, the two models complement each other in a useful way. EfficientNet handles the extraction of fine local structural patterns efficiently, while the transformer provides the global context. This balance seems especially beneficial when the dataset is small or contains noise, as is often the case in medical imaging. Together, the two approaches improve classification accuracy and lower the chance of false predictions, which helps make tumor detection more consistent. From a clinical perspective, this hybrid design not only boosts accuracy but also supports earlier diagnosis and may assist in shaping more personalized treatment strategies in neuro-oncology.

4. METHODOLOGY FOR BRAIN TUMOR DETECTION

The proposed methodology combines segmentation and classification in a single deep learning framework. Two datasets are used: multi-channel MRI scans with tumor masks for segmentation and labeled images for classification. Using both allows the framework to handle two important tasks, localizing tumors in detail and checking if a tumor is present. This reflects clinical needs, since doctors often rely on both detailed maps and overall diagnosis. The workflow runs through several steps. It begins with data collection, followed by preprocessing and augmentation. Preprocessing is critical here because it reduces noise and makes scans more consistent, which helps the models learn more effectively. After this stage, class imbalance is addressed before training begins. The final stages involve fine-tuning and evaluation. Setting up the pipeline this way keeps the process clear and makes it easier to reproduce in future work. Figure 6 illustrates the proposed framework for brain tumor detection.

4.1 Datasets Used for Brain Tumor Detection

This work relies on two publicly available datasets that complement each other in terms of scope and task: The BraTS 2025 (Bra, 2025) dataset for multimodal tumor segmentation and the Nickparvar (Nickparvar, 2020) Brain MRI dataset for binary classification. Together, they provide a robust foundation for developing and evaluating deep learning models for neuro-oncological imaging. Figure 6 demonstrates the proposed framework for detection of brain tumors using advanced hybrid deep learning models.

Figure 6. Proposed Framework for Brain Tumor Detection

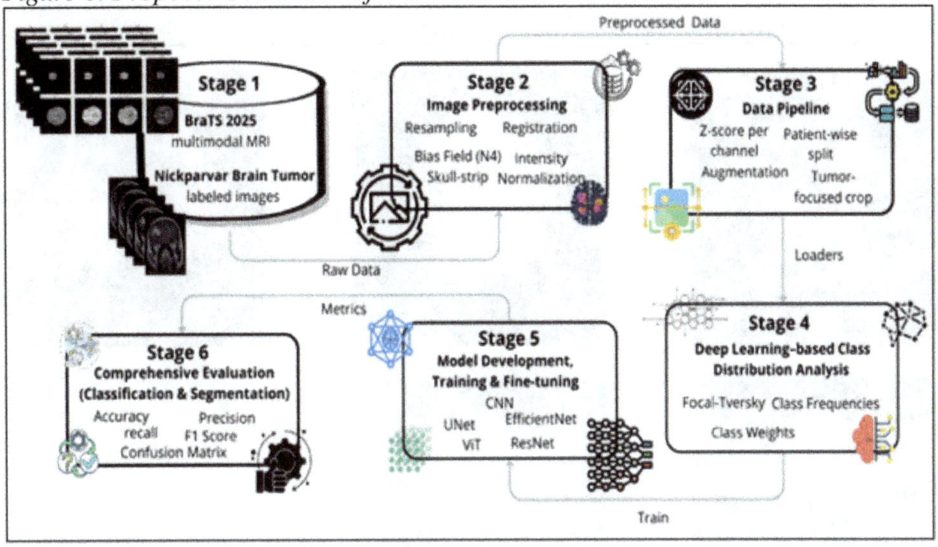

4.1.1 BraTS 2025 Multimodal MRI Images Dataset

The segmentation-oriented dataset is extracted from the BraTS 2025 challenge repository, which provides standardized multimodal MRI scans with expert annotations (Bra, 2025). Each 2D slice is represented as a 160 × 160 float32 tensor with four channels: T1-contrast (T1c), native T1 (T1n), T2-FLAIR (T2f), and T2-weighted (T2w). Corresponding segmentation masks are stored as single-channel integer maps (160,160,1) and converted on-the-fly to one-hot encoding with depth four. The full dataset comprises 34,539 slices, organized into 18 NPZ micro-shards. At the shard level, the data were divided into training (80%) and validation (20%) subsets using a fixed random seed (SEED = 42), yielding approximately 28,539 training slices and 6,000 validation slices. Data streaming was implemented using memory-mapped loading wrapped in a tf.data pipeline with shuffling, batching (batch size = 8), and prefetching. Figure 7 presents a sample of four MRI modalities and the corresponding tumor segmentation overlay.

Figure 7. Sample Multimodal MRI channels (T1c, T1n, T2f, T2w) and Tumor Segmentation overlay from the BraTS 2025 dataset

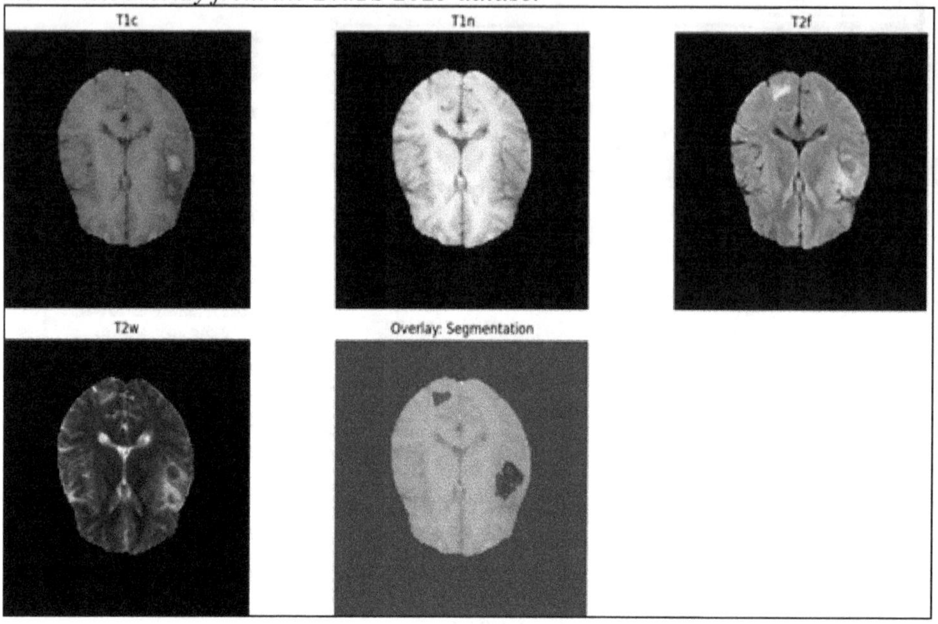

4.1.2 Nickparvar Brain Tumor MRI Dataset

The second dataset we assessed is the Brain Tumor MRI Dataset, curated by Masoud Nickparvar, and is publicly available on Kaggle (Nickparvar, 2020). This dataset consists of 7,023 MRI images annotated into four classes (meningioma, glioma, pituitary tumor, and no tumor). All images contain an associated segmentation mask delineating the tumor region. Table 1 illustrates the tumor types of in the Nickparvar dataset and a brief description of each is also presented.

Table 1. Brain Tumor Types

Tumor type	Description
Glioma	Malignant and aggressive tumor derived from the brain's glial cells.
Meningioma	Tumor in the protective membranes wrapping the brain
Pituitary Tumor	Tumor that caused by the hormone-producing pituitary gland
No tumor	Healthy brain without any sign of tumor

For this study, the dataset was constrained to a binary classification setup, focusing on glioma and no tumor. This simplification provides a clinically meaningful distinction between malignant tumors and healthy tissue while streamlining the classification task. All images were resized to 224 × 224. Pixel intensities were normalized, and data augmentation techniques were applied. These augmentations reduced overfitting and improved generalization.

4.2 Image Preprocessing

Preprocessing is essential to normalize heterogeneous MRI data and enhance learning consistency across scans. For the BraTS 2025 dataset, preprocessing steps included resampling to a standardized spatial resolution, registration across modalities, bias field correction (N4) to mitigate intensity inhomogeneity, skull striping to remove non-brain structures, and Z-score normalization applied per channel. Each slice was represented as a float32 tensor of size 160×160×4, with segmentation masks stored as single-channel integer arrays and converted to one-hot encodings for training.

For the Nickparvar dataset, all images were resized to 224×224 pixels to ensure compatibility with convolutional backbones. Intensity normalization was applied to standardize pixel distributions across varying scanners and acquisition conditions. To enhance robustness, data augmentation was applied, including horizontal/vertical flips, random rotations, and the MixUp technique, which interpolates pairs of images and their labels to generate synthetic training samples. These procedures collectively improved generalization and reduced overfitting.

4.3 Data pipeline

A robust and efficient data pipeline was implemented to handle large-scale input streams. For segmentation, the pipeline accesses memory-mapped NPZ shards and streamed slice-level samples through TensorFlow's tf.data API. Training batches were generated with random shuffling, prefetching, and caching to minimize I/O overhead and ensure high-throughput training. On-the-fly augmentations included random flips, 90° rotations, tumor-focused cropping, and random cropping of 85% of sliced dimensions (p=0.35). These operations increased the variability of tumor appearance while preserving spatial label alignment. For classification, the pipeline integrated preprocessing and augmentations into a coherent workflow that handled image resizing, normalization, and batch preparation. Automated loading and grouping facilitated efficient training and validation cycles. Patient-wise splitting ensured no data leakage between training and evaluation sets, thereby preserving clinical validity of the results.

The pipeline streamlines grouping, blending, and loading of data to achieve maximum computer performance and memory in training and testing processes. Automated procedures such as data handling are useful for dealing with large medical imaging data and enhancing reproducibility in deep learning experiments (Sasikumar et al., 2024). Furthermore, the pipeline allows one to combine data preparation procedures with model training activities in a coherent fashion. Such a structured methodology enhances consistent processing of data, removes potential inaccuracies, and increases overall computational velocity. This plays a crucial role in streamlining high-performance medical diagnostic cases.

4.4 Deep Learning-based Class and Distribution Analysis

Most of the MRI image datasets often suffer from the class imbalance issue during segmentation, where the healthy samples(background) dominate the tumor, or the lesions which are small (Pantelaios et al., 2024). This challenge in the deep learning models was confronted using targeted sampling. All slices containing tumor voxels were kept without exception, while purely background slices were retained at a probability of roughly 0.12. To further balance the learning signal, weighted class losses were introduced assigning lower penalties to background pixels and greater emphasis to tumor regions. A composite loss, combining weighted categorical cross-entropy with focal Tversky loss, was then applied (Abraham & Khan, 2019). This hybrid setup not only sharpened tumor boundary delineation but also increased sensitivity to subtle and small lesions that might otherwise be overlooked.

In classification, imbalance was approached from a different angle through the MixUp technique. By blending input samples and their labels, MixUp creates synthetic training examples that smooth the class decision boundaries. This augmentation alleviates bias toward majority categories and forces the model to generalize better under skewed distributions. As a result, the hybrid classifier became more robust and less prone to overfitting while maintaining improved responsiveness to tumor-positive cases. Importantly, these strategies contributed to stable convergence across training runs and reinforces the model's ability to detect clinically relevant minority samples and hence helps in overcoming the class imbalance and further it correctly classifies small tumors.

4.5 Model Development and Training

This phase illustrates deep learning models training through the implementation of hybrid architecture for accurate detection and classification of the brain tumors.

Furthermore, these hybrid model's performance ensures that variations are attributable to architecture decisions rather than handling of data. Five deep learning models (CNN, U-Net, ResNet, EfficientNet, and ViTs) were built and trained for extracting features from the BraTS 2025 multimodal dataset and Nickparvar Brain Tumor dataset. To enhance the performance for accurate segmentation of the tumor. Hybrid architectures were developed (CNN-U-Net, ResNet-U-Net, and EfficientNet-U-Net) which were trained and tested on the BraTS 2025 dataset, these hybrid models employ encoder–decoder variants that all share a U-Net-style decoder but differ in their choice of encoder. The first uses a plain CNN backbone, the second incorporates ResNet, and the third leverages EfficientNet. Model performance is assessed through pixel-wise accuracy, precision, recall, and F1-score, with results aggregated per case and then macro-averaged to produce a single score for each variant. This evaluation scheme reflects the scope of the study, enabling a direct comparison across CNN-U-Net, ResNet-U-Net, and EfficientNet-U-Net. The decision to standardize the U-Net decoder follows common practice in biomedical segmentation research, as it preserves fine lesion detail while offering a clear framework for encoder ablation studies (Isensee et al., 2021).

Similarly, for the Nickparvar Brain Tumor dataset, another hybrid approach-EfficientNetV2S with a Vision Transformer (ViT) design was adapted and was further fine-tuned trained and tested on similar settings employing the same patient-wise loaders and the rebalancing strategy. The EfficientNetV2S backbone provides efficient local feature extraction and benefits from large-scale pretraining, while the ViT head contributes global self-attention that captures long-range spatial dependencies, a property increasingly recognized as valuable in medical imaging (Tan & Le, 2021). During the model training, performance was monitored for accuracy and loss metrics. Furthermore, confusion matrix was produced, which illustrates the number of samples correctly classified and misclassified. The performance monitored through these metrics ensures the proposed advanced hybrid approaches are evaluated consistently and in a clinically interpretable manner.

4.6 Comprehensive Model Evaluation

The proposed hybrid approaches were assessed using several evaluation metrics, including precision, accuracy, recall, F1-score, and the confusion matrix. Additionally, validation accuracy and loss curves were analyzed. The results are presented in the following sections.

5. EXPERIMENTAL RESULTS AND COMPARATIVE EVALUATION

The experimental outcomes of the proposed deep learning approaches for brain tumor analysis using BraTS 2025(Bra, 2025), and Nickparvar dataset (Nickparvar, 2020) from kaggle are presented in this section.

5.1 Model Evaluation on BraTS 2025 Dataset

Experiments were conducted using our proposed hybrid U-Net, CNN-UNet, ResNet50-UNet, and EfficientNetB0-UNet models. All the models were trained under similar experimental conditions to ensure a fair comparison. These models were adapted to integrate both simple and advanced deep learning models for tumor segmentation and extraction for accurate extraction of tumor features. Hence the hybrid model not only facilitates quantitative comparison of the model's performance, it also shows how advanced hybrid architecture can have an impact on accurate detection and classification of tumors in practice.

Figure 8. Validation Accuracy Comparison of Segmentation Models

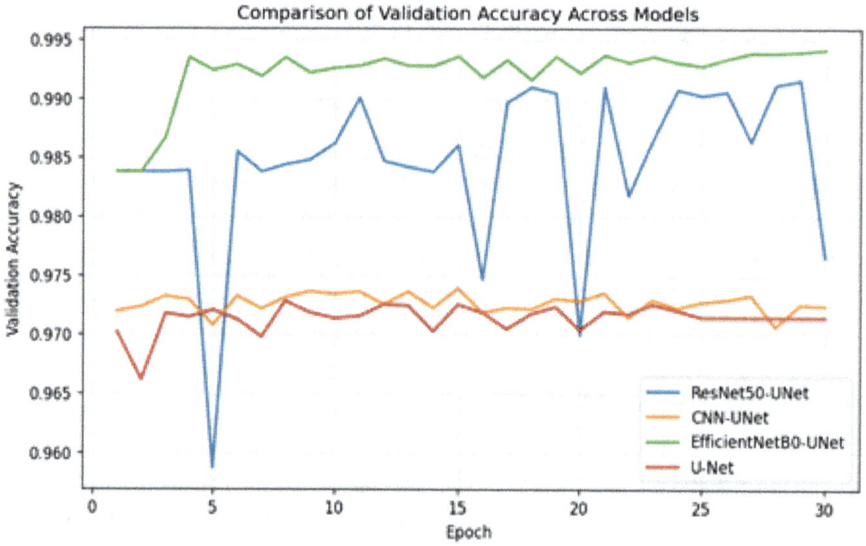

The model's evaluation was focused on metrics which include loss, validation accuracy, recall, precision, and F1-score, which are adequate to test the model's performance. Figure 8 illustrates the validation accuracy comparison among the four models. EfficientNetB0-UNet provided the best performance and achieved an of 0.99, which was much superior higher than the other models. The U-Net and CNN-UNet models reached an accuracy of 0.97. While the ResNet50-UNet was less predictable, it sometimes achieved strong scores, but its results fluctuated more than expected, likely because its deeper structure is trickier to fine-tune under this setup.

Figure 9. Validation Loss Comparison of Segmentation Models

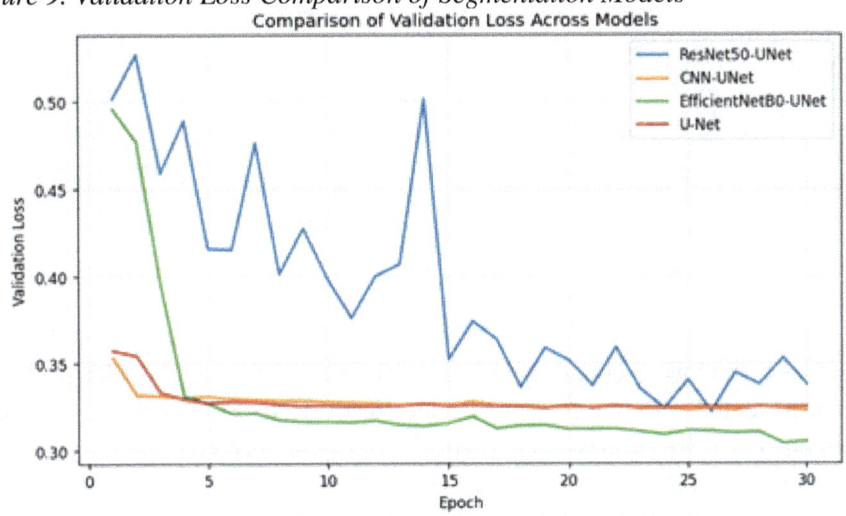

The loss curves largely reinforced these observations, shown in Figure 9. The validation loss with EfficientNetB0-UNet dropped quickly and kept it low, indicating more effective optimization. In contrast, ResNet50-UNet had noticeable inconsistencies, which reduced confidence in its stability. U-Net and CNN-UNet followed smoother paths, but they seemed to level off at higher loss values, implying that they were easier to train but less efficient overall compared with the EfficientNetB0-UNet.

Figure 10. Validation Precision Comparison of Segmentation Models

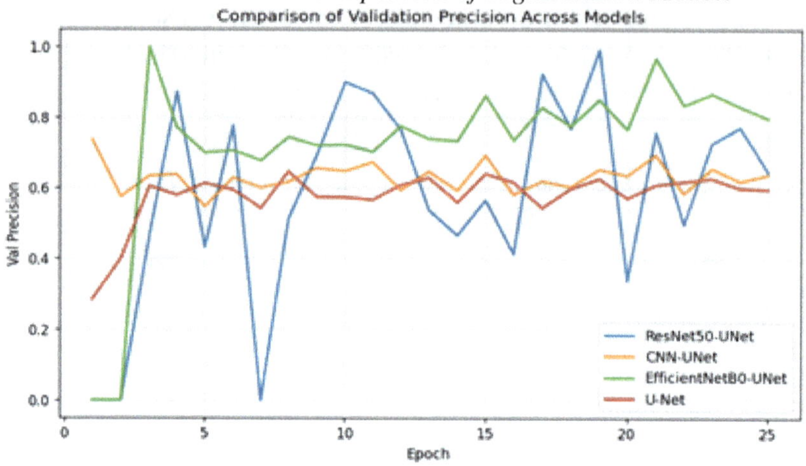

Similar results were obtained when the models were evaluated with precision metrics, presented in Figure 10. For EfficientNetB0-UNet a precision value of 0.80 was obtained, which indicates that the EfficientNetB0-UNet model correctly detected tumor regions while avoiding false alarms. Further with U-Net and CNN-UNet a precision value of 0.60 was obtained which was very low compared EfficientNetB0-UNet, suggesting more frequent misclassifications. These findings point to a clear trend: encoders designed with efficiency not only improve predictive accuracy but also tend to provide more stable and reliable training behavior. ResNet50-UNet displayed highly irregular precision values, underscoring its difficulty in consistently localizing tumors. Complementing to precision, the recall values in Figure 11 illustrate the capacity of each model to capture all positive tumor regions. Here, EfficientNetB0-UNet again outperformed others with a recall of 0.86, while CNN-UNet and U-Net performed comparably with recall values near 0.78 and 0.76, respectively. ResNet50-UNet struggled with unstable recall performance, averaging around 0.69.

Figure 11. Validation Recall Comparison of Segmentation Models

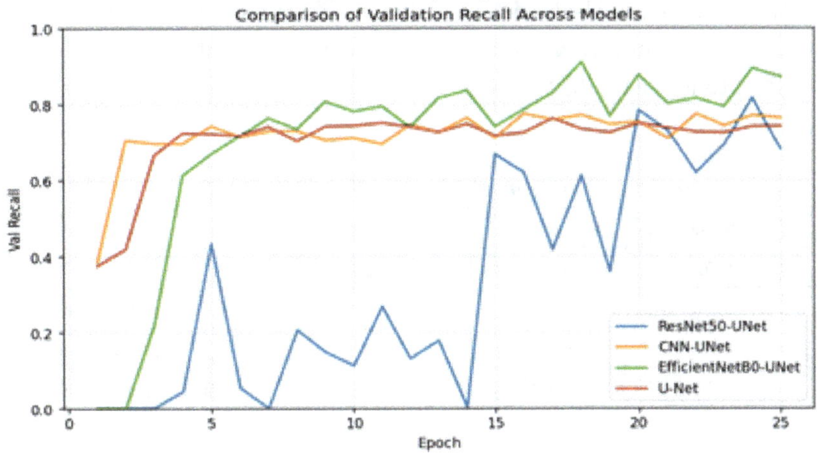

The balance between precision and recall is best represented by the F1-score, which is summarized in Figure 12. EfficientNetB0-UNet achieved the highest F1-score of 0.93, demonstrating a robust balance between sensitivity and specificity. CNN-UNet and U-Net followed with scores of 0.77 and 0.72, respectively, while ResNet50-UNet lagged at 0.69, primarily due to its unstable recall. These outcomes emphasize the advantage of efficient encoder designs in maintaining both accurate detection and comprehensive coverage of tumor regions.

Figure 12. Validation FG F1 Comparison of Segmentation Models

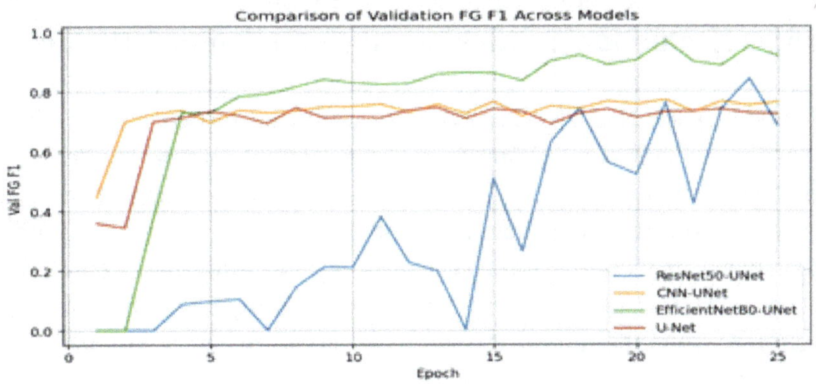

The performance of all four models across the key evaluation metrics is presented in Table 2. Consistent with the graphical analyses, the EfficientNetB0-Unet provided superior performance with the highest accuracy of 99.47%, precision of 80%, recall of 86%, and F1-score of 93%. CNN-UNet offered competitive recall but provided a lower precision, while U-Net delivered balanced yet moderate results. Despite its relatively strong accuracy, ResNet50-UNet underperformed in terms of recall and F1-score due to its instability.

Table 2. Performance Evaluation on BraTS 2025 Dataset

F1	Recall	Precision	Accuracy	Model
0.72	*0.76*	*0.6*	*0.9728*	U-Net
0.77	*0.78*	*0.64*	*0.9739*	CNN-Lite-UNet
0.69	*0.69*	*0.64*	*0.9764*	ResNet50-UNet
0.93	*0.86*	*0.8*	*0.9947*	EfficientNetB0-UNet

Overall, our experiments suggest that EfficientNetB0-UNet provides superior performance and is considered as the most reliable model for tumor classification on the BraTS dataset. In practice, it not only achieved consistently high accuracy but also trained in a smoother and more stable way than the others. While the baseline U-Net and the ResNet-based variant came close in some runs, they often struggled to keep a good trade-off between precision and recall. This gap may be linked to the efficiency of the encoder itself, which seems to help EfficientNetB0-UNet converge more steadily and avoid the sharp fluctuations seen in deeper models. From a practical standpoint, this combination of accuracy, stability, and reproducibility makes it particularly appealing for clinical settings, where reliable results are just as important as raw performance.

5.2 Model Evaluation on Nickparvar Brain Tumor MRI dataset

A hybrid EfficientNetV2S-ViT model was proposed, and experiments were conducted under a binary setup (glioma vs. no tumor) on the Nickparvar Brain Tumor MRI dataset (Nickparvar, 2020). The main purpose was to examine the model's predictive performance and generalization capacity. For both model training and validation two main metrics, loss and accuracy, were recorded for 15 epochs to provide a complete understanding of EfficientNetV2S-ViT hybrid model convergence. Accuracy represents the ratio of exact classifications, whereas loss indicates the variation between estimated and true labels. All these parameters present a comprehensive assessment of the classifier's ability to acquire discerning descriptions from medical imaging data.

Figure 13. Accuracy Curve of EfficientNetV2S+ViT Classifier

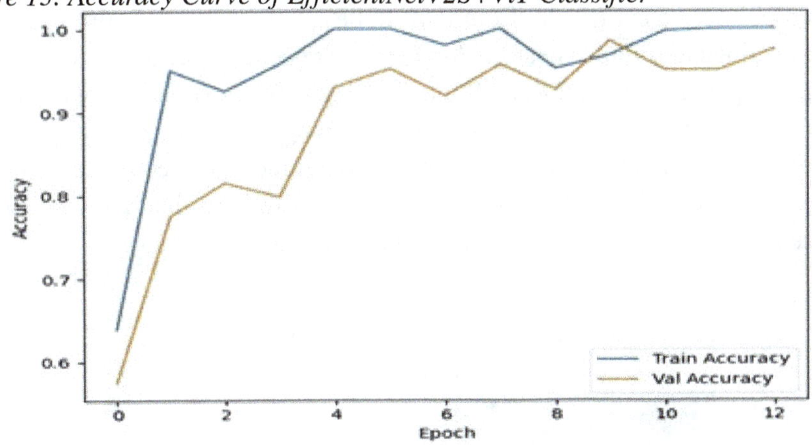

The evolution of accuracy across training epochs is presented in Figure 13. The training accuracy curve rose sharply from approximately 0.63 at initialization to exceed 0.90 by the second epoch and ultimately stabilized near 0.99 by the final epoch. The validation accuracy followed a similar trajectory, improving from an initial 0.57 to approximately 0.93 within the first four epochs, before converging around 0.97 with minor fluctuations during mid-training. This consistent upward trend across both curves presents the model's effective capability to generalize, with only slight instability observed in the intermediate stages of training.

Figure 14. Loss Curve of EfficientNetV2S+ViT Classifier

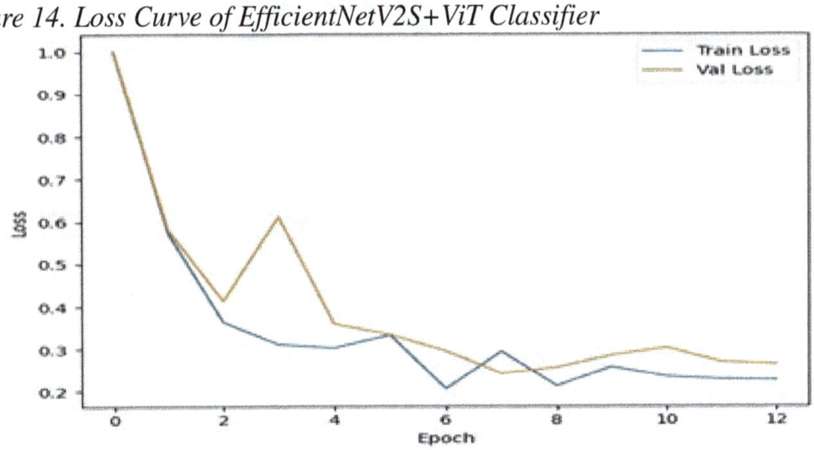

The corresponding validation and training losses are shown in Figure 14. The training loss decreased rapidly from 0.60 to around 0.30 for the third epoch and further declined to stabilize near 0.22 in the later epoch. Validation loss followed a comparable pattern, beginning at 1.0 and showing a sharp decline to approximately 0.26, albeit with more pronounced fluctuations, including a spike around epoch four. The general downward trend across both curves indicates effective learning and reduced prediction error, while the transient variability in validation loss suggests some sensitivity in generalization during the earlier training stages.

Figure 15. Confusion Matrix of EfficientNetV2S-ViT Classifier

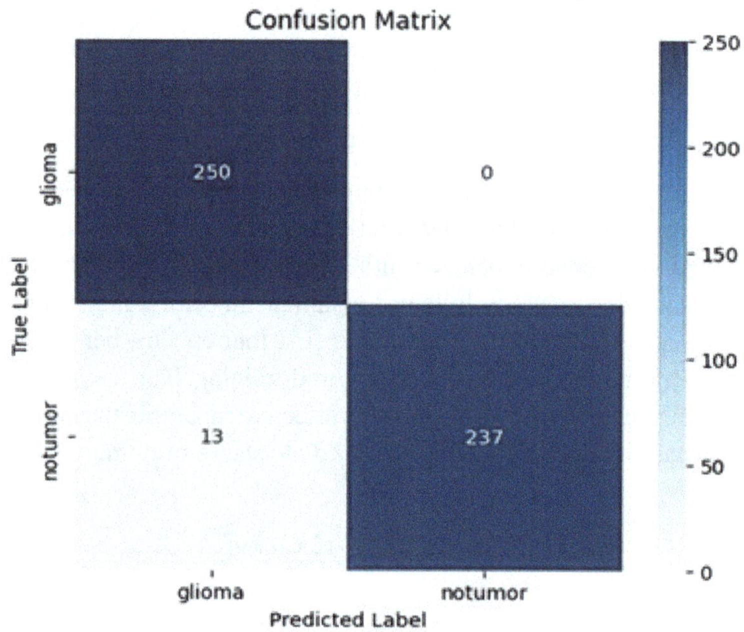

The model's performance was further validated through the confusion matrix metrics for the test set, the results obtained are presented in Figure 15. The model was able to classify 250 tumor cases correctly along with 237 cases without tumors. Although 13 non-tumor scans were mistakenly flagged as tumors, importantly, no tumor case was missed. This pattern highlights the model's high sensitivity, which is crucial because overlooking a tumor is far riskier than issuing a false alarm.

From the overall results, the EfficientNetV2S–ViT hybrid appears well-suited for the binary classification of glioma versus non-tumor MRI scans. Both training and validation curves for accuracy and loss showed steady convergence, a sign that the model learned consistently without obvious signs of overfitting. The confusion matrix backed this up, showing only a small number of errors or misclassifications. A likely reason behind the strong performance of EfficientNetV2S–ViT hybrid approach is the way EfficientNet captures detailed local image patterns, while the Vision Transformer complements this with its ability to model broader contextual information. Together, they seem to give the framework both robustness and precision. In practical terms, the fact that it maintains accuracy while avoiding false negatives makes it especially promising in clinical contexts, where consistency and safety are just as important as raw accuracy.

6. CHALLENGES AND FUTURE DIRECTIONS

In the sections to follow the challenges encountered while automatic detection of brain tumors using advanced deep learning models, and future directions are elucidated.

6.1 Challenges

The automated identification of brain tumors by deep learning has significant challenges and constraints which include

- **Data Scarcity:** Due to privacy issues and the requirement for annotation by professional radiologists obtaining high-quality annotated MRI or CT scans possess a significant challenge, which results in scarcity of data.
- **Data Annotation and Labelling**: For segmentation of the tumor, deep learning techniques utilize 3D images which need slice-by-slice annotations, this process is time-consuming and demands an extensive level of proficiency, hence poses difficulties in the brain tumors examination.
- **Class Imbalance:** Most datasets contain much less tumor samples compared to normal brain scans. New brain tumor images can be produced by applying data augmentation methods such as scaling and rotation, however, this may result in class imbalance. This discrepancy may bias the models towards the majority class, hence reducing sensitivity in detecting rare tumor types or small lesions.
- **Generalization presents a challenge**: models developed using data from a particular hospital, MRI scanner, or patient demographic frequently exhibit worse performance on data from other sources, attributable to discrepancies in imaging methods, resolution, and population attributes. Moreover, the computational requirements are significant, particularly for training deep neural networks on 3D MRI data, necessitating considerable GPU or TPU

resources, which may constrain experimentation and model refinement. The opaque aspect of several deep learning models, such as Vision Transformers and CNNs, impedes clinical adoption, since these models frequently yield predictions devoid of interpretable rationale, complicating radiologists' ability to accept and evaluate automated diagnostic conclusions (Ghorbian et al., 2025).

6.2. Future Directions

Future investigations in brain tumor detection will likely emphasize overcoming existing limitations while improving model precision, resilience, and clinical significance. A potential approach is the creation of extensive, diverse annotated datasets that encompass various patient demographics and imaging techniques, hence enhancing model generalization across populations. Data augmentation and synthetic data production by generative models, including GANs and diffusion models, can mitigate data scarcity and class imbalance. A crucial focus is the amalgamation of multi-modal imaging (MRI, CT, PET) with clinical data (genomic, histology, and electronic health records) to offer a comprehensive perspective on tumor features and facilitate precision therapy. The use of explainable AI (XAI) methodologies will be essential in enhancing transparency and confidence, enabling clinicians to comprehend and verify model judgments. Federated learning enables collaborative model training among institutions while safeguarding patient privacy. Ultimately, the integration of deep learning with sophisticated radiomics and personalized medicine methodologies may facilitate early identification, enhance treatment planning, and optimize patient outcomes.

7. CONCLUSION

This study explored advanced hybrid deep learning models for brain tumor detection. The relevant studies analyzed methodologies for brain tumor segmentation and classification, highlighting their advantages and disadvantages. The relevant studies illustrated the effectiveness of CNN-based models, SVM, Random Forest, and KNN in tumor classification from MRI images, while also emphasizing significant limitations such as restricted dataset sizes, data imbalance, and insufficient segmentation methodologies. To address these constraints, we have introduced hybrid deep learning models, encompassing CNN-U-Net, ResNet50-U-Net, EfficientNetB0-U-Net, and EfficientNetB0-Vision Transformers (ViTs), for precise detection and classification of brain cancers from multimodal MRI images. Deep learning has demonstrated significant promise in the diagnosis of brain tumors, especially in classification and segmentation tasks. The amalgamation of multimodal MRI imaging with advanced AI techniques has yielded promising results in improving the accuracy and effectiveness of brain tumor classification. The empirical evaluation demonstrates that the suggested hybrid approaches yielded higher performance in precise data extraction relative to existing methods. EfficientNetB0-U-Net obtained superior performance on the BraTS multimodal dataset with an accuracy of 99.47%, while EfficientNetV2S-ViT reached a validation accuracy of 97% on the Nickparvar Brain MRI dataset. The suggested method surpasses current techniques in detection and classification, producing enhanced outcomes for brain tumor identification utilizing MRI images.

REFERENCES

Abraham, N., & Khan, N. M. (2019, April). A novel focal tversky loss function with improved attention u-net for lesion segmentation. In *2019 IEEE 16th international symposium on biomedical imaging (ISBI 2019)* (pp. 683-687). IEEE. DOI: 10.1109/ISBI.2019.8759329

Alzubaidi, L., Zhang, J., Humaidi, A. J., Al-Dujaili, A., Duan, Y., Al-Shamma, O., Santamaría, J., Fadhel, M. A., Al-Amidie, M., & Farhan, L. (2021). Review of deep learning: Concepts, CNN architectures, challenges, applications, future directions. *Journal of Big Data*, *8*(1), 53. DOI: 10.1186/s40537-021-00444-8 PMID: 33816053

Azzarelli, R., Simons, B. D., & Philpott, A. (2018). The developmental origin of brain tumours: A cellular and molecular framework. *Development (Cambridge, England)*, *145*(10), dev162693. DOI: 10.1242/dev.162693 PMID: 29759978

Bra, T. S. 2025 Lighthouse Challenge. (2025). *BraTS 2025 lighthouse challenge* [Data set]. The Cancer Imaging Archive. https://www.synapse.org/brats2025- Retrieved April 20, 2025

Byeon, K., Lim, J., Lee, J., Han, C., Bay, S., Park, G., & Kwak, J. T. (2025, January). Lightweight Look-ahead Multi-context Vision Transformer. In *2025 International Conference on Electronics, Information, and Communication (ICEIC)* (pp. 1-6). IEEE.

Deepak, S., & Ameer, P. M. (2021). Automated categorization of brain tumor from mri using cnn features and svm. *Journal of Ambient Intelligence and Humanized Computing*, *12*(8), 8357–8369. DOI: 10.1007/s12652-020-02568-w

Dorfner, F. J., Patel, J. B., Kalpathy-Cramer, J., Gerstner, E. R., & Bridge, C. P. (2025). A review of deep learning for brain tumor analysis in MRI. *NPJ Precision Oncology*, *9*(1), 2. DOI: 10.1038/s41698-024-00789-2 PMID: 39753730

Dosovitskiy, A., Beyer, L., Kolesnikov, A., Weissenborn, D., Zhai, X., Unterthiner, T., . . . Houlsby, N. (2020). An image is worth 16x16 words: Transformers for image recognition at scale. *arXiv preprint arXiv:2010.11929.*

Febrianto, D. C., Soesanti, I., & Nugroho, H. A. (2020, March). Convolutional neural network for brain tumor detection. [). IOP Publishing.]. *IOP Conference Series. Materials Science and Engineering*, *771*(1), 012031. DOI: 10.1088/1757-899X/771/1/012031

Filatov, D., & Yar, G. N. A. H. (2022). Brain tumor diagnosis and classification via pre-trained convolutional neural networks. *arXiv preprint arXiv:2208.00768*. DOI: 10.1101/2022.07.18.22277779

Ghorbian, M., Ghorbian, S., & Ghobaei-Arani, M. (2025). Advancements in Machine Learning for Brain Tumor Classification and Diagnosis: A Comprehensive Review of Challenges and Future Directions. *Archives of Computational Methods in Engineering*, •••, 1–36. DOI: 10.1007/s11831-025-10340-6

Grant, R., Dowswell, T., Tomlinson, E., Brennan, P. M., Walter, F. M., Ben-Shlomo, Y., & Lawrie, T. A. (2020). Interventions to reduce the time to diagnosis of brain tumours. *Cochrane Database of Systematic Reviews*, 9. DOI: 10.1002/14651858.CD013564 PMID: 32901926

Han, K., Wang, Y., Chen, H., Chen, X., Guo, J., Liu, Z., Tang, Y., Xiao, A., Xu, C., Xu, Y., Yang, Z., Zhang, Y., & Tao, D. (2022). A survey on vision transformer. *IEEE Transactions on Pattern Analysis and Machine Intelligence*, *45*(1), 87–110. DOI: 10.1109/TPAMI.2022.3152247 PMID: 35180075

He, K., Zhang, X., Ren, S., & Sun, J. (2016). Deep residual learning for image recognition. In *Proceedings of the IEEE conference on computer vision and pattern recognition* (pp. 770-778).

Huang, J., Xiang, Y., Gan, S., Wu, L., Yan, J., Ye, D., & Zhang, J. (2025). Application of artificial intelligence in medical imaging for tumor diagnosis and treatment: A comprehensive approach. *Discover. Oncology*, *16*(1), 1–23. DOI: 10.1007/s12672-025-03307-3 PMID: 40856916

Hussain, S., Mubeen, I., Ullah, N., Shah, S. S. U. D., Khan, B. A., Zahoor, M., Ullah, R., Khan, F. A., & Sultan, M. A. (2022). Modern diagnostic imaging technique applications and risk factors in the medical field: A review. *BioMed Research International*, *2022*(1), 5164970. DOI: 10.1155/2022/5164970 PMID: 35707373

Hussain, T., Shouno, H., Hussain, A., Hussain, D., Ismail, M., Mir, T. H., & Akhy, S. A. (2025). EFFResNet-ViT: A fusion-based convolutional and vision transformer model for explainable medical image classification. *IEEE Access : Practical Innovations, Open Solutions*, *13*, 54040–54068. DOI: 10.1109/ACCESS.2025.3554184

Iqbal, A., Jaffar, M. A., & Jahangir, R. (2024). Enhancing Brain Tumour Multi-Classification Using Efficient-Net B0-Based Intelligent Diagnosis for Internet of Medical Things (IoMT) Applications. *Information (Basel)*, *15*(8), 489. DOI: 10.3390/info15080489

Isensee, F., Jaeger, P. F., Kohl, S. A., Petersen, J., & Maier-Hein, K. H. (2021). nnU-Net: A self-configuring method for deep learning-based biomedical image segmentation. *Nature Methods*, *18*(2), 203–211. DOI: 10.1038/s41592-020-01008-z PMID: 33288961

Jeong, J., Kim, S., Pan, L., Hwang, D., Kim, D., Choi, J., Kwon, Y., Yi, P., Jeong, J., & Yoo, S. J. (2025). Reducing the workload of medical diagnosis through artificial intelligence: A narrative review. *Medicine, 104*(6), e41470. DOI: 10.1097/MD.0000000000041470 PMID: 39928829

Manzari, O. N., Ahmadabadi, H., Kashiani, H., Shokouhi, S. B., & Ayatollahi, A. (2023). MedViT: A robust vision transformer for generalized medical image classification. *Computers in Biology and Medicine, 157*, 106791. DOI: 10.1016/j.compbiomed.2023.106791 PMID: 36958234

Martucci, M., Russo, R., Schimperna, F., D'Apolito, G., Panfili, M., Grimaldi, A., Perna, A., Ferranti, A. M., Varcasia, G., Giordano, C., & Gaudino, S. (2023). Magnetic resonance imaging of primary adult brain tumors: State of the art and future perspectives. *Biomedicines, 11*(2), 364. DOI: 10.3390/biomedicines11020364 PMID: 36830900

National Brain Tumor Society. (2023). *Brain tumor facts.* National Brain Tumor Society. https://braintumor.org/brain-tumors/about-brain-tumors/brain-tumor-facts/

Nickparvar, M. (2020). *Brain tumor MRI dataset [Data set].* Kaggle. https://www.kaggle.com/datasets/masoudnickparvar/brain-tumor-mri-dataset- Retrieved May 15, 2025.

Pantelaios, D., Theofilou, P. A., Tzouveli, P., & Kollias, S. (2024, May). Hybrid CNN-ViT models for medical image classification. In *2024 IEEE international symposium on biomedical imaging (ISBI)* (pp. 1-4). IEEE. DOI: 10.1109/ISBI56570.2024.10635205

Park, S., & Kim, J. (2024). Explainability of deep neural networks for brain tumor detection. *arXiv preprint arXiv:2410.07613.*

Rahman, A., Hayat, M., Iqbal, N., Alarfaj, F. K., Alkhalaf, S., & Alturise, F. (2025). Enhanced MRI brain tumor detection using deep learning in conjunction with explainable AI SHAP based diverse and multi feature analysis. *Scientific Reports, 15*(1), 29411. DOI: 10.1038/s41598-025-14901-4 PMID: 40790336

Rajatha, & Ashoka, D. V. (2025). EffiViT:: Hybrid CNN-Transformer for Retinal Imaging.

Razzaghi, P., Abbasi, K., Shirazi, M., & Rashidi, S. (2022). Multimodal brain tumor detection using multimodal deep transfer learning. *Applied Soft Computing, 129*, 109631. DOI: 10.1016/j.asoc.2022.109631

Ronneberger, O., Fischer, P., & Brox, T. (2015, October). U-net: Convolutional networks for biomedical image segmentation. In *International Conference on Medical image computing and computer-assisted intervention* (pp. 234-241). Cham: Springer international publishing. DOI: 10.1007/978-3-319-24574-4_28

Sarvamangala, D. R., & Kulkarni, R. V. (2022). Convolutional neural networks in medical image understanding: A survey. *Evolutionary Intelligence, 15*(1), 1–22. DOI: 10.1007/s12065-020-00540-3 PMID: 33425040

Sasikumar, P., Cherukuvada, S., Balmurugan, P., Anand, P. V., Brindasri, S., & Nareshkumar, R. (2024, May). An Efficient Brain tumor classification using CNN and transfer learning. In *2024 International Conference on Advances in Computing, Communication and Applied Informatics (ACCAI)* (pp. 1-5). IEEE. DOI: 10.1109/ACCAI61061.2024.10602391

Satushe, V., Vyas, V., Metkar, S., & Singh, D. P. (2025). AI in MRI brain tumor diagnosis: A systematic review of machine learning and deep learning advances (2010–2025). *Chemometrics and Intelligent Laboratory Systems, 263*, 105414. DOI: 10.1016/j.chemolab.2025.105414

Tan, M., & Le, Q. (2021, July). Efficientnetv2: Smaller models and faster training. In *International conference on machine learning* (pp. 10096-10106). PMLR.

Tan, M., & Le, Q. V. (2019). *EfficientNet: Rethinking model scaling for convolutional neural networks*. In *Proceedings of the 36th International Conference on Machine Learning (ICML 2019)* (Vol. 97, pp. 6105–6114).

Thaha, M. M., Kumar, K. P. M., Murugan, B. S., Dhanasekeran, S., Vijayakarthick, P., & Selvi, A. S. (2019). Brain tumor segmentation using convolutional neural networks in MRI images. *Journal of Medical Systems, 43*(9), 294. DOI: 10.1007/s10916-019-1416-0 PMID: 31342192

[] Thahiruddin, M. (2025). CNNs vs. Hybrid Transformers for Brain Tumor Classification on the BRISC Dataset. *Jurnal Aplikasi Teknologi Informasi dan Manajemen (JATIM), 6*(1), 24-33.

Zhou, A., Ma, Y., Ji, W., Zong, M., Yang, P., Wu, M., & Liu, M. (2023). Multi-head attention-based two-stream EfficientNet for action recognition. *Multimedia Systems, 29*(2), 487–498. DOI: 10.1007/s00530-022-00961-3

Chapter 6
Artificial Intelligence in Early Breast Cancer Screening:
A New Frontier

Shaheen Layaq
https://orcid.org/0000-0002-1785-610X
Singareni Collieries Women's Degree and PG College, India

S. K. Parvez Ahammad
Kavitha Memorial Degree College, India

Pakalapati Arpitha
Telangana Social Welfare Residential Degree College for Women, India

ABSTRACT

Breast cancer is a kind of malignant tumor that mostly found in women which grows around the tissue of breast. During the process of diagnosis the cancer cells and non cancer cells are been identified and their count is made. If the count of cancer cells is greater than non cancer cells then the patient undergoes the treatments. The early detection of breast cancer can save the life of patient. Now a day's AI is playing a vital role in classifying cancer and non cancer cells in a accurate way. Many of the earlier researchers had performed the work of classifying them but, most of them lack in the accuracy. To have good accuracy a new method EBCS (Early Breast Cancer Screening) is proposed which consists of four steps or phases-preprocessing, classifying, performance evaluation and providing clear understanding to human.. To implement the four steps python programming is been used and cancer data set was extracted from Breast Cancer Wisconsin (Diagnostic) data set. The proposed method EBCS gave an accuracy of 99 percentage and complexity is also reduced.

DOI: 10.4018/979-8-3373-4312-9.ch006

1. INTRODUCTION

One among the genetic diseases is cancer which occurs due to unusual cell growth and splitting. World Health Organization (World Health Organization, 2024) has predicted that by 2050 the growth rate of global cancer will be about 77 percentage and new cases will be of about 35 millions. There are various kinds of cancers such as

- Carcinomas cancer it develops in epithelial cells and tissues.
- Sarcomas cancer seen in bones and tissues.
- Leukemia cancer found in blood, lymphoma cancer found in lymphocytes.
- Brain and spinal cord cancer.
- Melanoma cancer seen in melanocytes (skin) and
- Some common cancers (kidney, skin, breast, lungs, colorectal, prostate, thyroid, myeloma, uterine).

Many factors may effects for cause of cancer like

- Inherit of genetics
- Disclosure to substances that source cancer
- Lifestyle choices and environment (Infections, diet, smoking, obesity).

The cancer can be confirm by performing many medical clinical tests and once it is been confirmed the patient undergoes the following treatments like

- Surgery,
- Chemotherapy,
- Radiation therapy and
- Other treatments.

To avoid painful treatments early detection and prevention can be done by following

- Regular checkups
- Good diet
- Healthy lifestyle and
- Awareness

Among the entire cancers breast cancer is most commonly seen and it is mostly found in women's. The Fig.1 shows four years from 2021 to 2024 statistics related to breast cancer and their death levels (Observer Research Foundation,) in India among females. The new breast cancer cases are increasing steadily from year 2021

(21,0714) to 2024 (31,0720) as well as death rates are also increasing steadily from year 2021(78,387) to 2024 (84,429).

Figure 1. Total Estimated Breast Cancer and Death of Breast Cancer Cases from

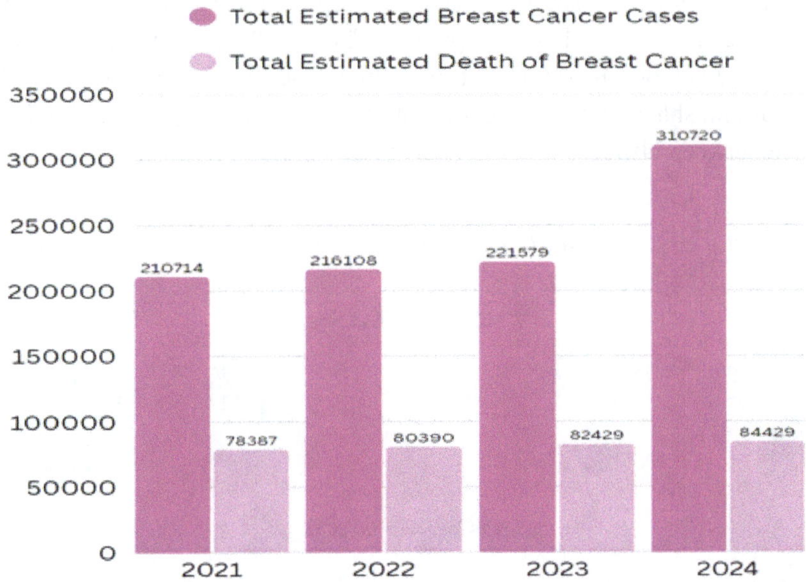

(2021 to 2024) in India

In lab studies the researchers in research experiments have divided the cell into two categories

1) Breast Cancer Cell (BCC)
2) Non Breast Cancer Cell (NBCC) or Normal cell

The Breast Cancer Cell (BCC) is known as malignant and Non Breast Cancer Cell (NBCC) is known as benign. The pictorial representation (Gupta & Bhavsar, 2019) of NBCC and BCC is given in Fig.2. The NBCC are not so dangerous as it does not represent or lead to cancer. It may be considered as cyst which does not lead to cancer. In very rare cases this NBCC may be turn to cancer cells. So, if it is found its better to take care by regular checkups and monitoring. NBCC needs attention if

- It is growing faster
- Change in size is observed
- Patient feels pain

- The structure of skin changes to discharge, dimpling or any other nipple problems
- Patient has family history of breast cancer

Generally doctors may suggest scans and biopsies for NBCC. Detecting breast cancer early can save the life of the patient. The NBCC are found under the area of capsule, are smooth, found to be round shape and grow slowly. Whereas BCC are not in round shape they are irregular or jagged and grow quickly. The detailed difference between NBCC and BCC is given in the Table 1 below.

Figure 2. Pictorial Representation of NBCC and BCC

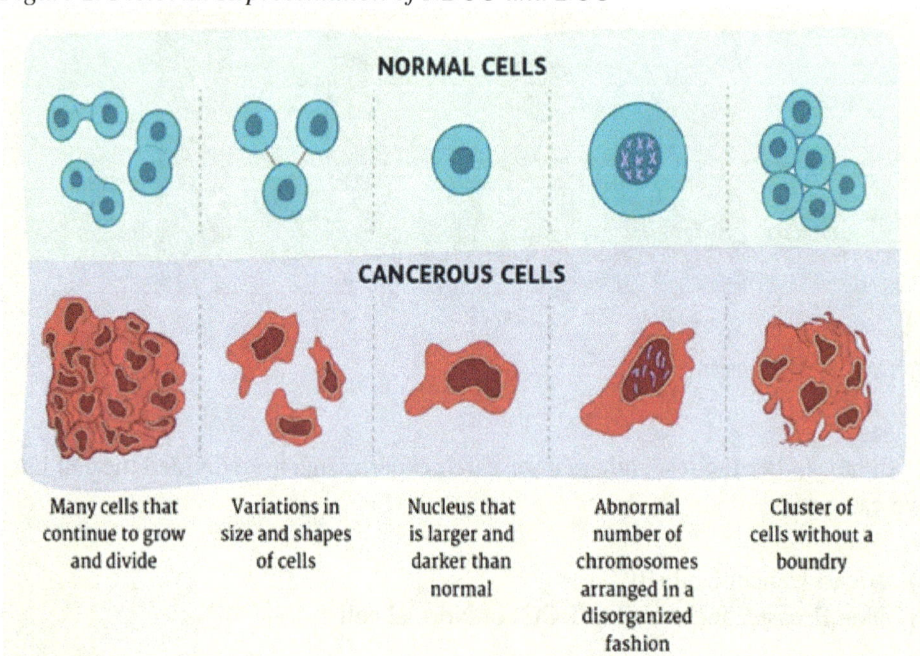

Table 1. Difference between Non Breast Cancer Cell and Breast Cancer Cell

	Non Breast Cancer Cell or Begin Tumor	**Breast Cancer Cell or Malignant Tumor**
Location	Restricted within the area of capsule	Extends with neighboring tissue
Shape	Smooth and round	Irregular and jagged
Growth	Slow	Quickly and undesirably
Danger	Low	High

To identify the breast cancer the count of BCC and NBCC are been made. If count of BCC is greater than NBCC then patient is confirmed as breast cancer. But, if count of BCC cell is less than that of NBCC cells then the patient is predicted as out of danger. Here, the less count of BCC cells must not be ignored there has to be taken seriously because patient might be at the early stage of cancer which must be identified and diagnosis. Actually, the less count of NBCC than BCC is concern with imbalance problem related to class. The figure 3 shows the imbalance between NBCC and BCC. The red color cross are considered as BCC and blue color cross are considered as NBCC. The imbalance between them is occurred as the count of NBCC is more than that of BCC cells. On this if patient's report is generated then the final result will be generated as she is out of danger. But, in the initial stage it must be identified and patient must be start treated early to overcome the problem. For this some sort of preprocessing has to be done to highlight the less count of BCC cells.

Figure 3. Class Imbalance of NBCC and BCC

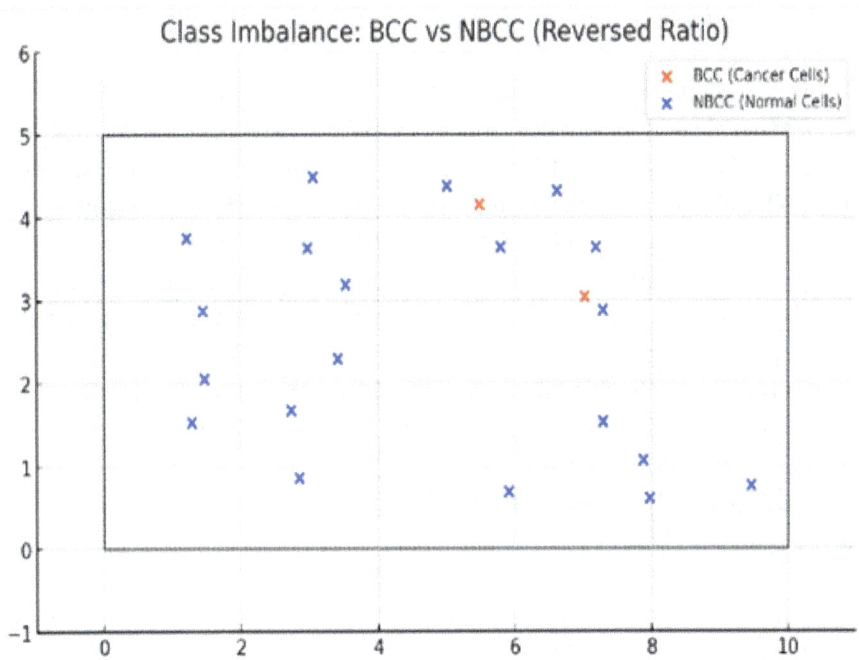

1.1 Preprocessing of NBCC and BCC

In preprocessing process the less count of NBCC are made balance with BCC so that they can be identified. For balancing the NBCC and BCC many balancing methods are present which can be broadly classified as

- Data Sampling strategies
- Algorithm related strategies
- Cost related strategies
- Ensemble related strategies

Among them data sampling strategies are more popular, proved as best and mostly used. In data sampling strategies the operation is performed on the data related to NBCC and BCC. The data sampling strategies are further divided into three types

- Oversampling
- Undersampling
- Hybrid Sampling

In oversampling strategy the count of BCC is increased by using various methods like ROS, CBOS (Jo & Japkowicz, 2004), SMOTE (Chawla et al., 2002), B-SMOTE (Han et al., 2005) and MWM(Barua et al., 2014). In Undersampling strategy the count of NBCC is decreased by using various methods like RUS (Prusa et al., 2015), CBUS (Yen & Lee, 2009), DSUS (Ng et al., 2015) and F-CBUS (Ofek et al., 2017). In hybrid strategy both oversampling and undersampling are used in which few BCC will be increased by using oversampling and few NBCC is decreased by using undersampling strategy so that finally there are balanced. Various hybrid strategies are present such as SMOTEENN, IDROUS and so on. Among them IDROUS is the best one for balancing NBCC and BCC with good accuracy and less complexity.

1.2 Traditional (Non AI) and AI Based Breast Cancer Detection Methods

The breast cancer can be identified in two ways traditional (Non AI) and AI based.

a) Traditional (Non AI) Breast Cancer Detection Methods: Traditional methods (Osareh & Shadgar, 2010) (Sahiner, Chan, Petrick, Helvie, Goodsitt, & Hadjiiski, 1996) (Quinlan, 1993) (El-Naqa, Yang, Galatsanos, Nishikawa, & Wernick, 2002) (Jain & Singh, 2007) (Elter & Horsch, 2009) (Nishikawa, 2007) (Street, Wolberg, & Mangasarian, 1993) depends on expertise of human, interpretation of manual images, and biological testing. It does not depend on intelligent and automated algorithms. The following are the traditional breast cancer detection techniques

- **Breast Self Check –** In this type of check the women manually checks her breast if any lumps are present, observing shapes, and pain.
- **Clinical Examination of Breast –** Doctor performs it by visual inspection or feeling for lumps.
- **By performing Mammography-** X-ray of breast is done to identify the masses, abnormal calcifications, lumps, and doubted tissues.
- **Ultrasound Imaging-** Here, sound waves are been used to identify lumps and also detect whether lumps are solid which means cancer or fluid which means cyst.
- **Magnetic Resonance Imaging-** Here, magnetic fields and radio waves are been used to identify high contrast images of lumps. It is mostly used for risky patient and if lumps are very dense.
- **Biopsy-** A small tissue sample is taken and tested under a microscope. For this Fine Needle Aspiration, Core Needle Biopsy and Surgical Biopsy methods are considered.
- **Histopathology and Cytology-** The tissue or cells detailed pathologist study is been done to identify the cancer cells.

Advantages of Traditional (Non AI) Breast Cancer Detection Methods-

- Medically proven and tested.
- Early detection of lumps or tissues may be happen.
- It is mostly used and easily available.
- Cost effective compare to other methods.
- Done and proved by medical experts.
- Maintains international standards.

Disadvantages of Traditional (Non AI) Breast Cancer Detection Methods-

- Performed by human so there are high chances of error.
- Late detection may be happen.
- Unnecessary testing may be performed some times.
- Time taken process.
- If lumps are dense then may be unable to identify.
- Tissue removal is painful.
- Different treatments have to be consider for different patients.

b) AI based Breast Cancer Detection Methods: Now a day's Artificial Intelligence (AI) and its tools (ML and DL) (Sahiner, Chan, Petrick, Helvie, Goodsitt, & Hadjiiski, 1996) (El-Naqa, Yang, Galatsanos, Nishikawa, & Wernick, 2002) (Jain & Singh, 2007) (Street, Wolberg, & Mangasarian, 1993) (Elter & Horsch, 2009) (Nishikawa, 2007) (Dheeba et al., 2011) (Dhungel et al., 2015) (Ribli et al., 2018) (Arevalo et al., 2016) (Cireşan et al., 2013) (Spanhol et al., 2016) (Nanni et al., 2012) (Kumar et al., 2017) (Abdel-Zaher & Eldeib, 2016) (George & Sahoo, 2020) (Gupta & Bhavsar, 2019) are playing a vital role in classifying BCC and NBCC in a very efficient and more accurate way. Machine Learning (ML) consists of many efficient classification techniques which produces more accurate result and which is more helpful in early detection of breast cancer. The following are the AI based breast cancer detection techniques

- **Machine Learning based Breast cancer detection-** from medical images features are extracted and passed to algorithms (SVM, random forest, decision tree, KNN, so on) to identify the cancer and non cancer cells.
- **Deep Learning based Breast cancer detection-** Automatically extracts the features and uses algorithms like CNN, ResNet, so on for identify the cancer and non cancer cells.
- **Computer Aided identification-** Uses CAD or CADx.
- **AI related Clinical Image Analysis-** AI is applied on Mammography, ultrasound, MRI, and so on.
- **AI related Personalized Screening and Risk Prediction methods-** Consider patient's personal information age, family history so on. Methods like neural methods, logistic regression methods are considered for customized screening planning.
- **AI based Segmentation methods-** Cancer cells and non cancer cells are been separated.

Advantages of AI Breast Cancer Detection Methods-

- AI based detection have high accuracy than traditional methods.
- Human errors can be eliminated or reduce.
- Efficient and quick identification.
- Dense lumps can be identified accurately.
- Personalized treatment can be done accurately.
- AI model keeps updating by learning from large medical dataset.
- AI models are more scalable.

Disadvantages of AI Breast Cancer Detection Methods-

- To implement it initially it is costly.
- Totally dependent on dataset . So, dataset must be accurate and clear.
- Technical knowledge and experts of AI are required.
- May be advised to unnecessary examination.
- May be raised to ethical and security issue problems as patients personal data is been used.
- AI cannot replace the expert doctor's suggestions.

1.3 AI Adoption and Global Disparities

AI adoption in breast cancer detection varies across regions as some regions are advancing quickly technology. The reasons for regional difference in AI adoption are that all region income is not same and it is divided into high, middle and low income regions.

- High income regions like Japan, Europe and U.S uses AI integrated tools more rapidly for breast cancer detection.
- Middle income regions like India, Brazil, South Africa adoption is growing but it is very slow.
- Low income regions like part of Africa, Southeast Asia adoption is minimal due to many reasons.

AI can act as potential to reduce inequalities in healthcare related to breast cancer by

- AI tools can be used in remote regions where medical help is rare and not quickly accessible.
- If AI tools are able to generate accurate then it reduces dependence on medical staff.
- AI related portable devices must provide digital screening of breast cancer in a affordable cost.
- If patient is living far away or remote area AI must provide Tele medicine and remote diagnosis.
- AI must also be able to improve the screening consistency.

1.4 Ethical and Privacy Issues in AI Based Breast Cancer Detection

As AI needs large volume of patient personal data related to breast cancer the following ethical and privacy must be consider

- **Data Privacy –** The large volume of personal data related to patients is used by AI for detection of cancer so it must be secure from misused, and leaked.
- **Data Security-** In hospitals the data must be stored securely so that it is been not stolen. Beyond this cyber security attacks strategies must also consider.
- **Patient Agreeing-** Patients must have knowledge how their data is been used either for training AI model or for research purpose.
- **Fair and Bias:** Results must be fair and bias as most of the results are dependent on one attribute.
- **Transparency –** AI tools must be able to explain why the particular result is been obtained instead of acting as a black box.
- **Concerns related to accountability and responsibility:** As AI is virtual the mistakes done by it must be targeted to either hospital, management, doctor or AI company it must be clear.
- **Federated Learning in AI-** It is a privacy securing machine learning based method where AI techniques learns from large data stored in various multiple different places without sharing or moving the authentic data.
- **FDA/EMA Approval –** AI systems must strictly follow the FDA/EMA ethical principles and privacy laws such as safe for patients, medically accurate, privacy patient is protected, ethically designed, transparent and accountable before adopting in health care system.
- Reducing of human medical skills and judgment capabilities by too much dependency on AI.

1.5 Policy Making Role in AI Based Breast Cancer Detection

Policy making plays a important part in deciding how AI based breast cancer identification tools are regulated, used and accepted in medical department. It defines the following

- The detection or screening guidelines.
- Rules related to data privacy.
- AI tools approval processes.
- Matter related to funding and resource allocation.

1.6 Impact of AI Based Breast Cancer Detection

a) **Impact of AI on Job Roles**-AI does not replace radiologists but AI changes the way of doing work like automation of tasks which are routinely done,specific roles related to AI are done, and radiologist can concentrate toward patient interaction.

b)**Training and skills**- Radiologist must be given training related to technical aspects, data literacy related to imaging data, collaboration and interaction between AI and human, and updated programs training.

c) **Impact on Decision Making**-AI can turn ass important decision making tool which helps radiologist in many ways-

- Quick and accurate treatment.
- Standard reports are generated with consistency.
- Decision related to time critical are taken faster.
- Predictive analysis and research analysis for patient survival can be done.

1.7 Cost Benefit Analysis in AI Adoption and Implementation Framework

- Before adopting AI in organization or medical field the management compares the cost and its benefits. Cost related to software, hardware, licensing, infrastructure, upgrades, training, maintenance, regulatory compliance and security cost. These cost analysis can be done using ROI, time saving analysis and so on.
- Implementation framework guides secure and effective deployment.

1.8 Challenges in AI for Breast Cancer Detection

For AI to be used perfectly in the medical environment it has to meet following challenges

- **Model Basis**- The training data from various different patient is not consider then AI systems become bias. It may lead to healthcare inequalities.
- **Interpretability**- Many AI's tools like DL system works like a black box means does not provide clear explaination but provides good prediction. By which it slows medical acceptance.
- **Integration with legacy systems** - most of the hospitals in middle and low income regions uses older medical software and hardware by which it is hard to integrate with modern AI.

- **Systematic Challenges-** integrating AI with older and out dated medical system leads to systematic challenges. So, changes is required in software, hardware,training must be given, regulations and workflow must be implemented.

1.9 Future Challenges for AI Based Breast Cancer Detection

- AI tools and technology must be provided at affordable cost.
- Different design structures must be considered to over come the bias and less accuracy.
- Federated learning and strategies must be used for ethical or privacy risk.
- Must be integrated with legacy system easily by using seamless integration.

1.10 Contribution of Work

To have good accuracy and precision a completely new frontier method Early Breast Cancer Screening (EBCS) is proposed which consists of four steps or phases- preprocessing, classifying, performance evaluation and providing clear understanding to human.

1) During the first step, the cancer data set is extracted from Breast Cancer Wisconsin (Diagnostic) data set and then preprocessing is been performed on cancer dataset to overcome the problems of missing values and imbalance.
2) In second step the preprocessed cancer data is been passed for classifying into BCC and NBCC. To classify it efficiently ML efficient algorithm Support Vector Machine (SVM) is been used.
3) In third step the classified data performance is been evaluated by using two performance measures accuracy and precision. It is also compared with the previous classification methods and the performance is presented in the form of charts and tables.
4) Finally, to give more understanding to human one of the XAI (Explainable Artificial Intelligence) approach SHAP (SHapley Additive explanations) is been used.

2. ASSOCIATED WORK

Many of the earlier researchers had performed their work of classifying breast cancer dataset to identify the BCC and NBCC. The list of earlier work is given in the below Table 2.

Table 2. Associated Work Related to Breast Cancer Dataset

S.No	Discussion	Classification Technique	Accuracy
1	Non surgical classification model to detect metastasis in breast cancer patients, using clinical data or blood profile data, rather than Using only biopsy or tissue examination (Botlagunta et al., 2023).	Decision Tree Classifiers.	83%
2	The main purpose was to build a robust deep learning based strategy to classify breast cancer benign vs malignant using medical images. Especially, they used the publicly available BUSI dataset (Breast Ultrasound Images) of breast lesions (Ali et al., 2023).	Meta-learning approaches and Convolutional Neural Networks.	90%
3	Subtypes of Breast Cancer (Orrantia-Borunda et al., 2022).	The four subtypes of breast cancers.	-
4	To surpass important challenges such as **imbalanced data** of benign and malignant images likely not evenly represented, **focal loss function** in training was used by them, which helps the system focus on ignored classes (Liu et al., 2024).	A Convolutional Neural Network applied to breast X-ray mammography image classification.	96%.
5	Authors suggested that with careful preprocessing, choosing model, and adaptive ensemble setup machine learning classifiers can provide high accuracy, which helps to suitable for use as complementary tools for diagnosis or decision support even though not a replacement for medical professionals(Batool & Byun, 2024).	Adaptive Voting Ensemble Learning Algorithm.	97.6%
6	The authors proposed an automated deep learning method to find out mammogram images, providing the classification of breast tissue as either normal or indicative of cancer(Meenalochini & Ramkumar, 2024).	Breast Cancer Classification System Using Deep Learning on Mammograms.	98.5%
7	The authors implemented a model using **Transfer Learning (TL)** with a modified version of AlexNet refer to a convolutional neural network (CNN) for identifying and classifying breast cancer from both ultrasound and histopathology images(Arooj et al., 2022).	Techniques in deep learning, machine learning, and transfer learning.	96.66% (Dataset A)
8	The authors proposed a hybrid breast cancer classification method that merges a convolutional neural network (CNN) with a meta heuristic optimization algorithm(Thirumalaisamy et al., 2023).	Synthesized deep learning framework utilizing a metaheuristic optimization method.	98.63%

2.1 Brief Overview of Drawbacks of Earlier Approaches

- Preprocessing was not done properly. Mostly it was done manually without using AI based technique.
- Imbalance problem was not considered.
- Latest AI tools were not considered for classification
- Accuracy is not same for all dataset or repository.
- Accuracy is also low.
- Not scalable with large volume of data.
- None of the previous papers or work considered about AI adoption, AI challenges, AI impact, cost benefit analysis, ethical and privacy issues, policy making, traditional and AI based differences for breast cancer detection.

The above mentioned problems can be overcome by using our proposed work.

3. PROPOSED WORK

Many of the earlier researchers had performed the work of classifying dataset of breast cancer cases to identify the BCC along with NBCC but, most of them lack in the accuracy and complexity was also too high. To have good accuracy and precision a new method EBCS (Early Breast Cancer Screening) is proposed. The detailed frame work of proposed work is given in Fig. 4. which consists of four steps or phases- preprocessing, classifying, performance evaluation and providing clear understanding to human. The detail of each steps are explained below.

Figure 4. A Detailed Framework of Proposed System

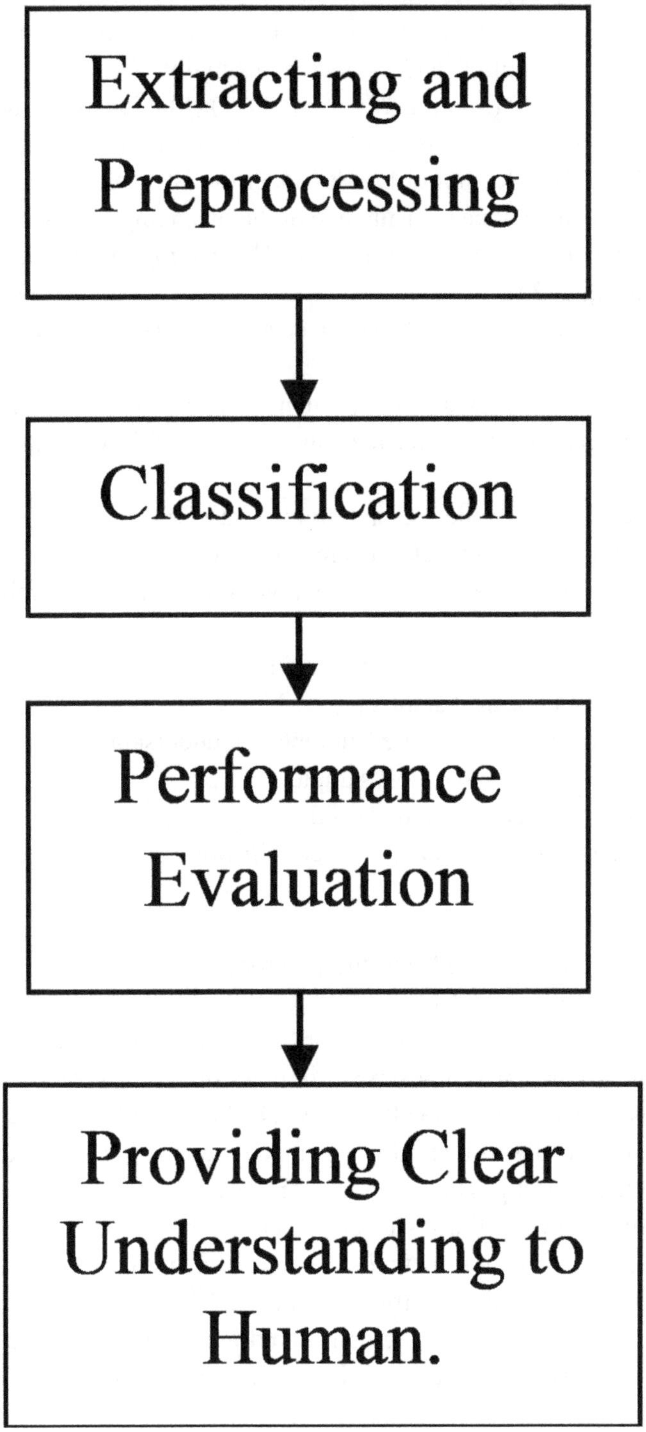

1) Extracting and Preprocessing- The cancer data set is extracted from Breast Cancer Wisconsin (Diagnostic) data set and then preprocessing is been performed on cancer dataset to overcome the problems of missing values and imbalance. The missing values are identified and corrected manually. The imbalance problem (Layaq & Manjula, 2020) (Manjula & Layaq, 2022) (Manjula & Layaq, 2022)[16] occurs when the count of BCC is less than NBCC, if ignored the patient life will be in threat. For early detection of breast cancer the BCC and NBCC count must be balance which can be done by using one of the balancing technique Imbalanced Dataset Reduction Using Oversampling and Undersampling method (IDROUS) (Manjula & Layaq, 2023).

Imbalanced Dataset Reduction Using Oversampling and Undersampling method (IDROUS) Process-

IDROUS is hybrid balancing method which balance the imbalance cancer dataset to balance cancer dataset. To perform balancing it does following steps-

- Imbalance dataset is collected and divided into BCC and NBCC dataset.
- Mean sample of the both datasets are calculated.
- From the mean sample the nearest sample or neighbor is identified for both dataset.
- For BCC dataset the required number of oversamples are created between mean sample and nearest sample.
- For NBCC dataset the required number of undersamples are dropped between mean sample and nearest sample.
- By which the cancer will be balanced.
- On this balanced cancer dataset if classification is done accurate result is obtained.

2) Classification- In second step the preprocessed breast cancer data is been passed for classifying into BCC and NBCC. To classify it efficiently machine learning efficient algorithm Support Vector Machine (SVM) is been used. SVM is a most efficient, accurate and supervised ML classification algorithm which works with numerous breast cancer data efficiently. The basic working principal of SVM is that it separates the classes by finding optimal hyperlane (decision boundary) and it aims to find the widest possible vectors from different classes.

3) Performance Evaluation- After classification the performance is determined using performance evaluation methods. There are many performance evaluation methods like accuracy, recall. Specificity, precision, F1 score, and confusion matrix. For our problem three measures are considered among them there are accuracy, precision which are shown in Equation 1-2 and confusion matrix in Table 3.

- **Accuracy-** Accuracy is calculated to know the ratio of right consideration by total consideration. It is done by adding the number of true positive and number of true negative divided by sum of number of true positive, number of true negative, number of false positive and number of false negative.

$$Accuracy = \frac{a+b}{a+b+c+d} \tag{1}$$

Where,
a=Number of True Positive
b= Number of True Negative
c= Number of False Positive
d= Number of False Negative

- **Precision-** precision is calculated when the chances of number of false positive is high. It is done by number of true positive divided by sum of number of true positive, and number of true negative.

$$Precision = \frac{a}{a+b} \tag{2}$$

Where,
a=Number of True Positive
b= Number of True Negative

- **Confusion Matrix-** Confusion matrix is used to know the performance of the classification. It is in table format consisting of rows and columns. The performance is known with the help of predicted and actual values.The column contain predicted positive and predicted negative values. The rows contain actual positive and actual negative values. By viewing the we can compare the predicted labels and actual labels. It consists the values as number of true positive,number of true negative,number of false positive, and number of false negative.

Table 3. Confusion Matrix

		Predicted	
		Pos	**Neg**
Actual	**Pos**	a	d
	Neg	c	b

Where,
a=Number of True Positive
b= Number of True Negative
c= Number of False Positive
d= Number of False Negative
Pos= positive
Neg= Negative

4) Providing Clear Understanding to Human- Finally, to give more understanding to human one of the XAI (Explainable Artificial Intelligence) approach SHAP (SHapley Additive explanations) is been used. SHAP is used to clear understanding of ML models and it is dependent on shapley values (concept of game theory).

3.1 Proposed Algorithm- Early Breast Cancer Screening (EBCS)

The breast cancer in women are becoming life threatening problem day by day. As the days are passing the breast cancer rate is increasing in women more quickly and along with them the death rate is also increasing simultaneously. To overcome it both traditional and AI based methods are been introduced. The traditional methods are done manually and continuous monitoring from doctors are been required. Breast cancer patients has to be completely under observation of doctors and they have to spend their time and lot of money for medical treatment. Due to drawbacks of traditional methods now a days AI based methods are becoming more predominant. Many researchers are also looking forward to work on this problem and proposed many AI based and non AI based algorithms for early detection of breast cancer by which the life of the patients can be saved. But, earlier methods faced with some problems like preprocessing was not done properly, mostly it was done manually without using AI based technique, imbalance problem was not considered, latest AI tools were not considered for classification, accuracy is not same for all dataset or repository,accuracy is also low, not scalable with large volume of data, none of the previous papers or work considered about AI adoption, AI challenges, AI impact, cost benefit analysis, ethical and privacy issues, policy making, traditional and AI based differences for breast cancer detection. The mentioned problems can be overcome by using our proposed work Early Breast Cancer Screening.

The main purpose of proposed algorithm Early Breast Cancer Screening (EBCS) is to do first preprocessing so that the accurate classification result may be obtained. By performing preprocessing the quality of the data gets improved. If quality of data is improved the classification can produce more efficient result. The major problem is that the large patient data is required to perform the AI based classification. This large patient data is almost imbalanced. That means the non cancer cells are predominating on the cancer cells by which the imbalance problem occurs. Imbalance is a case which occurs when data is in large in size but the required data is very less. Here, the less data is cancer cells and more data is non cancer cells which leads to inaccurate result. The less data cannot be ignored as it might be less but it is very important. This less data means non cancer cells are very life threatening and must not be ignored. At the initial stage itself when they count is less there must be identified, studied and elaborated so that the life can be saved by early detection and treatment. To, perform this preprocessing is required.

In preprocessing initially, the data of cancer is extracted and then preprocessing has to be done. After extracting if imbalance is observed then that data related to cancer is been send or performed the preprocessing. The preprocessing can be performed by using sampling techniques which are based on the data known as data sampling methods. As we perform sampling directly on the imbalanced data the accuracy of the result increases. This sampling related to data is again classified into over sampling, under sampling and hybrid sampling.

Over sampling tries to increase the count of cancer cells so that the cancer cells get equal priority as that of non cancer cell. Now on this balanced cancer and non cancer cells if classification is done, we get most accurate result. By which the prior identification of cancer in patient are noticed and she may get early treatment. But, by this the non cancer cells get ignored the size or count of cancer cell will be increases.

Under sampling tries to decrease the count of non cancer cells so that the cancer cells can be highlighted and may be more visible. By this also patient can be treated early. But, this method also has a problem that only non cancer cells are been considered and cancer cells are been ignored, and chances are that important cells may also be dropped.

Hybrid method gives important to both over sampling and under sampling. It can be said that it is the combination of over sampling and under sampling. To perform hybrid sampling the count of both cancer and non cancer cells are been made and the difference is been calculated. Then that difference count number is divided into half and hybrid sampling is performed. The half difference count of cancer cells are increased and simultaneously the other half difference non cancer cells are been dropped. By which the both cancer cells and non cancer cells are been balanced. Here, both cancer and non cancer cells are been given equal importance. Most of the time the accuracy of hybrid sampling is better than over sampling and under sampling. Many hybrid sampling methods are been proposed by the researchers but for our work IDROUS (imbalanced data reduction using over sampling and under sampling) hybrid sampling method is been considered. By using IDROUS method the preprocessing of cancer cells and non cancer cells are done efficiently. Then later classification is done, performance evaluation and clear understanding to human is done using XAI. The proposed algorithm EBCS is explained in Table 4 below. To implement the algorithm Python programming is been used.

Table 4. Algorithm for Early Breast Cancer Screening (EBCS)

Algorithm: Early Breast Cancer Screening(EBCS) **[Algorithm EBCS is used to predict breast cancer at early stage. EBCS consists of four steps preprocessing, classifying, performance evaluation and providing clear understanding to human which are explain below]**
Input: Breast Cancer Wisconsin (Diagnostic) data set. **Output:** Classification and clear understanding of Breast Cancer Dataset. **Step-1:** [Extract the Breast Cancer Wisconsin (Diagnostic) data set and store in Breast Cancer Data Set (BC_{DS})] BC_{DS} <- read_fwf(Wdbc.data) **Step-2**:[Balancing (Preprocessing) is been performed on BC_{DS} by using IDROUS method and stored in Bal_BC_{DS} Bal_BC_{DS} <- IDROUS(BC_{DS}) **Step-3:**[Pass Bal_BC_{DS} to SVM method for classification and store the result in Classi_ Bal_BC_{DS}] Classi_ Bal_BC_{DS} <-train_svm_classifier(Bal_BC_{DS}) **Step-4:**[Performance is evaluated for Classi_ Bal_BC_{DS}.] Accuracy (Classi_ Bal_BC_{DS}) Precision(Classi_ Bal_BC_{DS}) **Step-5:**[Use shap.Explainer() and shap_values() for clear understanding] explainer=shap.Explainer(model.predict,Classi_Bal_BC_{DS}) shap_values = explainer(Classi_Bal_BC_{DS}) shap.plots.waterfall(shap_values) **Step-6:**End.

In the above for Early Breast Cancer Screening (EBCS) algorithm consists of four steps preprocessing, classifying, performance evaluation and providing clear understanding to human. These four steps are very useful in early detection of breast cancer in women. As a input the Breast Cancer Wisconsin (Diagnostic) data set is been obtained. The output is classification and clear understanding of Breast Cancer Dataset.

In step - 1 breast cancer data set is retrieved and stored in Breast Cancer Data Set (BC_{DS}) variable. To extract the data set the read_fwf() method is been is used. The read_fwf() is pandas function which is used to read file of type fixed formatted type. The file may contain set of characters.The read_fwf() function takes one variable of file type. Here in our algorithm we had passed the file named Wdbc.data which consists of cancer data and it is cancer data set type.

In step - 2 balancing or preprocessing is been performed on BC_{DS} data set by using IDROUS method and stored in Bal_BC_{DS} data set. The IDROUS method takes one variable or parameter. Here, the obtained BC_{DS} is passed a argument to the IDROUS method which in turn performs the balancing and balanced breast cancer data set is been obtained which in turn is stored in Bal_BC_{DS} variable or data set.

In step - 3 the Bal_BC_{DS} is passed to Support Vector Machine method for classification and store the result in Classi_ Bal_BC_{DS} variable or data set. The train_svm_classifier trains the SVM on balanced breast cancer data set or $Bal\_BC_{DS.}$ The train_svm_classifier method takes only one parameter that is $Bal\_BC_{DS.}$

In step - 4 the performance is evaluated for Classi_ Bal_BC_{DS} output using both accuracy and precision functions. The accuracy function takes only one parameter Classi_ Bal_BC_{DS} and accuracy is been performed. The precision function takes only one parameter Classi_ Bal_BC_{DS} and precision is been performed. The output is generated for both.

In step - 5 the shap.Explainer() and shap_values() are been used for clear understanding. The output of it will be in the pictorial format. To generate pictorial format output shap.Explainer() method is used which automatically identifies the best SHAP method. The shap.Explainer() takes two parameters model.predict, and $Classi\_Bal\_BC_{DS.}$ To that selected model the $Classi\_Bal\_BC_{DS}$ is passed. The explainer() function generates shap values. The generated shap values are passed to shap.plot.waterfall() which generate the final output in waterfall model type or format. The shap.plots.waterfall() takes only one argument.

In step - 5 the algorithm ends.

4. EXPERIMENTAL RESULTS AND DISCUSSION

To predict BCC and NBCC and to evaluate the performance of EBCS a Diagnostic Wisconsin Breast Cancer Database (Wdbc.data) has considered which consists of 32 variables (Machine Learning Repository,) the details of the variables or attributes are shown below in Table 5. Table contains column values such as attribute name, function, data type, and missing entries.

Table 5. Diagnostic Wisconsin Breast Cancer Database Variable Table

S.No	Attribute Name	Function	Data Type	Missing entries
1	Identifier	Identifier	Nominal	None
2	Detection (M=malignant(BCC), B = benign (NSCC))	Goal	Nominal	None
3	Radius_1	Attribute	Quantitative	None
4	Texture_1	Attribute	Quantitative	None
5	Perimeter_1	Attribute	Quantitative	None
6	Area_1	Attribute	Quantitative	None
7	Smoothness_1	Attribute	Quantitative	None
8	Compactness_1	Attribute	Quantitative	None
9	Concavity_1	Attribute	Quantitative	None

continued on following page

Table 5. Continued

S.No	Attribute Name	Function	Data Type	Missing entries
10	concave_points_1	Attribute	Quantitative	None
11	Symmetry_1	Attribute	Quantitative	None
12	fractal_dimension_1	Attribute	Quantitative	None
13	Radius_2	Attribute	Quantitative	None
14	Texture_2	Attribute	Quantitative	None
15	Perimeter_2	Attribute	Quantitative	None
16	area_2	Attribute	Quantitative	None
17	Smoothness_2	Attribute	Quantitative	None
18	Compactness_2	Attribute	Quantitative	None
19	Concavity_2	Attribute	Quantitative	None
20	Concave2_points_2	Attribute	Quantitative	None
21	Symmetry2_2	Attribute	Quantitative	None
22	Fractal2_dimension_2	Attribute	Quantitative	None
23	Radius3_3	Attribute	Quantitative	None
24	Texture3_3	Attribute	Quantitative	None
25	Perimeter3_3	Attribute	Quantitative	None
26	Area3_3	Attribute	Quantitative	None
27	Smoothness3_3	Attribute	Quantitative	None
28	Compactness3_3	Attribute	Quantitative	None
29	Concavity3_3	Attribute	Quantitative	None
30	Concave3_points_3	Attribute	Quantitative	None
31	Symmetry3_3	Attribute	Quantitative	None
32	Fractal3_dimension_3	Attribute	Quantitative	None

The SVM (Support Vector Machine) classification is performed as it gives best accuracy result than other classification methods and the performance (accuracy and precision) of EBCS is shown in Table 6. It is observed that our proposed EBCS accuracy is 99% and EBCS precision is 96% and the Fig. 5 shows the pictorially representation of EBCS performance.

Table 6. EBCS Performance

Classification Method	Measures	EBCS
SVM	Accuracy	99%
SVM	Precision	96%

Figure 5. The Proposed method EBCS performance (Accuracy and Precision)

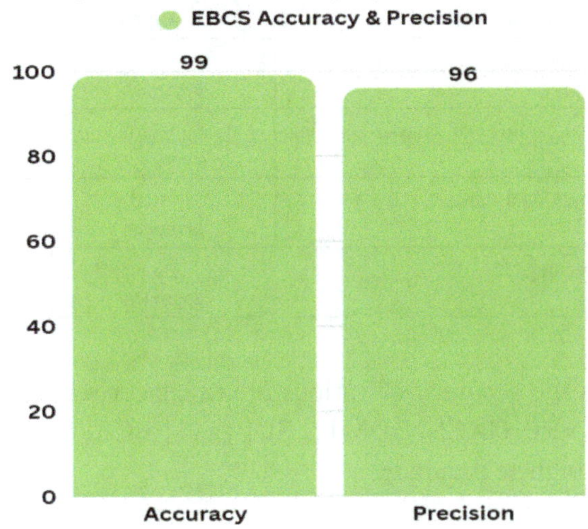

The comparative result analyzing of our proposed method EBCS with earlier seven classification methods such as decision tree classifiers, meta learning approach convolutional neural networks, convolutional neural network to classify breast X-ray (mammogram) images, adaptive voting ensemble learning algorithm, breast cancer classification using deep learning on mammogram images, deep learning, machine learning and transfer learning techniques, and Integrated deep learning model enhanced by meta heuristic optimization is also done by using performance measure accuracy and has presented in Table 7. The EBCS has superior accuracy of about 99%.

Table 7. Comparing EBCS Performance with Various Earlier Techniques for Screening Breast Cancer

Techniques for Screening Breast Cancer	Approach	Accuracy
Decision Tree Classifiers(DT).	Earlier approach	83%
Meta-learning approaches and Convolutional Neural Networks(MLCNN).	Earlier approach	90%
Using a Convolutional Neural Network (CNN) to classify breast X-ray (mammogram) images.	Earlier approach	96%
Adaptive Voting Ensemble Learning Algorithm(AVEL).	Earlier approach	97.6%

continued on following page

Table 7. Continued

Techniques for Screening Breast Cancer	Approach	Accuracy
Breast Cancer Classification Using Deep Learning on Mammogram Images (GACNN).	Earlier approach	98.5%
Deep Learning, Machine Learning and Transfer Learning techniques(DMTL).	Earlier approach	96.66%
Integrated Deep Learning Model Enhanced by Metaheuristic Optimization (SDL).	Earlier approach	98.63%
Early Breast Cancer Screening (EBCS).	Proposed approach	99%

The Figure 6 shows the accuracy of various breast cancer screening methods (DT, MLCNN, CNN, AVEL, GACNN, DMTL, SDL, and EBCS). The chart clearly shows that EBCS with highest accuracy.

Figure 6. Accuracy of Various Breast Cancer Screening Methods

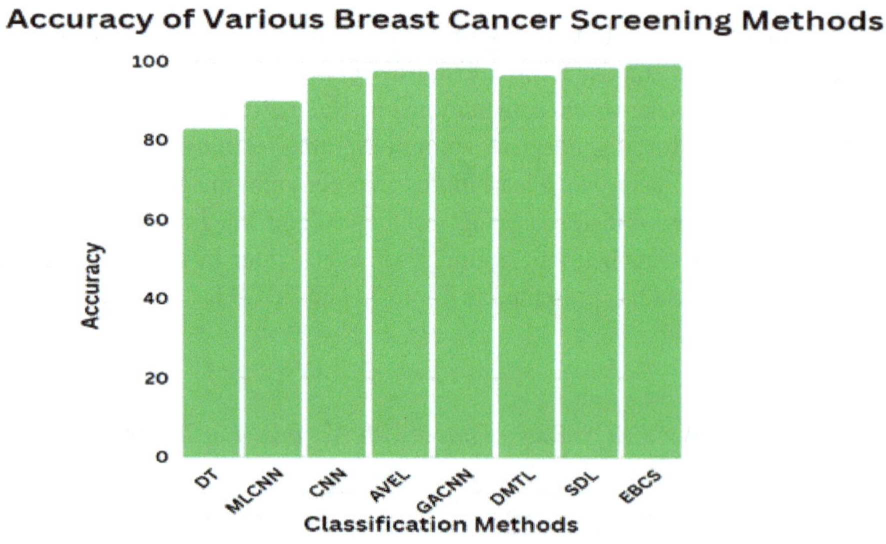

Further, one of the XAI tool SHAP (Shapley Additive exPlanations) is used to understand how individual variables involves in final outcome which is shown on the Fig.7. The SHAP summary plot provides an interpretable explanation of how each feature contributes to the classification decision in the breast cancer prediction model (EBCS method). Features are ranked from top to bottom based on their importance, with "concave points_mean," "perimeter_mean," and "concavity_mean" showing the highest influence on the model's output. The SHAP values on the x-axis represent the direction and magnitude of impact . Positive values indicate a higher likelihood of malignancy, while negative values contribute toward a benign prediction. Each point represents a sample, where red indicates a high feature value and blue represents a low value. For the most influential features, red points clustered on the positive side show that higher values strongly correlate with malignant tumors. Thus, the plot not only highlights feature importance but also shows how specific feature values drive decision outcomes, improving transparency and trust in the AI model.

Figure 7. SHAP Summary Plot for Breast cancer Screening using EBCS Method

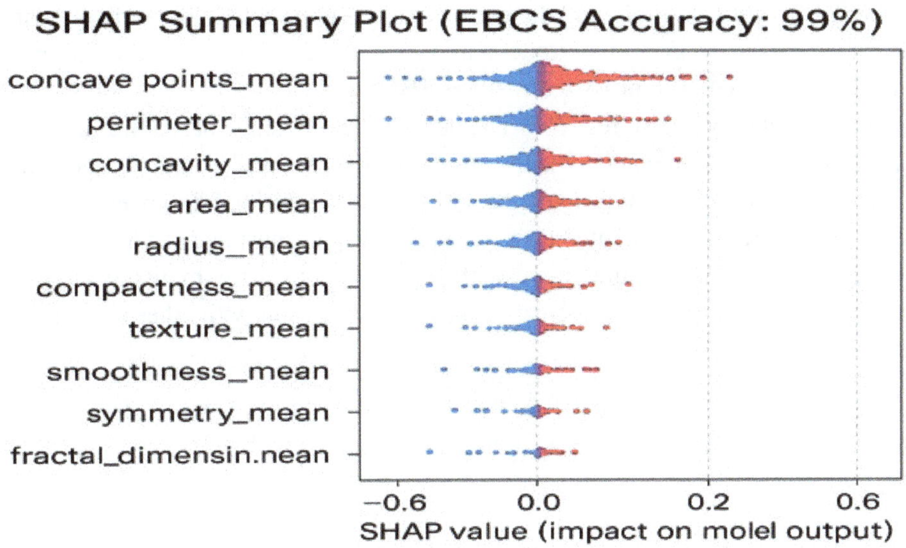

5. CONCLUSION AND FUTURE WORK

One of the genetic diseases is cancer which occurs due to unusual cell growth and splitting. Cancer related to breast is a kind of malignant (cancer) tumor which mostly found among women which grows around the tissue of breast. To confirm and diagnosis cancer the doctor performs different physical examinations. During the process of diagnosis the cancer cells and non cancer cells (lumps) are been identified and their count is made. If the count of cancer cells is greater than non cancer cells then the patient undergoes the treatments. Detecting breast cancer early can save the life of patient. Now a day's Artificial Intelligence is playing a vital role in classifying cancer and non cancer cells in a very efficient and more accurate way. To have good accuracy and precision a new method EBCS (Early Breast Cancer Screening) is proposed which consists of four steps or phases- preprocessing, classifying, performance evaluation and providing clear understanding to human. During the first step, the preprocessing is been performed on cancer dataset to overcome the problems of missing values and imbalance. In second step the preprocessed cancer data is been passed for classifying into cancer and non cancer cells. To classify it efficiently machine learning efficient algorithm Support Vector Machine (SVM) is been used. In third step the classified data performance is been evaluated by using two performance measures accuracy and precision. It is also compared with the previous classification methods and the performance is presented in the form of charts and table. Finally, to give more understanding to human one of the XAI approach SHAP is been used. The proposed method EBCS gave an accuracy of 99 percentage and complexity is also reduced. The artificial intelligence based breast cancer still has to face certain challenges like AI tools and technology must be provided at affordable cost, different design structures must be considered to over come the bias and less accuracy, federated learning and strategies must be used for ethical or privacy risk, and must be integrated with legacy system easily by using seamless integration. As, a future enhancement it has to be work out with other databases.

REFERENCES

Abdel-Zaher, A. M., & Eldeib, A. M. (2016). Breast cancer classification using deep belief networks. *Expert Systems with Applications*, *46*, 139–144. DOI: 10.1016/j.eswa.2015.10.015

Ali, M. D., Saleem, A., Elahi, H., Khan, M. A., Khan, M. I., Yaqoob, M. M., Khattak, U. F., & Al-Rasheed, A. (2023). Breast cancer classification through meta-learning ensemble technique using convolution neural networks. *Diagnostics (Basel)*, *13*(6), 1021. DOI: 10.3390/diagnostics13132242 PMID: 37443636

Arevalo, J., González, F. A., Ramos-Pollán, R., Oliveira, J. L., & López, M. A. (2016). Representation learning for mammography mass lesion classification with convolutional neural networks. *Computer Methods and Programs in Biomedicine*, *127*, 248–257. DOI: 10.1016/j.cmpb.2015.12.014 PMID: 26826901

Arooj, S., Rahman, A.-U., Zubair, M., Khan, M. F., Alissa, K., Khan, M. A., & Mosvi, A. (2022). Breast cancer detection and classification empowered with transfer learning. *Frontiers in Public Health*, *10*, 10. DOI: 10.3389/fpubh.2022.924432 PMID: 35859776

Barua, S., Islam, M. M., Yao, X., & Murase, K. (2014). MWMOTE—Majority weighted minority oversampling technique. *IEEE Transactions on Knowledge and Data Engineering*, *26*(2), 405–425. DOI: 10.1109/TKDE.2012.232

Batool, A., & Byun, Y.-C. (2024). Toward improving breast cancer classification using an adaptive voting ensemble learning algorithm. *IEEE Access : Practical Innovations, Open Solutions*, *12*, 12869–12882. DOI: 10.1109/ACCESS.2024.3356602

Botlagunta, M., Botlagunta, M. D., Myneni, M. B., Lakshmi, D., Nayyar, A., Gullapalli, J. S., & Shah, M. A. (2023). Classification and diagnostic prediction of breast cancer metastasis on clinical data using machine learning algorithms. *Scientific Reports*, *13*(1), 1045. DOI: 10.1038/s41598-023-27548-w PMID: 36627367

Chawla, N. V., Bowyer, K. W., Hall, L. O., & Kegelmeyer, W. P. (2002). SMOTE: Synthetic minority over-sampling technique. *Journal of Artificial Intelligence Research*, *16*, 321–357. DOI: 10.1613/jair.953

Cireşan, D. C., Giusti, A., Gambardella, L. M., & Schmidhuber, J. (2013). Mitosis detection in breast cancer histology images with deep neural networks. In *Medical Image Computing and Computer-Assisted Intervention* (pp. 411–418). DOI: 10.1007/978-3-642-40763-5_51

Dheeba, J., Selvi, S. T., & Singh, N. A. (2011). Computer-aided detection of breast cancer on mammograms. *Journal of Biomedical Informatics, 44*(4), 640–647. PMID: 24509074

Dhungel, N., Carneiro, G., & Bradley, A. P. (2015). Deep structured learning for mass segmentation from mammograms. In *IEEE International Conference on Image Processing* (pp. 2950–2954). DOI: 10.1109/ICIP.2015.7351343

El-Naqa, I., Yang, Y., Galatsanos, N. P., Nishikawa, R. M., & Wernick, M. N. (2002). A similarity learning approach to content-based image retrieval. *IEEE Transactions on Medical Imaging, 23*(10), 1233–1244. DOI: 10.1109/TMI.2004.834601 PMID: 15493691

El-Naqa, I., Yang, Y., Galatsanos, N. P., Nishikawa, R. M., & Wernick, M. N. (2002). A similarity learning approach to content-based image retrieval. *IEEE Transactions on Medical Imaging, 23*(10), 1233–1244. DOI: 10.1109/TMI.2004.834601 PMID: 15493691

Elter, M., & Horsch, A. (2009). CADx of mammographic masses and clustered microcalcifications: A review. *Medical Physics, 36*(6), 2052–2068. DOI: 10.1118/1.3121511 PMID: 19610294

Elter, M., & Horsch, A. (2009). CADx of mammographic masses and clustered microcalcifications. *Medical Physics, 36*(6), 2052–2068. DOI: 10.1118/1.3121511 PMID: 19610294

George, Y., & Sahoo, A. (2020). Hybrid CNN–SVM model for breast cancer classification using ultrasound images. *Pattern Recognition Letters, 140*, 1–7.

Gupta, V., & Bhavsar, A. (2019). Breast cancer histopathological image classification: A hybrid CNN and random forest approach. *Biomedical Signal Processing and Control, 52*, 271–280.

Han, H., Wang, W.-Y., & Mao, B.-H. (2005). Borderline-SMOTE: A new oversampling method in imbalanced data sets learning. In *Advances in intelligent computing* (pp. 878–887). DOI: 10.1007/11538059_91

Jain, S. K., & Singh, S. (2007). A fuzzy logic-based approach for breast cancer diagnosis. *International Journal of Computer Science Issues, 4*(2), 32–36.

Jain, S. K., & Singh, S. (2007). A fuzzy logic-based approach for breast cancer diagnosis. *International Journal of Computer Science Issues, 4*(2), 32–36.

Jo, T., & Japkowicz, N. (2004). Class imbalances versus small disjuncts. *SIGKDD Explorations, 6*(1), 40–49. DOI: 10.1145/1007730.1007737

Kumar, N., Verma, R., Sharma, S., Bhargava, S., Vahadane, A., & Sethi, A. (2017). A dataset and a technique for generalized nuclear segmentation for computational pathology. *IEEE Transactions on Medical Imaging*, *36*(7), 1550–1560. DOI: 10.1109/TMI.2017.2677499 PMID: 28287963

Layaq, S., & Manjula, B. (2020). A recapitulation of imbalanced data. *International Journal of Innovative Technology and Exploring Engineering*, *9*(3), 452–455. DOI: 10.35940/ijitee.B8120.019320

Liu, Z., Peng, J., Guo, X., Chen, S., & Liu, L. (2024). Breast cancer classification method based on improved VGG16 using mammography images. *Journal of Radiation Research and Applied Sciences*, *17*(2), 100885. DOI: 10.1016/j.jrras.2024.100885

Machine Learning Repository, U. C. I. (n.d.). *Breast cancer Wisconsin (diagnostic) dataset*. https://archive.ics.uci.edu/dataset/17/breast+cancer+wisconsin+diagnostic

Manjula, B., & Layaq, S. (2022). An integrated approach to reduce class imbalance. In *Intelligent systems* (Lecture Notes in Networks and Systems, Vol. 431, pp. 381–392). Springer. DOI: 10.1007/978-981-19-0901-6_35

Manjula, B., & Layaq, S. (2022). An innovative oversampling method for imbalanced data reduction. *Advanced Engineering Science*, *54*(1), 891–899.

Manjula, B., & Layaq, S. (2023). A new method for imbalanced data reduction using data-based under sampling. In *Proceedings of the 5th International Conference on Soft Computing & Signal Processing* (pp. 243–250). DOI: 10.1007/978-981-19-8669-7_22

Meenalochini, G., & Ramkumar, S. (2024). A deep learning-based breast cancer classification system using mammograms. *Journal of Electrical Engineering & Technology*, *19*(4), 2637–2650. DOI: 10.1007/s42835-023-01747-x

Nanni, L., Brahnam, S., & Lumini, A. (2012). A very high performing system to discriminate tissues in histopathology images. *Expert Systems with Applications*, *39*(12), 10465–10470.

Ng, W. W., Hu, J., Yeung, D. S., Yin, S., & Roli, F. (2015). Diversified sensitivity-based undersampling for imbalance classification problems. *IEEE Transactions on Cybernetics*, *45*(11), 2402–2412. DOI: 10.1109/TCYB.2014.2372060 PMID: 25474818

Nishikawa, R. M. (2007). Computer-aided detection and diagnosis in breast imaging: A review. *Breast Imaging*, *30*(1), 1–10.

Nishikawa, R. M. (2007). Computer-aided detection and diagnosis in breast imaging. *Breast Imaging*, *30*(1), 1–10.

Observer Research Foundation. (n.d.). *Rising breast cancer in India: Challenges and opportunities*. https://www.orfonline.org/expert-speak/rising-breast-cancer-in-india-challenges-and-opportunities

Ofek, N., Rokach, L., Stern, R., & Shabtai, A. (2017). Fast-CBUS: A fast clustering-based undersampling method. *Neurocomputing*, *243*, 88–102. DOI: 10.1016/j.neucom.2017.03.011

Orrantia-Borunda, E., Anchondo-Nuñez, P., Acuña-Aguilar, L. E., Gómez-Valles, F. O., & Ramírez-Valdespino, C. A. (2022). Subtypes of breast cancer. *Breast Cancer (Tokyo, Japan)*. PMID: 36122153

Osareh, A., & Shadgar, B. (2010). A computer-aided diagnosis system for breast cancer using SVM-based feature selection. *International Journal of Computer Theory and Engineering*, *2*(6), 883–887.

Prusa, J., Khoshgoftaar, T. M., Dittman, D. J., & Napolitano, A. (2015). Using random undersampling to alleviate class imbalance on tweet sentiment data. In *IEEE International Conference on Information Reuse and Integration* (pp. 197–202). DOI: 10.1109/IRI.2015.39

Quinlan, J. R. (1993). *C4.5: Programs for machine learning*. Morgan Kaufmann.

Ribli, D., Horváth, A., Unger, Z., Pollner, P., & Csabai, I. (2018). Detecting and classifying lesions in mammograms with deep learning. *Scientific Reports*, *8*(1), 4165. DOI: 10.1038/s41598-018-22437-z PMID: 29545529

Sahiner, B., Chan, H.-P., Petrick, N., Helvie, M. A., Goodsitt, M. M., & Hadjiiski, L. (1996). Classification of mass and normal breast tissue on digital mammograms. *Medical Physics*, *23*(7), 1065–1075.

Sahiner, B., Chan, H.-P., Petrick, N., Helvie, M. A., Goodsitt, M. M., & Hadjiiski, L. (1996). Classification of mass and normal breast tissue on digital mammograms. *Medical Physics*, *23*(7), 1065–1075.

Spanhol, F. A., Oliveira, L. S., Petitjean, C., & Heutte, L. (2016). A dataset for breast cancer histopathological image classification. *IEEE Transactions on Biomedical Engineering*, *63*(7), 1455–1462. DOI: 10.1109/TBME.2015.2496264 PMID: 26540668

Street, W. N., Wolberg, W. H., & Mangasarian, O. L. (1993). Nuclear feature extraction for breast tumor diagnosis. *IS&T/SPIE Proceedings, 1905*, 861–870.

Thirumalaisamy, S., Thangavilou, K., Rajadurai, H., Saidani, O., Alturki, N., Mathivanan, S. K., Jayagopal, P., & Gochhait, S. (2023). Breast cancer classification using synthesized deep learning model with metaheuristic optimization algorithm. *Diagnostics (Basel), 13*(18), 2925. DOI: 10.3390/diagnostics13182925 PMID: 37761292

World Health Organization. (2024, February 1). *Global cancer burden growing amidst mounting need for services.* https://www.who.int/news/item/01-02-2024-global-cancer-burden-growing--amidst-mounting-need-for-services

Yen, S.-J., & Lee, Y.-S. (2009). Cluster-based under-sampling approaches for imbalanced data distributions. *Expert Systems with Applications, 36*(3), 5718–5727. DOI: 10.1016/j.eswa.2008.06.108

Chapter 7
From Black Box to Glass Box Interpretable AI for Lung Cancer Radiomics

Bappaditya Das
https://orcid.org/0000-0001-6731-3659
Dr. B.C. Roy Engineering College, Durgapur, India

Anirban Bose
Dr. B.C. Roy Engineering College, Durgapur, India

ABSTRACT

Lung cancer is the leading cause of cancer mortality, with deaths due to the disease anticipated to exceed 4.6M new cases and 3.5 million lives each year by 2050. AI-based radiomics tools can potentially analyze the levels of pixel distribution and identify hidden biomarkers related to tumor aggressiveness. However, clinicians are reluctant to adopt these methodologies due to the lack of transparency in the DL models, known as the "black-box" phenomenon. The chapter "From Black Box to Glass Box: Interpretable AI for Lung Cancer Radiomics" aims to facilitate the transition of AI-based applications from laboratories to clinics. The protocol for AI-enhanced radiomics is systematically described. The core focus is on enhancing transparency through explainable AI (XAI) techniques. AI designs should be transparent (glass boxes) and have the purpose of assisting clinicians rather than replacing them. The roadmap to success and excellence in the diagnosis and treatment of lung cancer is clear, with data-driven insights.

DOI: 10.4018/979-8-3373-4312-9.ch007

1. INTRODUCTION: INTERPRETABLE RADIOMICS IN LUNG CANCER

Lung cancer is the deadliest and most difficult to treat (Sung et al., 2021) because of its aggressive and heterogeneous nature, progressive asymptomatic growth, and varying responses to therapy (Bade & Dela Cruz, 2020) (Herbst et al., 2018). Advancements have been made in diagnosing and treating tumors using radiomics (Gillies et al., 2016), a term that employs the "-omics" suffix commonly used in biomedicine to extract valuable information from large datasets (Lambin et al., 2017). Radiomics extracts measurable data from common medical images, such as CT scans and MRIs, uncovering hidden tumour patterns that reveal how the tumour behaves, without requiring invasive procedures (Aerts et al., 2014). These high-dimensional features may enhance diagnostic accuracy, predict outcomes, and optimize personalized treatment strategies (Kumar et al., 2012). The potential of radiomics increases even further when integrated with artificial intelligence (AI) technologies, particularly those based on deep learning (LeCun et al., 2015). These models can automate the identification of complex and highly tri-dimensional imaging features that human experts often miss (Esteva et al., 2021). However, one of the most critical problems remains: the "black box problem." Most AI systems provide no rationale for their predictions or insights (Samek et al., 2017). This issue renders the clinical implementation of such systems problematic because the absence of explanation makes them unreliable, impossible to interpret, and difficult to validate in practices (Holzinger et al., 2019). Addressing these concerns, the focus is gradually shifting towards more transparent and logical models, also known as 'glass box' systems, that clarify the reasoning behind their operations in a way that boosts confidence and trust (Rudin, 2019). Such systems are needed as trust is essential, particularly with radiomics in lung cancer and patient-centric care (Vellido, 2020). This introduction allows us to examine how radiomics with explainable AI can transform lung cancer care toward trust-based analytics.

1.1 Lung Cancer: A Persistent Global Health Burden

The magnitude of lung cancer's impact globally highlights the necessity for solutions. Data from GLOBOCAN 2022 shows that Lung cancer remains at the top of statistics. It is responsible for a significant portion of newly diagnosed cases and an even greater portion of deaths across the world. For example, 2.5 million new cases of lung cancer were diagnosed around the world in 2022, which came with an estimated 1.8 million deaths (Ferlay et al., 2024). The number of people who have lung cancer is alarmingly high compared to other forms of the disease. Different parts of the world see dissimilar rates of lung cancer due to different social factors such as the number of smokers, environmental exposure as well as the availability of modernized screening programs. Even so, low and middle-income countries are expected to have these numbers rise steadily in the future due to poorly constructed tobacco control laws and little to no infrastructure for diagnosing patients with cancer (Bray et al., 2024).

Looking ahead, the trends projected for 2050 are alarming. While progress in preventive measures may mitigate some aspects of the epidemic, the aging global population, along with persistent risk factors, indicate that the total count of lung cancer cases and fatalities is likely to continue climbing. If highly accurate and targeted treatment options, along with timely diagnosis, breakthroughs are made in these areas, the socioeconomic toll from lung cancer could be reduced (Liu et al., 2023). In tackling this multifaceted crisis, combining comprehensive public health policies alongside profound medical innovation and the calculated deployment of sophisticated technologies such as radiomics and AI is essential to lessen its catastrophic impact. The focus should shift from treating the ailment to comprehensively understanding its pathophysiology for timely intervention and more precise treatment pathways (Herbst et al., 2018).

1.2 Clinical Challenges in Lung Cancer Management

The effective management of lung cancer continues to face several fundamental challenges, even with decades of clinical innovation and research. These issues are complex and span every stage of the treatment process, from the first appointment to ongoing follow-up.

First and foremost, late diagnosis is still an issue that requires improvement. A considerable number of lung cancer patients are diagnosed only after the disease progresses to its advanced stages (Stage III or IV) when it has spread to other regions of the body (Goldstraw et al., 2016). This late diagnosis significantly reduces the available treatment options. The late presentation is because early-stage lung cancer is usually slow to develop, typically masked with vague or absent symptoms, and does not exhibit distinct clinical symptoms (Bray et al., 2018). When symptoms do show up, they are often labelled as mild and non-serious, which further delays the diagnosis. Although Screening using LDCT (low-dose computed tomography) has been effective for high-risk populations (National Lung Screening Trial Research Team, 2011), there are still practical, economical, and logistical challenges to consider. Thus, the primary difficulty is designing low-risk, non-invasive, and cost-effective screening tools that can accurately identify lung nodules at the earliest and most treatable stages, ideally at a sub-symptomatic stage.

The second complication is that nodule heterogeneity poses a complex diagnostic and prognostic problem. Lung nodules, often found incidentally in imaging studies, span many diseases, from simple inflammatory processes to complex and aggressive cancers (Gould et al., 2013). It is tough to differentiate benign and malignant nodules, and further classifying the malignant ones (e.g., adenocarcinoma vs. squamous cell carcinoma and indolent vs. aggressive) is a significant challenge relying on only imaging (Travis et al., 2015). Within a single tumor, there is often substantial heterogeneity in spatial and temporal factors such as the cellular composition, genetic mutations, and the microenvironment (Jamal-Hanjani et al., 2017). This heterogeneity can create diverse clinical outcomes, different response rates to treatment, and difficulty obtaining accurate biopsies. Traditional imaging techniques do not capture this important subtle heterogeneity, and this deficiency requires more advanced analytical approaches (Kumar et al., 2012).

Variability in treatment response remains a significant barrier for personalized oncology. Patients with clinical and pathological similarities undergo different reactions to the same treatment regimen (Chemotherapy, Radiation therapy, Targeted therapy, Immunotherapy), and their response patterns can differ dramatically (Tsimberidou et al., 2020). Predicting which patients will respond positively, experience toxicity, or be neutralized is almost impossible (Prasad, 2016). The current model often resorts to trial-and-error methods, leading to unnecessary side effects, treatment delays, and suboptimal results in the case of non-responders (Hyman et al., 2017). Predictive modelling that can accurately forecast the efficacy of therapy pre-therapy commencement is required, enabling tailored intervention plans to be designed for the individual profiles of patients (Jiang et al., 2022), thus improving outcomes while reducing adverse events. Addressing these issues requires a more precise approach based on data instead of relying solely on images (Topol, 2019).

Figure 1. Lung Cancer: Key Clinical Challenges

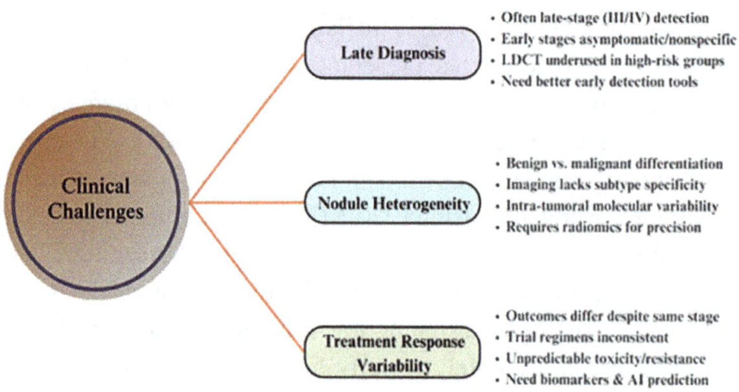

Before constructing an AI-enhanced radiomics pipeline, designing a thorough clinical framework is essential. The report outlines the steps, from initial assessment to follow-up, as per recommendations by the Fleischner Society (MacMahon et al., 2017), NCCN (National Comprehensive Cancer Network, 2024) and IASLC (Goldstraw et al., 2016). By organizing care in this structured manner, the algorithm balances the need for prompt diagnosis with the prudent use of limited resources, while identifying precise opportunities for AI-driven tools to enhance diagnostic accuracy or treatment selection.

The pseudocode provided incorporates every aspect of a complete clinical decision support system for identifying, diagnosing, staging, and managing potentially malignant lung cancer. It includes the patient's risk factors, imaging studies, AI interpretation of the images, pathology reports, and treatment formulation aligned with the stage of the disease. The system is all about speed and ensuring that no precious time is wasted when a patient's life is on the line. It is also about consistency and quality, ensuring everyone gets the best care possible. This systematic approach allows prompt identification and prolonged monitoring for the high-risk patients.

Table 1.

Step 1: Initial Risk Stratification and Triage		
IF ((Age > 50 AND Male) OR (Hemoptysis OR Weight loss > 10% OR Persistent cough) OR (Smoking history ≥ 20 pack-years OR occupational exposure) OR (First-degree relative with lung cancer))		
	THEN	
		RISK_STATUS ← ``High-Risk"
		Perform LDCT.
	ELSE	
		RISK_STATUS ← ``Low-Risk"
		Perform CXR (PA + LAT)
		IF CXR is NORMAL **THEN**
		Discharge patient. Schedule routine follow-up.
		ELSE Perform LDCT.
		ENDIF
ENDIF		

1.3 Radiomics in Clinical Oncology: A Physician's Perspective

From a clinical perspective, radiomics transforms conventional medical imaging such as CT scans, MRIs, and PET scans into quantitative datasets that can be processed and analyzed, allowing oncologists to visualize and assess tumors quantitatively (Gillies et al., 2016) (Liu et al., 2017). On a broader level, this technology solves some of the fundamental issues in everyday oncology practice by offering objective biomarkers for assessing tumor malignancy grade, estimating the likelihood of aggressive behavior and response to treatment, metastasis, and invasion (Aerts et al., 2014) (Trebeschi et al., 2019). Most importantly, these include prognostication of immunotherapy response in non-small cell lung carcinoma (NSCLC), distinguishing radiation necrosis versus recurrence in glioblastoma, and uncovering hidden metastatic lesions in head and neck cancers (Unterrainer et al., 2020) (Mayerhoefer et al., 2020). Still, caution must be exercised, considering the lack of standardization and validation as barriers to widespread utilization (Parmar, Grossmann, Bussink et al, 2015) (Barragán-Montero et al., 2021). When combined with genomic and clinical knowledge, radiomics augments but does not replace clinical decision-making in oncology (Lambin et al., 2017) (Li & Zhou, 2022).

1.4 The Interpretability Imperative in Radiomics AI

Even though AI-enhanced radiomics offers remarkable prospects for managing lung cancer, it faces a significant barrier to clinical use due to the "black box problem." This problem stems from complex deep learning algorithms, which use processes entirely inaccessible to the user for decision-making, decreasing clinician confidence and making validation difficult (Arrieta et al., 2020). This lack of transparency raises three fundamental problems (Coeckelbergh, 2020):

(a) It is impossible to check the accuracy of the predictions based on biological systems.
(b) There is no systematic way to identify and resolve inaccuracies, and
(c) The processes for determining responsibility are insufficient (Felder, 2021).

These challenges require a change in the approach to XAI, which will be discussed in Section 4.

2. AI-DRIVEN RADIOMICS PIPELINE

AI-based radiomics is a transformative computational approach for analyzing medical images, which utilizes advanced ML algorithms to obtain numerous quantitative features from standard radiographic tests (Hosny et al., 2018). Recent breakthroughs in deep radiomics have established its supremacy over traditional models for lung cancer characterization, especially in decoding the complex molecular subtypes and immunotherapy responses from regular CT imaging (Yadav et al., 2024) (Balbi et al., 2025). It permits non-invasive tumor phenotyping beyond the qualitative visual interpretation and decreases observer variability (Aerts et al., 2014),(Pei et al., 2022).

From the "black box" to the "glass box," AI implementation requires efforts in technical and clinical standardization (Zwanenburg et al., 2020). Emerging techniques in 2024 utilize physics-informed neural networks to eliminate scanner-specific distortions while maintaining biologically significant details (Zarei et al., 2024),(Xie et al., 2022). The latest IBSI-2.0 guidelines on 4DCT focus on dynamic radiomics to analyze temporal variations in tumor heterogeneity (Lei et al., 2021).

Figure 2. Process flow for lung cancer detection

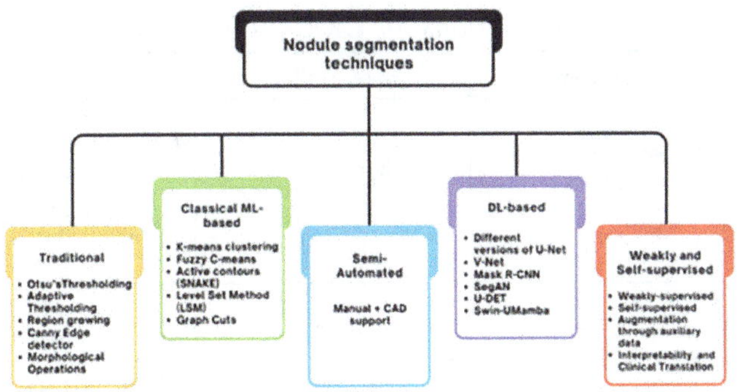

2.1 Image Acquisition and Preprocessing

High-performing radiomics frameworks for lung neoplasms depend critically on the fidelity of the source images. The selection of modality, the specific machine settings during acquisition, and post-capture fixes shape the statistical landscape from which features are mined. The following discussion reviews the main imaging techniques, X-ray, and advanced tomographic methods, with their comparative advantages and trade-offs. It then enumerates basic preprocessing routines to align the datasets for valid analysis.

2.1.1 Radiography (Chest X-Ray)

Chest X-ray (CXR) is the most accessible and affordable preliminary lung cancer screening imaging technique (Bradley et al., 2019). It is beneficial in identifying large tumors, fluid buildup in the pleural cavity (pleural effusion), and metastasis (Kakeda et al., 2004). However, due to the poor soft-tissue contrast and low sensitivity for small nodules (< 1 cm), the method has a high rate of missed diagnoses (false negatives) of early-stage cancer (Oudkerk et al., 2017). Recent advancements in digital radiography (DR) and dual-energy subtraction (DES) techniques have enhanced the capability of detecting nodules. However, CXR still falls short compared to cross-sectional imaging when performing detailed radiomic analysis (Schaefer-Prokop et al., 2008).

Standardized acquisition protocols are key to ensuring the highest possible diagnostic yield. Table 2 lists technical parameters for CXR in the evaluation of lung cancer.

Table 2. Key Technical Specifications for CXR in Lung Cancer

Parameter	PA View	Lateral View	Clinical Rationale
Patient Position	Upright, PA projection; chest in contact	Upright, LL projection; LT thorax in contact	PA ↓ cardiac magnification; lateral localizes lesions
Beam Direction	PA	Lateral	Standard projections ↓ anatomical overlap
Source-to-Image Distance	SID: 180 cm (72″)	SID: 180 cm	↓ geometric distortion & magnification
kVp	110–130 kVp	110–130 kVp	High kVp → better mediastinal penetration; ↓ bone overlap
mAs	1–5 mAs	2–6 mAs	Balances dose/noise per body habitus
Exposure Time	< 0.03 s	< 0.05 s	↓ motion artifacts
Grid Use	Yes (anti-scatter)	Yes	↓ scatter, ↑ contrast (especially in adults)
Detector Type	Digital (FPD/CR)	Digital (FPD/CR)	Enables post-processing (e.g., windowing, enhancement)
Effective Dose	0.02–0.04 mSv	0.1–0.15 mSv	Equivalent to 2–4 days background exposure (ICRP, 2017)

2.1.2 LDCT

LDCT is considered the gold standard for lung cancer screening methods because it offers high spatial resolution (~0.5–1.0 mm) and fast image acquisition (Bach et al., 2012). It minimizes radiation exposure (1–2 mSv) without compromising the ability to identify nodules. However, the anatomical structures' characterization and motion artifacts due to respiration limit LDCT efficacy (Rizzo et al., 2018). Table 3 lists technical parameters for LDCT in the evaluation of lung cancer.

Table 3. Key Technical Specifications for LDCT in Lung Cancer Detection

Parameter	LDCT Protocol	Clinical Rationale
Patient Position	Supine, arms ↑	↓ artifacts; better apical lobe viz.
Breath-Hold Time	5–10 s	↓ resp. motion artifacts
Scan Mode	Helical CT	Volumetric data in single BH (National Lung Screening Trial Research Team, 2011)(Gierada et al., 2020)
Tube Voltage	100–120 kVp	Sufficient penetration; ↓ dose, preserve contrast (MacMahon et al., 2017)
Tube Current	30–80 mAs (w/ AEC)	AEC → dose balance + IQ (Gierada et al., 2020)
Pitch	1.0–1.5	High pitch ↓ scan time & blur; ↑ dose efficiency (National Lung Screening Trial Research Team, 2011)
Slice Thickness	1.0–1.25 mm	↑ nodule detection & 3D recon (MacMahon et al., 2017)
Reconstruction Interval	0.5–1.0 mm	Ensures isotropic res. For 3D/multiplanar eval (Willemink et al., 2020)
Recon Kernel	Med-sharp (B50f/ B60f)	Edge enhances for nodules (Willemink et al., 2020)
FOV	300–400 mm	Lung-focus; ↓ excess radiation.
Nodule Threshold	≥ 4 mm	↑ sensitivity/specificity (MacMahon et al., 2017)
Radiation Dose	1.0–1.5 mSv	5–10× ↓ than std CT; NLST aligned (National Lung Screening Trial Research Team, 2011)
Contrast Use	None	Avoid contrast risks; nodules/masses visible in lung window

2.1.3 PET-CT

PET-CT combines metabolic (18F-FDG uptake) and anatomical imaging, improving tumor staging and treatment response assessment (Fletcher et al., 2008). The standardized uptake value (SUV) quantifies glucose metabolism, aiding in distinguishing malignant from benign lesions (Wahl et al., 2009). However, PET-

CT has lower spatial resolution (4–5 mm) than CT, is costly, and exposes patients to higher radiation (~7–10 mSv) (Kumar et al., 2012).

Table 4. PET-CT Protocol for Lung Cancer Evaluation

Parameter	PET-CT Protocol	Clinical Justification
Patient preparation	NPO 4–6 hrs; glucose <150 mg/dL	↓ Physiologic FDG uptake; ↑ SUV reliability
Radiotracer	^{18}F-FDG IV	Tags metabolically active lesions
Dose	3.7–5.5 MBq/kg (0.1–0.15 mCi/kg)	Balances image quality vs radiation dose
Uptake Time	60 ± 10 min post-FDG	Standardizes SUV comparability
Positioning	Supine; arms above head	↓ Attenuation; reproducible FOV
Scan Extent	Skull base → mid-thigh	Captures primary + metastatic sites
CT Component	Low-dose CT ± contrast	For attenuation correction + anatomy
CT Params	120 kVp; 30–80 mAs; 3–5 mm slices	Low-dose for staging; contrast CT for diagnosis
PET Acq. Time	2–3 min/bed position (3D mode)	Ensures count density, especially in ↑ BMI
Reconstruction	OSEM (2–3 iterations, 16–24 subsets); TOF + PSF	↑ Lesion detectability; accurate SUVmax, TLG
Attenuation Correction	CT-based algorithm	Enables quantitation (SUV, MTV)
SUV Normalization	SUVBW, SUL (SUVLBM)	SUL preferred in obese patients
Spatial Resolution	4–6 mm FWHM	Detects nodules ≥8 mm
Artifacts	Respiratory motion, inflammatory uptake	May mimic malignancy; gated/delayed imaging advised
Optional Add-ons	IV contrast CT, brain PET, respiratory gating	Refines staging; detects metastasis

2.1.4 MRI

MRI offers superior soft-tissue contrast without ionizing radiation, making it valuable for assessing tumor vascularity (via DCE-MRI) and cellularity (via diffusion-weighted imaging) (Meier-Schroers et al., 2018). Ultra-short echo time (UTE) sequences improve lung signal detection. However, MRI has longer acquisition times, susceptibility to motion artifacts, and lower availability in screening settings (Biederer et al., 2012).

Table 5. MRI Protocol for Lung Cancer Staging

Parameter	Protocol	Rationale
Scanner/Coil	1.5T/3T; 12–32 ch thoracic coil	3T: ↑SNR; 1.5T: ↓motion artifact
Preparation	No fasting; remove metal	Artifact ↓; safety ↑
Position	Supine; arms ↑/alongside	↓Motion; reproducibility
Resp. Control	Breath-hold (10–20s) or navigator	Blur ↓ in thoracic structures
ECG Gating	Optional; if cardiac invasion suspected	↓Cardiac motion artifact
T1W Seq.	Ax/cor FSE/SPGR/VIBE; 3–5 mm	Fat plane, invasion
T2W Seq.	Ax/cor STIR/HASTE; FS; ≤1 mm gap	Necrosis, edema, cysts
DWI	b = 0–800 s/mm^2; EPI; ADC map	Diffusion restriction; nodes
Dynamic MRI	Gd 0.1 mmol/kg; art–ven–delayed	Perfusion, angiogenesis
MRA	3D GRE post-Gd; resp-gated	Vascular encasement
FOV/Res.	300–400 mm; in-plane ≤1.5 mm	Lesion margin clarity
Slices	3–5 mm; gap ≤1 mm; 3D pref.	Res–coverage balance
Resp Tools	Navigator, bellows, ext. trigger	Motion-free acquisition

Standardization and Preprocessing

Radiomic features, which quantify a tissue's phenotype, are susceptible to differences in image acquisition parameters. Differences in acquisition parameters such as slice thickness, pixel spacing, reconstruction kernels, scanner manufacturers' magnetic field strength (MRI), and tube current and voltage (CT) will significantly affect image intensity, noise contrast, and spatial resolution. The subtle differences directly affect the first-order (e.g., mean, standard deviation), shape- and texture-based (e.g., GLCM or GLRLM matrices) radiomic features and cause significant variability. Therefore, a radiomic signature derived using one specific imaging protocol may not be replicable or applicable if different acquisition parameters are used. Thus, for the radiomic features to be stable across multiple sites and scanners, rigorous standardization of imaging acquisition parameters or practical post-acquisition harmonization approaches is needed.

- **Digital Imaging and Communications in Medicine (DICOM)** is an international standard that governs the storage of metadata in medical imaging to harmonize multicentre research studies (Clunie, 2001). DICOM also specifies the parameters for the pixel data, such as pixel spacing and bit depth, which are necessary to ensure that images display correctly and consistently. This means that medical images can be easily shared between hospitals and medical systems, essential when researchers want to extract radiomic features from many images.

- Variability in voxel dimensions can have a substantial impact on radiomics feature extraction. When texture features are extracted from images with anisotropic voxels (e.g., 0.5×0.5×2~mm^3), the resulting texture features may be biased because of the distorted sample space. Isotropic resampling directly addresses the problem of inconsistent voxel dimensions in lung cancer imaging, reduces the influence of differing acquisition settings, and improves the stability of derived radiomic features. Such consistency becomes essential because tumors can shift with each breath, and reliable metrics are mandatory for any feature-based clinical decision (Lee et al., 2019) (Mackin et al., 2018). The voxel dimension is a dominant factor driving reproducibility as larger voxels (3×3×3~mm^3) result in poorer reproducibility compared to smaller ones (2×2×2~mm^3). Moreover, the measurements taken by the same radiologist on a given slice were more consistent than those between different observers, underlining the importance of independently having an individual outline a region of interest (Zhong et al., 2024). In medical practice, isotropic resampling is indispensable for radiomic model generalization (across CT and MRI scans) and precise tumor motion estimation (in 4D imaging) (Bortolotto et al., 2024). However, it is not a standalone solution. To achieve optimal reliability in radiomic studies, other parameters, including segmentation variability, need to be considered in addition to isotropic resampling and adequate filtering.
- Most radiomic features in PET/CT are sensitive to respiratory motion. In ^{18}F-FDG PET, over 96% of features were respiratory motion-sensitive (ICC >0.9 and COV <5%), even post-correction using a data-driven gating algorithm, thus categorizing them as nonviable for subsequent ML modelling (Chen et al., 2023). Feature stability varies across respiratory phases, with shape features proving most stable (COV ≤10%) compared to others during 4D CT imaging (Du et al., 2019). Furthermore, motion amplitudes exceeding 2.5~mm cause a sharp deterioration in feature consistency (Adachi et al., 2022). Numerous motion-correction strategies have been developed for hybrid imaging. Joint Correction frameworks for PET/CT target the dual problems of motion blur and partial-volume loss (Chang et al., 2010). Local Respiratory Motion Correction (LRMC) confines adjustments to user-defined regions and often relies on elastic modeling to track shifting tumors (Lamare et al., 2015). The Motion Freeze Technique couples deformable image registration with gated data sets to mitigate discrepancies in tumor shape between PET and CT (Huang et al., 2014).

The datasets listed below (Table 5) are extensively utilized in radiomics research.

Table 6. Summary of Public Lung Imaging Datasets

Dataset	Type	Number of Images/ Samples	Format	Annotated
ANODE09	CT	NA/55	Meta	
BMIRDS	FFPE	143/143	Pyramidal TIFF	✓
ChstX-ray14	DX	112,120/30,805	PNG	✓
CheXpert	CT	224,316/65,240	JPEG	✓
CPTAC-LAUD	CT, MR, PT	43,333/25	DICOM	✓
DeepLesion	CT	32,120/10,594	PNG	✓
I-ELCAP	CT	NA/50	DICOM	✓
IQ-OTII/NCCD	CT	1190/110	PNG	✓
JSRT	CR	247/247	PGM	✓
LC25000	H&E	15000/NA	JPEG	✓
LIDC-IDRI	CT, DX, CR	244,527/1018	DICOM	✓
LNDb	CT	294/NA	Meta	✓
LungCT-Diagnosis	CT	4682/61	DICOM	
Lung TIME	CT	NA/157	DICOM	✓
Lung-PET-CT-Dx	CT, PT	251,135/355	DICOM	✓
LUNA 16	CT	888/888	Meta	✓
MIMIC-CXR	CR	377,110/227,835	DICOM	✓
NELSON	CT	7557/NA	DICOM	✓
NLST	CT	26254/451	DICOM	✓
NSCLC-Radiomics	CT	52073/422	DICOM	✓
PadChest	CR	160868/67625	DICOM	✓
P4-LUCAT	Clinical	NA/1242	CSV	✓
PN9	CT	8,798/NA	DICOM	✓
QIN LUNG CT	CT	3,954/47	DICOM	✓
RIDER Lung CT	CT	81548/32	DICOM	✓
Rider Lung PET-CT	PT, CT	266,280/243	DICOM	✓
SPIE-AAPM Lung CT Challenge	CT	22,489/70	DICOM	✓

2.2 Nodule Segmentation for Lung Cancer Radiomics

Widely prevalent semi-automated CAD-assisted lung nodule segmentation remains time-consuming, labour-intensive, and challenging. Divergence in opinion among radiologists undermines reproducibility. Moreover, the shortage of experienced radiologists also increases workload and the risk of errors. Even an expert's eye can overlook small lesions or subtle nodules, particularly those attached to vessels, the parenchymal wall, or the diaphragm, and that misses prove fatal for early-stage cancer intervention. Traditional methods like Otsu's thresholding often fail to segment these nodules accurately. DL methods, such as U-Net and Mask R-CNN, use CNNs to detect and segment nodules better, improving accuracy in medical imaging.

To accurately segment nodules from medical images, a variety of computational techniques—differing in their level of complexity and automation—are illustrated in the Fig. 3 below.

Figure 3. Categorization of nodule segmentation techniques

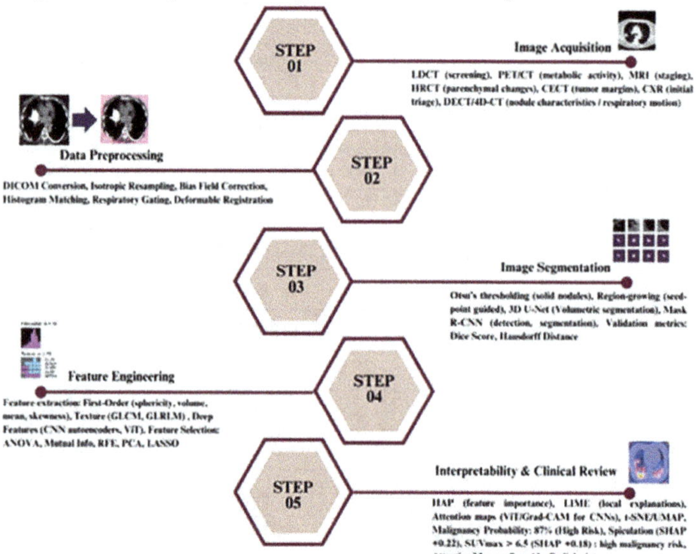

2.2.1. Traditional Techniques

Otsu's Thresholding (Otsu, 1975)

Key concept: An unsupervised global thresholding algorithm separates grayscale images into two parts: the foreground and background. The algorithm identifies the optimal threshold that minimizes the combined variance within each class (foreground and background) or equivalently maximizes the inter-class variance over the intensity histogram. This method works under an assumption that the histogram contains two distinct peaks corresponding to objects of interest and background objects respectively.

Otsu's method is becoming the best performer for well-defined, high-contrast solid nodules appearing as distinctly brighter or darker regions in CT scans, creating a prominent bimodal intensity histogram. Otsu's method fulfils two primary roles. First, it generates an initial binary mask through more sophisticated techniques such as region-growing algorithms, active contour models, or watershed transforms (Ying et al., 2009). Second, it provides an approximate region of interest (ROI) that helps constrain subsequent high-precision segmentation methods to relevant areas, thereby improving computational efficiency. The method also proves valuable in computer-aided detection (CAD) systems by facilitating preliminary identification of suspicious nodule candidates before applying morphological operations or advanced feature extraction techniques (Arimura & Suzuki, 2017).

Limitations: It struggles with juxta-pleural and juxta-vascular nodules (where there is an overlap of intensity distributions between the nodule and adjacent structures), subsolid nodules (where there is no sharp enough contrast difference), or noisy images (Zhang, Zhang, Zhao et al, 2017).

Adaptive Thresholding

Key Concepts: Adaptive thresholding enhances the lung nodules' segmentation by locally adjusting the image background to improve the subsolid/GGO nodules and juxta-pleural/vascular nodules. Local Otsu (applying Otsu's method to sliding windows), Niblack/Sauvola (adapting to local mean/standard deviation), and block-based thresholding (processing subregions independently). Adaptive methods are also more advantageous regarding intensity inhomogeneity and low dose/noisy CT scans, which significantly affect global methods and allow better segmentation of small, irregular, and low-contrast nodules (Lavanya et al., 2020) (Li et al., 2016).

Limitations: Block-level methods or local Otsu struggle when the nodule brightness is similar to the surrounding lung tissue. Even though the adaptive methods (e.g., Niblack Sauvola) can deal with non-uniform illumination, they still need careful parameter tuning to obtain satisfactory results. Traditional methods are inferior to cutting-edge deep-learning pipelines in segmenting challenging lesions such as juxta-pleural nodules or ground-glass opacities (Rocha et al., 2020) (Kido et al., 2022).

Region Growing

Key Concepts:

- The region-growing (Adams & Bischof, 1994) begins with a chosen seed point and, step by step, pulls in neighboring pixels that meet a user-set similarity score. Researchers appreciate the method because its algorithm is simple to code, runs relatively quickly, and produces unbroken patches, provided the target object exhibits strong contrast against its background.
- The adaptive region growing technique (Ren et al., 2020) dynamically modifies the similarity threshold during the region's expansion. The adaptation relies on the growing region's local image characteristics (mean intensity and standard deviation), making it more robust to the intensity variation within the object to be segmented.
- Multi-seed region growing (Heizmann et al., 2020) initiates the segmentation process from several points, which can be either manually placed or automatically identified. It then combines the individual regions that arise from the seeds. It is particularly effective for cases where the nodule to be segmented is complex and highly broken because it does not rely heavily on the accuracy of one seed point.
- 3D Region Growing (Cui et al., 2017) applies the region growing method across several CT scan slices for the volumetric segmentation of nodules. This method utilizes the spatial information of connected voxels to extract precise information regarding the entire circumference of a nodule in CT/PET-CT images for consequent analysis.
- Fuzzy Region Growing applies several sophisticated strategies to improve the segmentation of nodules from CT images. Such resilience is vital when radiologists must quickly decide whether a lesion is malignant or benign (Manikandan & Bharathi, 2011). An alternative method known as Adaptive Sphericity Oriented Contrast Region Growing leverages a fuzzy connectivity map to prune background clutter around vessels and other complex anatomy. In addition, a method based on fuzzy c-means clustering and region growing technique was proposed to reduce false positives for accurate lung nodules segmentation (Wang et al., 2015).
- Hybrid methods (Lu et al., 2015) combine the watershed or morphological operations for better nodule boundary smoothness and minimal leakage to adjacent structures. Advanced hybrid techniques combine several algorithms, typically regional growth and active contours, sometimes adding a machine learning module to improve the selection of initial points.

Limitations:

- Over-segmentation or under-segmentation might occur because the region-growing method relies heavily on the precise selection of seed points and an exact predefined intensity threshold. It can fail in cases where there is intensity variation within the object, low contrast between the object and background (e.g., ground-glass opacities), or "leakage" into adjacent structures (e.g., juxta-pleural nodules) (Kumar et al., 2012).

- The adaptive region growing method can still leak if the object of interest is tightly connected to surrounding structures with similar intensity profiles. Moreover, finding the best rules for this adjustment is not trivial (Dehmeshki et al., 2008).
- An efficient technique for selecting multiple seeds and definition of merging criterion is necessary to avoid possible leakage in (Heizmann et al., 2020).
- The method (Cui et al., 2017) still struggles with precise boundary identification in noisy images and distinguishing nodules from adjacent tissues of similar intensity. Moreover, it is computationally expensive since precise registration is a prerequisite for volumetric inter-slices nodules analysis.
- The fuzzy region growing approach is more computationally complex and requires careful consideration and tuning of the fuzzy membership functions, and the obtained results may be harder to interpret. This mainly arises from its high computational cost and parameter setting sensitivity when applied to GGO and other subsolid nodule analyses.
- Implementation of (Lu et al., 2015) requires precise adjustments to all algorithm parameters.

Canny Edge Detector

Key Concepts: The widely used Canny edge-detection procedure begins with a Gaussian filter to minimize high-frequency noise. It then estimates the gradient and eliminates all non-maximum gradient points, yielding a precise local maximum. Two thresholds (high and low) categorize edges into strong, weak, and non-edges. Gradients are generated via the derivative of the Gaussian filter, ensuring directional consistency. While it is reliable on single-channel grayscale images, extending this procedure to RGB images requires additional color-space conversions, complicating adaptive thresholding across multiple channels (Jadwaa, 2022).

Limitations: Subtle medical images are highly vulnerable to misdiagnosis due to being highly susceptible to noise and poor handling of various nodule sizes with its fixed scale. In complex medical imaging, blood vessels and bones can generate considerable gradients and may disrupt the actual boundaries of lung nodules. As a consequence, these structures can obstruct the actual contours of lung nodules, resulting in erroneous gradient-based localization where the algorithm perceives fragments of blood vessels or bones as nodule boundaries and fails to accurately characterize the nodule's boundary (McIlhagga, 2011). Canny Edge Detector is inconsistent with nodule complexity (size, shape, and texture).

Morphological Operations (Gonzalez, 2009)

Key Concepts: Morphological operations (i.e., dilation, erosion, opening, and closing) are frequently applied to improve the clarity and reliability of lung-nodule segmentation in CT scans. Dilation expands the objects while erosion shrinks. Opening (erosion followed by dilation) is utilized to smooth the boundaries of objects and remove thin protrusions, while closing (dilation followed by erosion) is used to join narrow gaps and eliminate small holes. The shape and dimensions of the structuring element (kernel) utilized to scan the image determine which pixels will be impacted. More sophisticated techniques, such as morphological gradients and top-hat transformations, further focus on nodule edges and eliminate background non-uniformity.

Limitations: Classical morphological operators rely solely on the predefined shape and size of the structuring elements. Nodule morphological mismatching could also lead to over/under-segmentation. It utterly fails to differentiate the boundaries of adjacent structures when the nodules are irregular or have low contrast and sometimes miss the entire lesion. Preprocessing is obligatory because the subsequent operations are highly susceptible to any form of noise or irrelevant structural information known as artifacts. Therefore, traditional methods usually combine DL or thresholding techniques to achieve accurate segmentation.

2.2.2 Classical Machine Learning-Based Methods

K-means Clustering

Key Concepts (Flores Cuautle et al., 2024): K-means clustering is an unsupervised ML approach that sorts CT scan pixels based on their grayscale intensities. It is optimal for use in the preliminary lung nodule segmentation. As the algorithm allocates each pixel to one of the k nearest cluster centers, brighter and denser regions (i.e., nodules) are separated from the lung tissue background. K-means works best for solid nodules when a distinct separation exists. Later versions, like k-means++ (Arthur & Vassilvitskii, 2006), aim to improve the speed and stability of initial centroid selection while retaining a measure of efficiency. K-means++ offers near real-time execution for preliminary segmentation compared to more advanced techniques due to its relatively low computational demands. The technique has barriers as it can precisely identify the borders only if there is a substantial difference in intensities.

Limitations: K-means segmentation often stumbles when a lung nodule and the adjacent tissues display nearly identical grayscale levels, as the algorithm is fully intensity-dependent. The manual selection of clusters remains a time-consuming process and is susceptible to various errors. Combining K-means with CNN and a few morphological tweaks can lift overall segmentation performance by a substantial margin.

Fuzzy C-Means (FCM)

Key Concepts: FCM is an effective method for segmenting lung nodule images as it deals with uncertainty, a common problem in medical image diagnosis. Traditional methods categorize pixels into discrete groups with rigid boundaries. FCM assigns pixels to clusters based on the degree of membership rather than using a hard threshold. The flexibility of this technique to better classify the nodules and surrounding lung structures when there is an overlap in intensity values between these two different tissues. Several advanced variants are being developed to address the shortcomings of the traditional FCM. Self-adaptive FCM (SA-FCM) (Liu et al., 2015) integrates ML with spatial and grayscale information in the image space, particularly those with vascular attachments and ground-glass opacities. Robust FCM (rFCM) (Liu et al., 2015) incorporates a penalty term to mitigate noise and intensity inhomogeneity effects. Intelligent FCM (IFCM) (Kavitha et al., 2019) employs the firefly algorithm to optimize initial cluster centers for faster convergence—this scheme achieves significant accuracy improvements when coupled with AI-based classifiers. These advanced FCM approaches collectively provide a more flexible and accurate framework for nodule segmentation, thereby helping to enable earlier and more dependable lung cancer screening in routine clinical practice.

Limitations: First, it is misled by image noise and artifacts, which results in incorrect nodule contour modeling. Secondly, for the nodules with a similar appearance to adjacent anatomical structures such as blood vessels, the algorithm may merge or separate them inaccurately.

Moreover, the method is slow with detailed scans, limiting its applicability in time critical medical settings. It ignores the proximity of pixels to one another, which can lead to a patchy appearance. Doctors and technicians also struggle because precise settings have to be selected manually. If poor choices are made, parts of nodules can either be missed or non-existent ones can appear (Li et al., 2020).

And perhaps most critically, FCM struggles with the faint and tiny nodules that do not protrude well from the images.

Active Contours (Snakes)

Key Features: Active contour models, also known as snakes, progressively adjust an initial contour model to the target boundary by minimizing a defined energy function (Itai et al., 2005). The energy model in the active contour algorithm has two basic components: image forces, which are external energies that move the snake toward the target image feature, and internal energies, which preserve smoothness and continuity. Together, these elements enable the snakes to conform to the detailed and frequently jagged outlines of lung nodules while guarding against random noise and misleading edges that can appear in medical scans.

Limitations: If the model is poorly initialized, it will not converge and find the object of interest. Manual corrections were needed to precisely trace the contours of the juxta-pleural nodule because the algorithm could "leak" into adjacent structures.

Level Set Methods (LSMs) (Biswas & Hazra, 2022)

Key Concepts: LSMs are a powerful mathematical tool for implementing geometric deformable models. Osher and Sethian (1988) proposed that the LSMs represent contours as the zero-level set of a higher-dimensional function $\phi(x,y,t)$, which allows them to handle cases when the tracked contour splits or merges naturally. For better visualization, Fig. 4 shows the simplified process flow of the LSM.

Figure 4. LSM flow

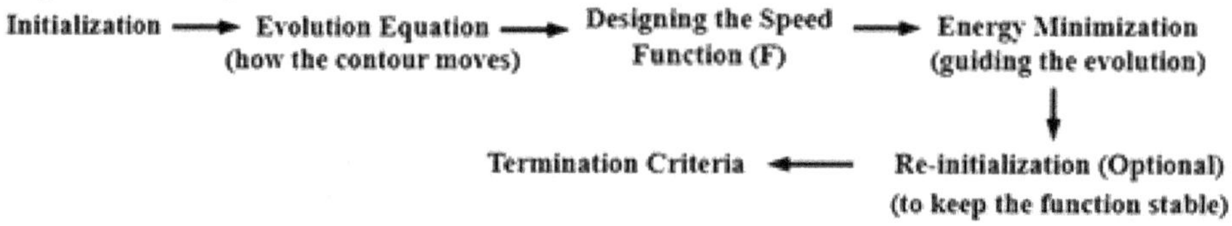

Limitations: LSMs require the initial contour to be placed near the actual boundary; otherwise, it might evolve into an incorrect solution and need several reinitializations or significant parameter tuning (Liu, Bai, Li et al, 2018). The second challenge relates to the nodules that exhibit low contrast with surrounding structures and are difficult to delineate, particularly when the lesion topology shifts from solid to juxta-pleural or ground glass (Roy et al., 2020). The third limitation is that the level set evolution and reinitialization are computationally expensive because multiple iterations are required, which makes this method time-consuming. Another issue is the tendency to misclassify blood vessels as nodules, leading to false positives, a problem highlighted by (Krishnamurthy et al., 2016).

Graph Cuts (Dai et al., 2015)

Key Concepts: Modelling the image into a weighted connected graph and applying the graph cut theorem is an elegant approach to image segmentation. It regards an image as a graph with pixels as nodes and edges connecting neighboring pixels. The approach has two terminal nodes. One is called a source node, and the other is a sink node. The source node indicates the foreground, and the sink node indicates the background. The weights are determined not only by the pixel similarity but also by the penalties when there is a sudden change of intensity in pixels that are supposed to be joined.

The approach finds the minimum-cost cut to partition the graph into two distinct regions, effectively separating the foreground from the background. It guarantees a globally optimal outcome for the specified energy function, eliminates the need for iterative fine-tuning, and readily handles irregular contours. In lung nodule segmentation, seed points placed within the lungs (foreground) and the adjacent thoracic regions (background) allow the algorithm to generate an accurate lung mask without any subsequent adjustment.

Limitations: Perfect manual foreground/background seed initialization produces optimum outcomes, whereas a poor seed selection model leads to under-segmentation. 3D CT volumes add another layer of difficulty because they consume considerable memory and run noticeably slower than simpler thresholding approaches. It struggles with familiar features of pulmonary nodules, including low-contrast ground-glass opacities, uneven margins, and the frequent false positives triggered by adjacent vessels. If nodules are attached to the lung wall, very tiny growths under 5mm, or if the nodules contain solid and somewhat hazy components, graph cut is the least efficient choice.

2.2.3. Semi-Automated Approaches

Manual + CAD Support

Key Concepts: The semi-automated approach (ReGANS model (Ren et al., 2020)) for segmenting lung nodules fuses the proficiency of skilled clinicians and intelligent computer-aided design systems. The process starts with the radiologist placing a single marker or "seed" in the center of a suspected nodule. That tiny seed initialized by the user acts as an input for the algorithm, which will automatically expand and outline the desired lesion area based on sophisticated region-growing techniques. It simply injects the expert's intuition into the system, thus maintaining human control while leveraging the machine's speed and consistency. The final objective is to minimize the time healthcare experts need to spend on segmentation while enhancing precision beyond achievable through entirely manual approaches.

Limitations (Girvin & Ko, 2008): This technique still suffers from a reliance on user-defined initialization, requiring exact seeds or contours from radiologists.

2.2.4. Deep Learning-Based Techniques

Studying the evolution of DL techniques for medical-image segmentation helps trace the path from the origins to modern approaches. The following timeline (Fig.

5) lists the architectural evolution, i.e., the transition from basic CNN to current transformer-based hybrid models.

A review of the developmental history of DL medical-segmentation networks shows that many leading models continue to build on, or draw inspiration from, the original U-Net architecture. First presented in 2015 as a solution for segmenting biomedical images, U-Net quickly became the benchmark encoder–decoder structure for two- and three-dimensional tasks. Its flexible, modular layout and the ability to learn effectively from relatively few labelled samples make it particularly attractive for real-world clinical settings.

Segmentation performance is typically measured using the Dice coefficient (Dice Similarity Coefficient, DSC), with scores above 0.7 viewed as clinically acceptable for nodule boundary delineation in radiological practice (Taha & Hanbury, 2015), and the Intersection-over-Union (IoU, or Jaccard index), where values larger than 0.6 signal solid spatial overlap (Yeghiazaryan & Voiculescu, 2015). Sensitivity, or recall, remains critical for detecting actual nodule voxels. In contrast, precision curbs the number of false-positive inclusions, and together these metrics underlie any trustworthy diagnostic claim (Armato et al., 2011). Boundary accuracy, critical in longitudinal monitoring, is usually quantified via the Hausdorff Distance (HD), with estimates below 5 mm widely considered acceptable in lung-nodule studies (Hofmanninger et al., 2020). The accompanying Fig. 6 depicts the standard U-Net design, emphasising the symmetric contraction and expansion pathways linked by skip connections.

Figure 5. Timeline of deep learning innovations in medical image segmentation over a decade.

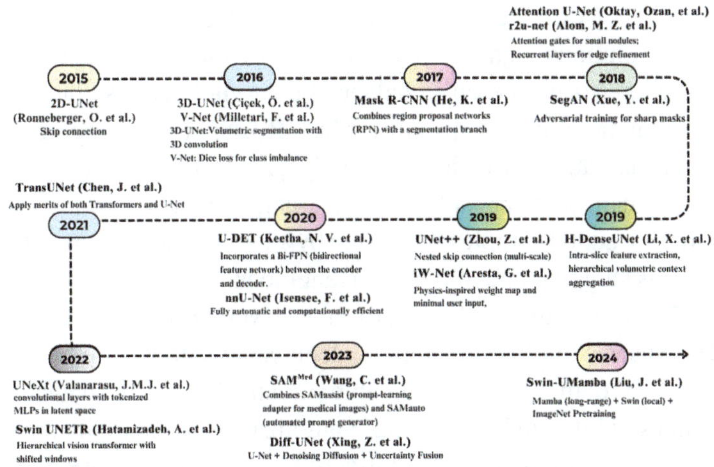

Figure 6. U-Net architecture with encoder–decoder structure and skip connections

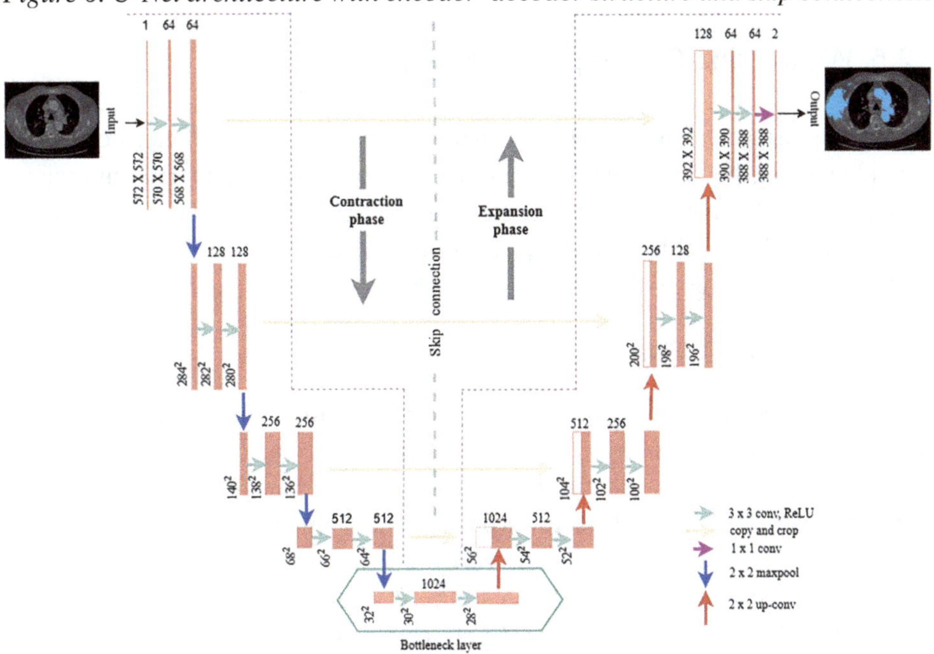

Limitations: Although medical image segmentation has advanced rapidly in the last decade, every new deep-learning model still has distinct drawbacks.

The plain vanilla 2D U-Net (2015) has an intrinsic limitation of not being able to capture 3D context and is thus suboptimal for segmenting volumetric medical images like CT or MRI. Meanwhile, 3D U-Net (2016) extended it by introducing volumetric convolutions, significantly increasing GPU memory requirements. V-Net (2016) boosted performance on imbalanced data via Dice loss but was still hard to train and computationally expensive. Mask R-CNN (2017) requires meticulous bounding box annotations, which are typically unavailable in medical imaging datasets since they mainly offer pixel-level mask annotations. Attention U-Net (2018) cannot handle the added complexity created by attention mechanisms. The R2U-Net (2018) model is sluggish due to the recurrent blocks.

SegAN (2018) struggles with stability and convergence during adversarial training, and H-DenseUNet (2019) cannot be deployed due to a huge parameter count. TransUNet (2021) demands an unattainable amount of annotated data for implementation in clinics, while nnU-Net's (2021) automated setups are incomprehensible. Swin UNETR (2022) requires prohibitively high amounts of VRAM (> 24GB), making it inaccessible for most hospitals, and Diff-UNet's (2023) diffusion-based refinement is computationally expensive. While SAM-Med (2023) minimizes the requirement for annotations due to its general-purpose nature, it tends to over-segment neighboring structures. Swin-UMamba (2024), while purportedly efficient, has not been tested on clinical applications because it is still new.

2.2.5. Weakly and Self-Supervised Learning

Annotating medical images for fully supervised learning is a significant bottleneck in implementing powerful segmentation techniques. Weakly and self-supervised learning methods have shown that it is possible to significantly cut down the annotation costs and still achieve an adequate performance level. These models require little supervision, ranging from image-level labels to entirely unannotated datasets.

Weakly Supervised CNNs

The weakly supervised ones show impressive flexibility in learning from incomplete annotations. Authors (Feng et al., 2017), who utilized a classification-trained CNN for segmentation by identifying discriminative regions from activation maps with only image-level labels. It achieved performance comparable to fully supervised methods while reducing annotation efforts by orders of magnitude. Later, researchers added spatial limits to the traditional fuzzy C-means method (Liu, Geng, Guo et al, 2018). The approach considered grayscale and spatial likenesses for better identification of nodule boundaries. A 3D CNN based on supervoxels could analyze nodules of different shapes using only one coordinate per nodule (Feng et al., 2023).

Self-Supervised Paradigms

Self-supervised strategies remove the need for explicit annotations by mining supervisory information directly from the inherent organisation of the data. For example, authors (Zhang et al., 2018) proposed an iterative self-learning pipeline in which an initial segmentation prediction is repeatedly updated by later iterations, reinforcing a positive feedback loop that improves detection of cystic lesions. This method can be straightforwardly extended to nodule segmentation tasks. More recently, contrastive-learning systems (Djahnine et al., 2024) have demonstrated notable success, with networks pretrained on extensive, unlabelled collections of chest CT images localising disease better after only minimal, task-oriented fine-tuning. By structuring pretext objectives around data augmentation and instance discrimination, these pipelines extract rich, latent features specific to nodules.

Augmentation Through Auxiliary Data

Weakly and self-supervised systems significantly benefit if the designers exploit any available auxiliary information. Authors (Yang et al., 2021) demonstrated this in a medical imaging task by enriching a training pipeline with linked electronic medical records (EMR). The system automatically locates lung nodules by generating risk scores and indicating the exact axial slice number, thus eliminating the need for manual bounding boxes. This work emphasizes the power of simple and modest metadata and its substantial effect on the performance of cutting-edge segmentation architectures in radiological applications.

Interpretability and Clinical Translation

A key improvement in these techniques is their rising interpretability. Models such as WSUnet (O'Shea et al., 2023) generate voxel-level probability maps from image-level annotations, giving clinicians clear decision boundaries. When paired with Dice coefficients nearing 0.75 in independent evaluations, this clarity reinforces the models' suitability for prospective clinical deployment.

Challenges and Future Directions

However, there is still a performance disparity between the discussed and fully supervised models, especially in the independent test set for sub-3 mm nodules, where adequate feature representation remains challenging. Current studies focus on hybrid approaches that aim to close the gap between fully automatic and interactive methods and make algorithms more robust toward different acquisition parameters. If these directions sustain their current momentum, they could make reliable, fine-grained segmentation widely available in clinics with limited computing or annotation resources.

2.3 Feature Extraction and Selection

Radiomic analysis takes medical images and, through a standardized process, pulls out a wide range of numbers that each describe something specific about the tissues' physical and biological properties. Doctors and researchers then use these numbers as the foundation for predictive models, guiding diagnosis, treatment, and follow-up decisions. The specific features can vary widely depending on the imaging technology used and the type of tumor examined, covering everything from simple brightness measurements to complex calculations of texture and three-dimensional shape. Table 6 lists the key radiomic features scientists often use when looking at lung nodules.

Table 6. Radiomic Feature Categories and Clinical Significance in Lung Nodule Evaluation

Category	Key Features	Clinical Significance
Shape / Morphological (Zwanenburg et al., 2020)	Volume, Sphericity, Surface/Volume Ratio, Compactness, 3D Diameter, Solidity	Irregular shape/spiculation → invasive; Sphericity < 0.7 → malignancy
First-Order Statistics (Parmar, Leijenaar, Grossmann et al, 2015)	Mean, MAD, Entropy, Energy, Uniformity	Entropy ↑ → necrosis; Energy ↑ → cellularity
GLCM (Song et al., 2023)	Contrast, Correlation, Cluster Prominence, IMC	High Cluster Prominence → chaotic texture (e.g., SCC)
GLSZM / GLRLM (Song et al., 2023)	Zone/Run Emphasis, GLNU	GLNU > 2.0 → heterogeneity (e.g., adenocarcinoma)
NGTDM (Wilson & Devaraj, 2017)	Coarseness, Busyness, Complexity	Coarseness < 0.1 → ground-glass opacity (early ADC)
Wavelet (Oneda et al., 2020)	HHH_Entropy, LLL_Skewness, HLH_IMC2	Captures multiscale texture; HHH_Entropy → microstructure
LoG (Oneda et al., 2020)	LoG_GLDM_NonUniformity, LoG_GLCM_Idmn	Highlights edges/spiculation; 3mm filter suits 5–10 mm nodules
DCE (De Visschere et al., 2017)	Wash-In Rate, TTP, SIR, K^{trans}	SIR > 1.5 → malignant perfusion (via DCE-MRI)
Diffusion (De Visschere et al., 2017)	ADC_Mean, ADC_P10, DKI Kurtosis, Restricted Fraction	ADC < 1.1×10^{-3} mm^2/s → high cellularity (e.g., SCLC)

The high-dimensional radiomic features (e.g., shape, texture, wavelet) are often highly interrelated and redundant. While these features capture clinically relevant heterogeneity, models that directly use them are prone to overfitting and lack interpretability, especially in lung nodules where the number of patients is often small compared with the number of features. Dimensionality reduction plays an essential role in three aspects: (1) identifying features that are biologically relevant and interpretable, (2) excluding noise that is not reproducibly measurable, and (3) ensuring algorithmic feasibility. Table 7 displays the comparison of methods that are typically used to reduce the dimensionality of the data or select features in radiomics. Collectively, these methods help manage high dimensionality without discarding the clinical insights needed for reliable patient diagnosis.

Table 7. Comparison of Dimensionality Reduction and Feature Selection Methods in Radiomics

Method			Mechanism	Use Case	Limitations	Clinical Utility
PCA (Zhang, Oikonomou, Wong et al, 2017)	US	L	Linear ⟶ max-var features	Denoising, feature decorrelation	Feature meaning lost	Survival stratification
ICA (Zhang, Oikonomou, Wong et al, 2017)	US	M	Source separation via ICs	Non-Gaussian texture patterns	Computaional load, order issues	DCE-MRI heterogeneity
ZV/NZV (Zhang, Oikonomou, Wong et al, 2017)	F	H	Remove low-var. features	Quick prefiltering	May drop rare but key traits	Multicentre harmonization
CC (Zhang, Oikonomou, Wong et al, 2017)	US	M	Consensus from multi-clusters	Subtype stability	Metric-sensitive	LUAD subtype profiling
LASSO (Yang et al., 2023)	S	H	L1 shrinkage (sparse selection)	Biomarker reduction	Struggles w/ collinearity	EGFR mutation prediction
t-SNE (Tunali et al., 2021)	US	N	Non-linear local manifold	Visualizing complex data	No back-mapping	GGN subtype exploration
RF (Parmar, Grossmann, Bussink et al, 2015)	S	M	Tree-based feature ranking	Non-linear dependency	Bias to high-cardinality	Shape features for IO response
UMAP (Yousefi et al., 2019)	US	N	Topology-aware embedding	Speedy cluster/ visualization	Param-sensitive	SCLC subtype clustering
mRMR (Yang et al., 2022)	S	H	↑Relevance, ↓Redundancy	Small, interpretable panels	Sub-optimal global search	12-feature benign/ malignant ID
sPLS-DA (Zhou et al., 2024)	S	M	Sparse latent projection	Multiclass, collinear data	Complex tuning	Histology-level classification
AE (Li et al., 2024)	US	L	Neural latent compression	Deep/high-D radiomics	Black-box, data hungry	Prognostic CT texture encoding

S = Supervised, US = Unsupervised, F = Filter; ITP = Interpretability: H = High, M = Medium, L = Low, N = None; RF = Random Forest, CC = Consensus Clustering, AE = Autoencoders.

3. INTERPRETABLE MODEL TRAINING AND VALIDATION

Transforming unprocessed medical images into meaningful recommendations for lung cancer care relies on artificial intelligence systems that combine high accuracy with clear explainability. Clinicians will only trust and routinely use a prediction if they can see, in understandable terms, the reasoning behind it. To build that trust, a step-by-step strategy for training and testing these systems, one that balances strict statistical checks with design choices that make the inner workings visible.

3.1. Data Preparation and Partitioning

The reliability of a high-performing AI model depends mainly on the quality and preparation of the underlying data. In lung cancer radiomics studies, this means assembling labeled datasets in which extracted radiomic features are paired with definitive ground-truth markers such as histopathology results, molecular assay findings (for example, EGFR or KRAS mutation status), or agreements reached among expert radiologists regarding tumor malignancy.

Before training an ML model, researchers need to split the dataset carefully so that the model produces an unbiased performance estimate and avoids unintentional data leakage. Stratified sampling plays a central role at this stage because it maintains the same proportion of malignant and benign cases in each subset, thus avoiding bias caused by uneven class distributions. Typical split ratios fall in the range of 70-30 or 80-20, with smaller datasets usually opting for the 80-20 division so that as many examples as possible contribute to training. Nested five-fold cross-validation has become a gold-standard practice in radiomics studies to minimize overfitting and a model's predictive excellence.

3.2. Model Selection

In contexts where interpretability is key, selecting the appropriate model structure becomes the defining step. Sophisticated deep-learning architectures may squeeze out slight improvements in predictive performance, yet that incremental accuracy usually comes with a significant drop in clarity. Because of this, researchers and practitioners often turn to so-called glass-box methods:

- Linear models with LASSO regularization are a robust technique for predictive modeling. LASSO will shrink the less important predictors' coefficients toward zero while leaving more substantial variables in the model. Consequently, one can easily determine which radiomic features predominantly drive the outcome and in which direction (positive or negative).

- Explainable Boosting Machines (EBMs) would be another possibility. EBMs are additive and thus highly interpretable, but allow the model to learn and elegantly present interactions when they matter. One can visualize the effect of each feature independently and see how it affects the prediction.
- For methods such as random forests or gradient boosting, one should restrict the number of levels in trees (forest) to at most five. Deep trees are cumbersome as clinicians cannot easily trace the decision logic.

3.3. Model Validation: Beyond Basic Accuracy

Validating a predictive model in healthcare requires much more than checking one accuracy number. Analysts look at multiple tests to confirm that the model is useful and that doctors will trust the results.

- Researchers typically evaluate discriminative power by calculating the Area Under the Receiver Operating Characteristic Curve (AUC-ROC). An AUC-ROC above 0.85 is usually viewed as demonstrating intense discrimination and may signal practical usefulness in clinical settings such as cancer detection or classification of histological subtypes.
- The Brier score evaluates how well a probabilistic model's forecasts match what happens. A score under 0.10 is rated excellent because it reflects ground reality; a score around 0.25 shows the same performance level as flipping a coin. Doctors rely on these numbers daily, and a well-calibrated model gives them confidence to act on the percentages they see, reducing the risk of needless tests or missed diagnoses. When the system cites a 70 percent chance of cancer, sound calibration means we should find about 70 of those hundred cases do have the disease.
- In multi-site clinical setups, the stability of extracted features frequently gets inadequate attention, though it forms the basis of interpretable and trustworthy clinical workflows. Researchers derive this score by calculating the Intraclass Correlation Coefficient (ICC) (Zhang et al., 2023) on data obtained from multiple scan sessions. An ICC threshold above 0.8 is conventionally accepted as indicating good reproducibility. The model must perform well when implemented in different hospitals with varying scanners.
- Testing the model on outside datasets, such as The Cancer Imaging Archive (TCIA) and the Lung Image Database Consortium and Image Database Resource Initiative (LIDC-IDRI), is key to ensuring it works well regardless of the scans.

Recent studies indicate that it is possible to obtain high accuracy using a hybrid model of interpretable models with other approaches. For example, (Kodete et al., 2024) demonstrated the effectiveness of interpretability by obtaining an AUC of 0.91 in lung-nodule evaluation using LASSO feature selection along with EBMs and generating decision rules comprehensible to clinicians.

3.3. Addressing Bias and Enhancing Explainability

To make radiomic models credible and useful in clinical practice, researchers must actively identify and correct biases while making the models easier for clinicians to understand.

- ComBat (Zhang et al., 2023) harmonization is a well-established preprocessing method that reduces batch effects from differences in imaging hardware and protocols across multiple hospitals and research centers. By adjusting the distribution of radiomic features, ComBat helps ensure that predictive models behave consistently, whether tested on data from an old scanner, a new one, or something in between.
- After data preprocessing, post-hoc explanation tools such as SHAP (SHapley Additive exPlanations) become essential for observing the model's behaviour. SHAP gives each feature a score for every prediction, helping doctors and researchers spot surprise patterns or confirm what they already expected. This clear peek into the model's reasoning links complicated code with everyday clinical choices, builds trust, and encourages radiology teams to welcome AI into their workflows (Zhang et al., 2023).

4. CLINICAL AI FOR LUNG CANCER SCREENING

Moving AI from the research arena to everyday lung cancer screening faces two significant challenges: passing rigorous regulations and proving real value in practice. Although hundreds of imaging algorithms claim impressive accuracy under controlled conditions, only a handful have earned FDA or CE marks that clear the regulatory bar. Such certification is not merely a paperwork formality; it signals that the technology is safe, effective, and can exchange data smoothly with existing clinical systems. The following subsection analyzes this first wave of approved solutions along two dimensions: the certified capabilities that enabled clinical implementation and the remaining shortcomings that still call for more transparent and interpretable approaches—the key concern of this chapter.

An increasing number of FDA- and CE-approved AI tools aimed at thoracic imaging have been developed. These tools facilitate automated detection, segmentation, and quantification across various modalities. The systems have been validated in multi-center clinical trials and have been approved by regulatory authorities, which means they are ready for implementation in radiology practice. The following tables (8-14) display the key attributes and architectural features of some of the commercially available solutions.

Table 8. Summary of DeltaView Model 2.1 (Riverain Technologies)

Attribute	Details
Submission Date	June 21, 2011
FDA 510(k)	K111776 (Cleared: Dec 28, 2011) [Link]
Developer	Riverain Technologies (Now part of Siemens Healthineers)
Type	CAD software for CXR
Regulation Class	Class II, 21 CFR §892.2050
Product Code	LLZ — Radiological Computer-Assisted Detection Software
Purpose	Detect lung nodules via temporal comparison of prior & current CXRs
Algorithm	ML with bone suppression, image registration, residual subtraction
Key Functions	Suppress static anatomy; enhance nodules; generate residual map
Validation	LROC: AUC ↑ from 0.477 to 0.536 (+12.4%); sensitivity increased significantly (p = 2.9E-05)
Predicate Device	SoftView (K092363), also by Riverain Technologies
Integration	PACS-compatible; used as second-read adjunct to conventional PA/AP CXR
Users	Radiologists, thoracic imaging teams
Primary Market	United States
Limitations	Adults only; prior + current image needed; quality dependent; radiologist interpretation required

Table 9. Summary of AVIEW LCS (Coreline Soft Co.)

Attribute	Details
FDA Submission	June 23, 2020
FDA 510(k)	K201710; Cleared Oct 16, 2020 (Link)
Developer	Coreline Soft Co., Ltd. (South Korea)
Type	CAD for thoracic CT
Purpose	AI-based nodule detection/tracking across single or serial CTs for lung cancer screening
Key Functions	3D size, volume, density (HU); Lung-RADS scoring
Advanced Metrics	VDT, solid/non-solid segmentation, CAC scoring, LAA analysis
AI/Algorithm	Deep CNNs for auto segmentation and quantification
Integration	Mevis CAD (K043617) compatible; structured reports
Primary Market	South Korea, EU (CE-marked), U.S. (FDA-cleared)
Users	Radiologists, LCS programs, hospitals
Limitations	Needs LDCT; sensitive to artifacts; limited interpretability

Table 10. Summary of AVIEW Lung Nodule CAD (Coreline Soft Co.)

Attribute	Details
Submission Date	May 19, 2022
FDA 510(k)	K221592 (Cleared: March 20, 2023), (Link)
Developer	Coreline Soft Co., Ltd. (Seoul, South Korea)
Type	CAD software for thoracic CT (DICOM-compatible)
Purpose	Assist radiologists in detecting pulmonary nodules (3–20 mm) from non-contrast chest CTs for lung cancer screening
Key Functions	Automatic nodule detection (solid/part-solid), centroid & bounding box localization, multiplanar slice visualization
Advanced Metrics	Nodule size (3D volume, major/minor axis); lung lobe-level anatomical classification; false positive reduction (FPR)
AI/Algorithm	Deep convolutional neural networks (multi-view)
Validation	Clinical reader study:
	AUC ↑ from 0.73 (unaided) to 0.92 (aided); Sensitivity ↑ from 0.68 to 0.91; FP/scan ↓ from 0.48 to 0.28
Integration	Integrates with AVIEW platform and PACS; results shown via AVIEW LCS Viewer; output formats: GSPS, XML
Hosting Platform	Siemens SOMATOM CT (validated); slice thickness ≤ 1.25 mm recommended

continued on following page

Table 10. Continued

Attribute	Details
Primary Market	South Korea, U.S. (FDA-cleared), CE-marked for EU
Users	Radiologists, lung cancer screening clinics, pulmonary specialists
Limitations	Not intended for nodules < 3 mm; dependent on CT resolution; Siemens CT series recommended; radiologist review required

Table 11. Summary of Veolity Lung Nodule CAD (MeVis Medical Solutions)

Attribute	Details
Submission Date	June 3, 2020
FDA 510(k)	K201501 (Cleared: Feb 23, 2021), (Link)
Developer	MeVis Medical Solutions AG (Bremen, Germany)
Type	CAD software for thoracic CT (PACS-integrated or stand-alone)
Purpose	Detection and characterization of solid pulmonary nodules (4–30 mm); supports temporal comparison and structured reporting in screening/diagnostic CT
Key Functions	Temporal side-by-side scan comparison; auto-segmentation of nodules with manual override; automatic quantification (diameter, volume, density, mass); Lung-RADS prefill; malignancy risk estimation (McWilliams model)
Advanced Metrics	Mass/volume doubling time; nodule type classification (solid, part-solid, non-solid); location/lobe segmentation; nodule spiculation
AI/ Algorithm	Hybrid pipeline with rule-based and machine learning modules; includes optional CAD engine for second-read detection of solid nodules (4–30 mm)
Validation	Benchmarked on multi-center CT datasets; CAD performance equivalent to ImageChecker CT (K043617); sensitivity and false positive rates matched
Integration	Supports server-client deployment; compatible with DICOM (GSPS, SR); exports structured reports; designed for lung cancer screening workflows
Hosting Platform	PC-based or server deployment; supports multi-vendor CT input with slice thickness ≤ 1.5 mm recommended
Primary Market	Germany, U.S. (FDA-cleared), EU (CE-marked), Canada, South Korea
Users	Radiologists, lung cancer screening centers, pulmonary clinics
Limitations	Only detects solid nodules (≥ 4 mm); CAD engine excludes part-solid/non-solid nodules; adjunct use only after primary read

Table 12. Summary of AI-Rad Companion Chest CT (Siemens Healthineers)

Attribute	Details
FDA 510(k)	K183271 (Pulmonary – Cleared July 26, 2019): Lung lobe segmentation, nodule analysis, emphysema quantification; K183272 (Engine – Multi-organ pipeline); K183268 (Cardiovascular – Coronary calcium scoring); FDA Link
Developer	Siemens Healthineers (Erlangen, Germany)
Type	AI-based CAD and quantification platform for thoracic CT; cloud/PACS hybrid via teamplay
Purpose	Automated segmentation, quantification, and reporting of lung lobes, emphysema burden, nodules, coronary artery calcium, and vertebral body attenuation
Key Features	**Lung:** 5-lobe segmentation (error: 1.5–3.5%), %LAV950 emphysema scoring; **Cardiac:** Agatston CAC scoring (syngo.CT Lung CAD); **Spine:** Vertebral density (HU), aortic diameter
AI Architecture	Deep CNN (ResNet/U-Net hybrid); Dice = 0.95–0.98 for lobe segmentation; vendor-neutral (Siemens, GE, Philips CT with FBP & IR)
Performance Metrics	Mean surface distance: 0.5–1.0 mm; 95% Hausdorff: 2.6–5.2 mm; 30% faster reporting than manual methods (Siemens, 2021)
Validation	4,500+ CT scans (multi-center); DICOM PS 3.1–3.20; ISO 14971, IEC 62304, IEC 80001 compliant
Integration	DICOM GSPS/SC; PACS/Cloud deployment; teamplay-enabled enterprise workflow
Primary Market	FDA-cleared (USA), CE-marked (EU), deployed in Asia-Pacific
Users	Radiologists, cardiothoracic specialists, lung screening programs
Limitations	Requires CT slice thickness ≤ 3 mm; not validated in pediatrics; cloud dependency may impact speed in low-bandwidth settings

Table 13. Summary of Lunit INSIGHT CXR (Lunit Inc.)

Attribute	Details
Developer	Lunit Inc. (Seoul, South Korea)
Type	AI-based CAD software for chest radiographs (CXR)
Purpose	Detects 10 radiologic abnormalities (e.g., nodule, pneumothorax, effusion); used for triage, screening, and prioritization
AI Architecture	**Dual-branch ResNet-152:** Branch 1 – Classification (10 abnormalities); Branch 2 – Localization (Attention-gated U-Net). **Uncertainty Estimation:** Monte Carlo dropout (p = 0.3)
Training Data	207,894 PA/AP CXRs (Lunit v4.1); 79,113 abnormal; 8,712 CT-confirmed; annotated by 18 radiologists (5 per test case). Lunit Whitepaper 2023. Multi-continent dataset (Korea, Europe, U.S.)
Performance Metrics	Nodule: AUC 0.971, JAFROC 0.918; Pneumothorax: AUC 0.997, JAFROC 0.994; TB: AUC 0.993, JAFROC 0.987

continued on following page

Table 13. Continued

Attribute	Details
Clinical Validation	Multi-center trials confirm AUC > 0.95 across Korea (SNUH: AUC 0.98, JAFROC 0.94), U.S. (UCSF: AUC 0.92), and international TB cohort (Montgomery: AUC 1.00). External validation in 5+ hospitals. Reader studies: 20% sensitivity boost for non-radiologists; 94.1% sensitivity for drainable pneumothorax
Integration	DICOM GSPS overlays (bounding boxes, heatmaps); HL7 FHIR API for EHR integration (triage prioritization, structured reporting with Lung-RADS/Fleischner). PACS/cloud compatible. Latency: 2.3 sec/image (NVIDIA T4). Scalable to enterprise deployments
Clinical Impact	Deployed in 3,000+ hospitals across 40+ countries. 34% faster emergency triage reads. Reduced missed nodules and subtle lesion oversight
Limitations	12% performance drop in portable CXRs due to artifacts; lower sensitivity for subpleural nodules (67%) vs. central (89%); FDA clearance pending

Table 14. Summary of Arterys MICA (Arterys Inc.)

Attribute	Details
Submission Date	December 17, 2020
FDA 510(k)	K203744 (Cleared: March 14, 2022); FDA Link
Developer	Arterys Inc. (San Francisco, CA, USA)
Type	Cloud-native CAD software for multimodal imaging (CT/MRI); DICOM and non-DICOM compatible
Purpose	Assists with visualization, segmentation, quantification, and follow-up assessment of thoracic (lung) and cardiac abnormalities from diagnostic imaging
Key Functions	AI-assisted segmentation and measurement of pulmonary lesions; longitudinal tracking; interactive visualization (2D/3D/MIP); radiomics-ready export; clinician-edited overlays
Advanced Metrics	Morphological change tracking; global/local T1/T2 myocardial mapping; volume/time-series lesion follow-up; multi-lesion support
AI/Algorithm	Modular AI architecture using deep convolutional networks for segmentation, contouring, mapping (e.g., cardiac, lung); integrated deep learning + rule-based workflows
Validation	Verified against predicate (K192437); IEC 62304 and ISO 14971 compliant; Global T1/T2 accuracy within ±30ms/4ms vs. OEM maps
Integration	Cloud-based viewer (app.arterys.com); supports PACS, HL7, and structured reporting; AWS-based secure hosting
Hosting Platform	Fully SaaS via web browser; HIPAA-compliant; global access over VPN
Primary Market	United States (FDA-cleared), Europe (CE-marked), Asia-Pacific deployments
Users	Radiologists, oncologists, cardiologists, image analysis teams

continued on following page

Table 14. Continued

Attribute	Details
Special Features	4D volumetric lesion analysis; tumor heterogeneity maps; radiogenomic links to EGFR/KRAS mutation probability; guideline-driven reporting (NCCN v3.2024 aligned); deployed in 200+ oncology centers
Limitations	Dependent on internet bandwidth; requires radiologist confirmation; non-diagnostic if internet interrupted or data incomplete

4.1. Emerging Research Models

Although state-of-the-art DL models now identify lung cancer with near-expert precision, hospitals are still reluctant to use them because many physicians cannot visualize the reasoning behind the predictions. This section reviews stateof-the-art methods that deliver top performance while offering clear, built-in, or afterward-visible insight, consistent with the chapter's glass-box vision.

Numerous studies acknowledge the advances in the methodology of interpretable AI. One utilizes stack-ensemble models (Ahmed et al., 2021), which incorporate multiple machine learning algorithms such as GLM, Random Forests, GBM, XG-Boost, and DNNs. This ensemble approach enhances prediction accuracy while retaining interpretability, essential in radiomics where accuracy and transparency are critical. Moreover, model-agnostic interpretability tools such as Permutation Feature Importance (PFI), Partial Dependence Plots (PDP), and breakdown plots reveal fine-grained influence of features. PFI has identified smoking as an important predictor of LBC mortality, and PDPs showcase nonlinear relationships. These methods can be applied directly to radiomics, thus explaining how imaging features like tumor texture, shape, and even metabolic activity are implicated in cancer diagnosis or prognosis, making radiomics less of a "black box" and more clinically interpretable.

A spatial interpretability framework goes beyond feature-level analysis by illustrating how risk factors contribute to mortality rates in specific geographic areas. This method reveals inequities that are often hidden in average or aggregate evaluations. In radiomics, a similar spatial analysis could identify differences in tumor characteristics across patient groups or specific tumor locations and guide personalized treatment approaches. The DNNs used in radiomics pose a challenge due to their "black-box" nature. XAI techniques like LIME and GradCAM can explain pre-trained models, striking a balance between complexity and transparency, thus offering a way out. The Lightweight Multi-Scale CNN (LWMS-CNN) model (Hasan et al., 2024) classifies lung and colon cancer with high accuracy while incorporating Grad-CAM and SHAP for visual and quantitative explanations. DeepXplainer, a hybrid CNN-XGBoost model, also attained high accuracy in lung cancer detection and applies

SHAP to provide local and global explainability, specifying the influential features driving model predictions.

The impacts of XAI in healthcare are deep and multifaceted. Interpretable models can guide targeted interventions like anti-smoking campaigns centered around specific, high-risk regions. In addition, within radiomics, models that classify tumors as malignant or predict certain prognoses enact reasoning clin icians should understand. This builds trust and speeds up the adoption of new AI technologies. Clinician interaction with AI technologies and visualization of predictions through intuition is now possible due to the development of web applications with Gradio. Meeting clinical AI application needs requires timely and accurate diagnoses, especially in resource-poor healthcare settings. The focus on computational efficiency, as demonstrated by DeepXplainer's (Wani et al., 2024) optimized hybrid architecture, is critical in these scenarios. Advancements that provide accurate results with strong interpretability and practical deployment elevate the radiomics of lung cancer from an enigmatic appendage to a lucid, reliable, and actionable clinical instrument.

These developments highlight the near future of AI in clinical practice. It is not about just being accurate; trust, transparency, and reliability are equally important. The road from "black box" to "glass box" is still long, with major obstacles that prevent the appropriate use and full-scale adoption of AI in oncology's precision medicine paradigm, demanding thoughtful approaches.

5. KEY BARRIERS TO AI ADOPTION IN CANCER TREATMENT

From initial screening to customized treatment approaches, artificial intelligence can potentially transform cancer treatment, but its integration is limited by a web of factors spanning numerous fields. These factors require critical examination and intervention to set free AI's full potential in oncology.

5.1 Healthcare System Challenges

- **Resource limitations:** Shortages of infrastructure and trained personnel continue to obstruct fair access to cancer care and delay diagnosis in many healthcare systems. Across numerous countries, specialized staff and basic imaging equipment such as MRI or PET-CT scanners are unevenly distributed, producing marked regional inequities and gaps even within single nations such as Greece, Italy, the UK, Cyprus, Serbia, and Spain. Clinicians report that these shortages disrupt screening programs and lengthen the time from initial visit to definitive diagnosis. The result is a higher proportion of cancers found at an advanced stage, narrower treatment choices, and worse overall survival, illustrating why a more strategic, equitable policy for allocating resources is urgent (Hesso et al., 2024).

- **Economic barriers:** High expenses remain a significant obstacle to incorporating AI into clinical cancer care across the healthcare system. Hospitals and clinics must first allocate significant capital to cover licensing fees for advanced AI programs, purchase upgraded servers and workstations, and run extensive training sessions for doctors and staff members (Silva et al., 2022) (Chapla et al., 2024). Even after these initial costs are paid, facilities must budget for routine maintenance, software patches, and occasional hardware refreshes if they want their systems to preserve performance and be trustworthy.
- **PACS Interoperability:** One significant benefit of Picture Archiving and Communication Systems (PACS) is that clinicians from different departments can view medical images virtually anywhere. Despite this flexibility, the software behind most PACS is still proprietary and closed-source, making it hard to plug in new artificial-intelligence tools. Because of that limited interoperability, many AI applications run separately, forcing staff to export data manually and import it again. This cumbersome transfer adds to radiologists' daily tasks and short-circuits the time savings AI was supposed to deliver (Theriault-Lauzier et al., 2024).
- **Fragmented perspectives:** Conflicting views among radiologists, oncologists, and surgeons about the role of AI keep its use uneven across hospitals. Because there are no standard clinical guidelines, these tools feel like an add-on instead of a must-have part of everyday patient care. Building that agreement is complicated, since every discipline expects different kinds of data, unique analyses, and varying levels of transparency from an AI system (Hesso et al., 2023).

5.2. Healthcare Professional (HCP) Concerns

- **Limited AI expertise:** Inadequate training to interpret AI reports remains a significant barrier to adding this technology to lung-cancer care. Many pulmonologists and thoracic-radiology specialists have a shallow grasp of algorithmic output, especially when cases involving subsolid nodules or probabilistic cancer scores that stray from familiar patterns. Because key features and model confidence are rarely explained in plain terms, clinicians often cannot see how an AI's conclusion fits their judgment. The problem worsens without widely accepted benchmarks for competence in AI-aided diagnosis. As a result, some doctors either trust the machines blindly or toss the idea out altogether, both of which slow down meaningful use of AI in spotting lung cancer (Hesso et al., 2023).

- **Fear of job displacement:** HCPs worry that AI might replace them in roles like image review and test analysis, which machines do more efficiently. This thinking poses a challenge to successfully introducing AI technologies in clinical practice. Many clinicians, however, acknowledge that with proper training, these systems can rational record-keeping, enhance search queries for complex treatment decisions, and free up mental bandwidth for more advanced patient interactions. In order to fully address unresolved fears, developers need to collaborate with the providers during the design and evaluation stages to ensure systems target the use of AI in lung-cancer care as a supporting technology rather than as a replacement for human expertise.
- **Work-pressure:** Overloaded HCPs cannot find time to learn new technology apart from their daily tight schedule. The shortage of sufficient training sessions and poor IT support also contributes to the reluctance to use the AI tools.

5.3. Clinical and Ethical Challenges

- **Black-Box models:** A major roadblock for putting AI into everyday clinical work remains the poor explainability and interpretability of many models, leaving front-line staff uneasy about so-called black-box systems. In practice, health professionals insist that they grasp how an algorithm arrives at its judgment and which variables matter before they trust a new digital tool, much less partner with it. Without that level of visibility, practitioners often feel uncertain, even uneasy, about the recommendations generated, raising questions about consistency, bias, and patient safety.
- **Ethical and legal risks (Chau, 2024):** Mistakes by AI in diagnosing or treating patients can harm health and even prove fatal. This raises challenging legal issues: Are doctors answerable for accepting the AI's recommendation? Or do developers bear the blame when their software fails? Because existing statutes and cases lack explicit guidance, hospitals, clinicians, and vendors tread cautiously yet anxiously as they adopt AI tools.

Although Australia has advanced its Therapeutic Goods Administration (TGA) framework for medical devices and updated the Privacy Act 1988, the nation still lacks specific, formal rules that directly address the trustworthiness of AI and the assignment of liability. As a result, healthcare professionals are in a legal grey area, leaving many uncertain about their responsibilities if the technology fails. At the global level, the European Union's General Data Protection Regulation (GDPR) outlines robust requirements for patient consent and promotes explainable AI. In contrast, the US Health Insurance Portability and Accountability Act (HIPAA) primarily safeguards sensitive data. These uneven yet overlapping regulatory landscapes make worldwide deployment of healthcare AI far more complicated than many technologists realise, reinforcing the urgent call for harmonised rules that clarify ethical and operational expectations.

Emphasizing the responsible use of AI again, the World Health Organization (WHO) released complete guidelines in January 2024 outlining more than 40 recommendations for governments, tech companies, and healthcare providers on the ethics and governance of LMMs. These recommendations focus on the ethical considerations of LMMs in healthcare. However, the persistent development of the legal landscape and the absence of well-defined responsibility frameworks for AI diagnosis systems still hinders widespread adoption.

- **Bias and transferability (Carter et al., 2020):** Being free from bias and transferability issues makes an AI tool more accountable. It must have consistent performance across clinics and patient groups. AI models typically absorb and even magnify the biases embedded in the training dataset. The algorithms may underperform if data from certain demographic groups is less represented in the training dataset. The net effect is a biased and unequal diagnostic performance, deepening existing health disparities and undermining the confidence among clinicians and patients.

Transferability describes how well an artificial intelligence model stays accurate when it encounters fresh, previously unseen data collected from other hospitals, different types of imaging machines, or patient groups that were not included in the original training sample. When a predictive model is developed using data collected at a single clinical site, it often fails to generalize to other settings. As a result, deploying the model in a different hospital or region usually involves costly and time-consuming procedures to tune or rebuild the system from scratch.

- **Inconsistent screening policies:** Demographic factors, such as ethnicity, age, and the prevalence of diseases, differ across populations (Fernandes et al., 2024). Thus, AI models will need additional investments to calibrate them for particular regions if the training data is not inclusive enough. The distinct regulatory mandates concerning AI validation (such as the FDA or EU-MDR) impede swift implementation since a given model must secure independent endorsements in each market, thus postponing its introduction. Additionally, constantly evolving screening guidelines—such as the recent USPSTF update on lung cancer screening—necessitate periodic AI model retraining to incorporate new criteria, which threatens sustainability (Hardavella et al., 2024).

5.4. Data Challenge

Although XAI promises to enhance trust and facilitate the clinical uptake of AI systems for lung cancer detection, several data-related barriers undermine its reliability and broader applicability. One major hurdle is the scarcity of sufficiently large, well-annotated lung-imaging datasets- including high-resolution CT scans and chest X-rays- constraining training DL architectures that can reliably perform across varied demographic and clinical backgrounds (Zhu et al., 2025). In addition, the intrinsic complexity of medical images coupled with the subtle differences between lung cancer subtypes demands meticulous, uniform labeling by experienced radiologists, a process that is time-consuming and still subject to considerable inter-observer disagreement (Zhu et al., 2025). Even though combining different types of data, like medical images, clinical notes, gene sequences, and patient lifestyle records, could make predictions smarter and give valuable background for explainable artificial intelligence, doing so consistently is still a major technical hurdle (Niu et al., 2025).

5.5. Patient-Centric Obstacles

- **Lack of human touch:** A significant barrier to adopting artificial intelligence in healthcare is patient discomfort with the idea of machines making decisions about their care. Many people trust face-to-face contact more than they trust lines of code, especially when their health is at stake. Research backs up this intuition, showing that customers only welcome new tools when they feel personal talk is possible. Because healthcare questions often carry higher emotional and physical stakes than other services, patients still demand to speak directly with staff before, during, and after treatment to ask questions, report problems, and build the rapport they assume an algorithm cannot offer.
- **Financial and compliance burdens:** Patients' out-of-pocket expenses typically rise as the new AI-assisted diagnostic tests require additional implementation and equipment costs. The low literacy level among patients is a potential barrier to comprehending independent AI analysis and suggested next steps. Furthermore, the intricate technical aspects that need to be acknowledged and comprehended regarding AI-based decisions can easily perplex patients if they do not have ample knowledge in data-driven diagnostics.

6. FUTURE DIRECTIONS

The real test of XAI in lung cancer radiomics is when it is fully integrated into clinical care pathways, enabling real-time decision-making and not just being viewed as a research tool. In treatment monitoring and personalization, upcoming XAI models will be able to detect subtle changes on serial CT or PET/CT scans, and they will be able to explain why tumors respond or progress by associating the imaging changes with biological processes or genomic alterations and thus giving a causal explanation for therapy changes (Cilla et al., 2025) (Prencipe et al., 2023). Survival and recurrence prediction models will need to evolve into transparent systems, displaying radiomic features that influence risk predictions, enabling clinicians to trust AI-predictive models in the long-term management (Martell et al., 2025). One area where XAI can accelerate discovery is in drug development, as it exposes mechanistic links between radiomics phenotypes and direct affections or therapeutic targets, e.g., CT/PET features with EGFR and KRAS mutations in lung adenocarcinoma (Zuo et al., 2024) (Huang et al., 2024) within explainable radiogenomic frameworks. This foundation supports true personalisation by providing access to interpretations. Instead of unexplained scores, models would be clear enough to explain the reasons underlying treatment suggestions, given the patient's particular radiological and molecular profile. This brief explanation suggests that the high likelihood of clinical integration necessitates that such models be explainable, i.e., they should be capable of being audited so that one can understand why a given decision was made. Success in AI and radiomics hinges on models achieving a balance among interpretability, fairness, and other operational criteria, rather than merely avoiding or meeting any of these (Van der Velden et al., 2022) (Batra et al., 2024).

7. CONCLUSIONS

Lung cancer radiomics has advanced significantly from the traditional "black box" approaches to more sophisticated and interpretable models. Utilizing XAI methods (e.g., SHAP values, attention maps, and decision paths) helps to understand AI-based diagnosis. This allows medical professionals to understand the basis of the model's predictions. Each step toward XAI earns the AI system more trust and empowers radiologists to use AI, which results in corroboration with clinical reasoning. Thus, it reduces the reluctance toward AI technology implementation.

Although XAI is widely recognised as the backbone of reliable and equitable clinical algorithms, real-world deployment requires more than simply refining the underlying models. Meaningful interpretability depends on three interlocking steps: first, adopting consistent, multi-site protocols for data gathering so that training sets truly reflect the patient population; second, embedding tools that detect and correct bias at every stage of development; and third, subjecting models to thorough, independent testing in varied health-care settings. Federated-learning techniques further protect patient privacy while exposing algorithms to diverse cases, and fairness-oriented design patterns systematically reduce imbalances linked to age, race, or gender. However, technical improvements will matter little unless they are matched by updated regulatory pathways for testing and real-world reporting and by extensive educational programs that equip clinicians to critique and trust what these interpretable systems promise.

Ultimately, the AI-assisted future of lung cancer detection is bound to become a reality. This means that radiologists and algorithms will work hand in hand. XAI will ensure this collaboration is possible by building a bridge between radiologists and AI algorithms. By turning AI into a "glass box," we equip clinicians with the tools to derive maximal benefits, boost diagnostic precision, and ensure that the care delivered is equitable and centered around the patient. The path forward is clear: interpretability is not merely a desirable attribute but an essential requirement for the ethical and successful implementation of AI tools in oncology.

REFERENCES

Adachi, T., Nagasawa, R., Nakamura, M., Kakino, R., & Mizowaki, T. (2022). Vulnerabilities of radiomic features to respiratory motion on four-dimensional computed tomography-based average intensity projection images: A phantom study. *Journal of Applied Clinical Medical Physics, 23*(3), e13498. DOI: 10.1002/acm2.13498

Adams, R., & Bischof, L. (1994). Seeded region growing. *IEEE Transactions on Pattern Analysis and Machine Intelligence, 16*(6), 641–647. DOI: 10.1109/34.295913

Aerts, H. J. W. L., Velazquez, E. R., Leijenaar, R. T. H., Parmar, C., Grossmann, P., Carvalho, S., Bussink, J., Monshouwer, R., Haibe-Kains, B., Rietveld, D., Hoebers, F., Rietbergen, M. M., Leemans, C. R., Dekker, A., Quackenbush, J., Gillies, R. J., & Lambin, P. (2014). Decoding tumour phenotype by noninvasive imaging using a quantitative radiomics approach. *Nature Communications, 5*(1), 4006. DOI: 10.1038/ncomms5006

. Ahmed, Z. U., Sun, K., Shelly, M., & Mu, L. (2021). Explainable artificial intelligence (XAI) for exploring spatial variability of lung and bronchus cancer (LBC) mortality rates in the contiguous USA. *Scientific Reports, 11*(1), 24090. Nature Publishing Group UK. DOI: 10.1038/s41598-021-03198-8

Armato, S. G.III, McLennan, G., Bidaut, L., McNitt-Gray, M. F., Meyer, C. R., Reeves, A. P., Zhao, B., Aberle, D. R., Henschke, C. I., Hoffman, E. A., Kazerooni, E. A., MacMahon, H., van Beek, E. J. R., Yankelevitz, D., Biancardi, A. M., Bland, P. H., Brown, M. S., Engelmann, R. M., Laderach, G. E., & Clarke, L. P. (2011). The lung image database consortium (LIDC) and image database resource initiative (IDRI): A completed reference database of lung nodules on CT scans. *Medical Physics, 38*(2), 915–931. DOI: 10.1118/1.3528204

Arrieta, A. B., Díaz-Rodríguez, N., Del Ser, J., Bennetot, A., Tabik, S., Barbado, A., García, S., Gil-López, S., Molina, D., & Benjamins, R.. (2020). Explainable Artificial Intelligence (XAI): Concepts, taxonomies, opportunities and challenges toward responsible AI. *Information Fusion, 58*, 82–115. DOI: 10.1016/j.inffus.2019.12.012

Arthur, D., & Vassilvitskii, S. (2006). *k-means++: The advantages of careful seeding* (Technical Report). Stanford University. https://dl.acm.org/doi/10.5555/1283383.1283494

Bach, P. B., Mirkin, J. N., Oliver, T. K., Azzoli, C. G., Berry, D. A., Brawley, O. W., Byers, T., Colditz, G. A., Gould, M. K., Jett, J. R., Sabichi, A. L., Smith-Bindman, R., Wood, D. E., Qaseem, A., & Detterbeck, F. C. (2012). Benefits and harms of CT screening for lung cancer: A systematic review. *Journal of the American Medical Association, 307*(22), 2418–2429. DOI: 10.1001/jama.2012.5521

Bade, B. C., & Dela Cruz, C. S. (2020). Lung cancer 2020: Epidemiology, etiology, and prevention. *Clinics in Chest Medicine, 41*(1), 1–24. DOI: 10.1016/j.ccm.2019.10.001

Balbi, M., Mazzaschi, G., Leo, L., Dalla Tor, L. M., Milanese, G., Marrocchio, C., Silva, M., Mura, R., Favia, P., & Bocchialini, G.. (2025). Longitudinal changes of CT-radiomic and systemic inflammatory features predict survival in advanced non–small cell lung cancer patients treated with immune checkpoint inhibitors. *Journal of Thoracic Imaging, 40*(1), e0801. DOI: 10.1097/RTI.0000000000000801

Barragán-Montero, A., Javaid, U., Valdés, G., Nguyen, D., Desbordes, P., Macq, B., Willems, S., Vandewinckele, L., Holmström, M., Löfman, F., Michiels, S., Souris, K., Sterpin, E., & Lee, J. A. (2021). Artificial intelligence and machine learning for medical imaging: A technology review. *Physica Medica, 83*, 242–256. DOI: 10.1016/j.ejmp.2021.04.016

Batra, U., Nathany, S., Nath, S. K., Jose, J. T., Sharma, T., Pasricha, S., & Rawal, K. (2024). AI-based pipeline for early screening of lung cancer: Integrating radiology, clinical, and genomics data. *The Lancet Regional Health. Southeast Asia, 24*, 100352. Advance online publication. DOI: 10.1016/j.lansea.2024.100352

Biederer, J., Mirsadraee, S., Beer, M., Molinari, F., Hintze, C., Bauman, G., Both, M., Van Beek, E. J. R., Wild, J., & Puderbach, M. (2012). MRI of the lung (3/3)—Current applications and future perspectives. *Insights Into Imaging, 3*(4), 373–386. DOI: 10.1007/s13244-011-0142-z

Biswas, S., & Hazra, R. (2022). State-of-the-art level set models and their performances in image segmentation: A decade review. *Archives of Computational Methods in Engineering, 29*(4), 2019–2042. DOI: 10.1007/s11831-021-09646-y

Bortolotto, C., Pinto, A., Brero, F., Messana, G., Cabini, R. F., Postuma, I., Robustelli Test, A., Stella, G. M., Galli, G., Mariani, M., Figini, S., Lascialfari, A., Filippi, A. R., Bottinelli, O. M., & Preda, L. (2024). CT and MRI radiomic features of lung cancer (NSCLC): Comparison and software consistency. *European Radiology Experimental, 8*(1), 71. DOI: 10.1186/s41747-024-00468-8

Bradley, S. H., Abraham, S., Callister, M. E. J., Grice, A., Hamilton, W. T., Rodriguez Lopez, R., Shinkins, B., & Neal, R. D. (2019). Sensitivity of chest X-ray for detecting lung cancer in people presenting with symptoms: A systematic review. *The British Journal of General Practice*, *69*(689), e827–e835. DOI: 10.3399/bjgp19X706853

Bray, F., Ferlay, J., Soerjomataram, I., Siegel, R. L., Torre, L. A., & Jemal, A. (2018). Global cancer statistics 2018: GLOBOCAN estimates of incidence and mortality worldwide for 36 cancers in 185 countries. *CA: a Cancer Journal for Clinicians*, *68*(6), 394–424. DOI: 10.3322/caac.21492

Bray, F., Laversanne, M., Sung, H., Ferlay, J., Siegel, R. L., Soerjomataram, I., & Jemal, A. (2024). Global cancer statistics 2022: GLOBOCAN estimates of incidence and mortality worldwide for 36 cancers in 185 countries. *CA: a Cancer Journal for Clinicians*, *74*(3), 229–263. DOI: 10.3322/caac.21834

Carter, S. M., Rogers, W., Win, K. T., Frazer, H., Richards, B., & Houssami, N. (2020). The ethical, legal and social implications of using artificial intelligence systems in breast cancer care. *The Breast : Official Journal of the European Society of Mastology*, *49*, 25–32. DOI: 10.1016/j.breast.2019.10.001

Chang, G., Chang, T., Pan, T., Clark, J. W.Jr, & Mawlawi, O. R. (2010). Joint correction of respiratory motion artifact and partial volume effect in lung/thoracic PET/CT imaging. *Medical Physics*, *37*(12), 6221–6232. DOI: 10.1118/1.3512780

Chapla, D., Chorya, H. P., Ishfaq, L., Khan, A., Subrahmanyan, V. R., & Garg, S. (2024). An artificial intelligence (AI)-integrated approach to enhance early detection and personalized treatment strategies in lung cancer among smokers: A literature review. *Cureus*, *16*(8). Advance online publication. DOI: 10.7759/cureus.66688

Chau, M. (2024). Ethical, legal, and regulatory landscape of artificial intelligence in Australian healthcare and ethical integration in radiography: A narrative review. *Journal of Medical Imaging and Radiation Sciences*, *55*(4), 101733. DOI: 10.1016/j.jmir.2024.101733

Chen, Y.-H., Kan, K.-Y., Liu, S.-H., Lin, H.-H., & Lue, K.-H. (2023). Impact of respiratory motion on 18F-FDG PET radiomics stability: Clinical evaluation with a digital PET scanner. *Journal of Applied Clinical Medical Physics*, *24*(12), e14200. DOI: 10.1002/acm2.14200

Cilla, S., Romano, C., Macchia, G., Pezzulla, D., Lepre, E., Buwenge, M., Donati, C. M., Galietta, E., Morganti, A. G., & Deodato, F. (2025). Radiomics-based explainable artificial intelligence to predict treatment response following lung stereotactic body radiation therapy. *The British Journal of Radiology*, *98*(1175), tqaf043. Advance online publication. DOI: 10.1093/bjr/tqaf043

Clunie, D. A. (2001). DICOM structured reporting: An object model as an implementation boundary. In *Medical Imaging 2001: PACS and Integrated Medical Information Systems: Design and Evaluation* (Vol. 4323, pp. 207–215). DOI: 10.1117/12.435478

Coeckelbergh, M. (2020). Artificial intelligence, responsibility attribution, and a relational justification of explainability. *Science and Engineering Ethics*, *26*(4), 2051–2068. DOI: 10.1007/s11948-019-00146-8

Cui, Q., Qiang, Z., Zhao, J., Qiang, Y., & Liao, X. (2017). A 3D segmentation method for pulmonary nodule image sequences based on supervoxels and multimodal data. *International Journal of Performability Engineering*, *13*(5), 682. DOI: 10.23940/ijpe.17.05.p12.682696

Dai, S., Lu, K., Dong, J., Zhang, Y., & Chen, Y. (2015). A novel approach of lung segmentation on chest CT images using graph cuts. *Neurocomputing*, *168*, 799–807. DOI: 10.1016/j.neucom.2015.05.044

De Visschere, P. J. L., Vral, A., Perletti, G., Pattyn, E., Praet, M., Magri, V., & Villeirs, G. M. (2017). Multiparametric magnetic resonance imaging characteristics of normal, benign, and malignant conditions in the prostate. *European Radiology*, *27*(5), 2095–2109. DOI: 10.1007/s00330-016-4479-z

Dehmeshki, J., Amin, H., Valdivieso, M., & Ye, X. (2008). Segmentation of pulmonary nodules in thoracic CT scans: A region growing approach. *IEEE Transactions on Medical Imaging*, *27*(4), 467–480. DOI: 10.1109/TMI.2007.907555

Djahnine, A., Jupin-Delevaux, E., Nempont, O., Si-Mohamed, S. A., Craighero, F., Cottin, V., Douek, P., Popoff, A., & Boussel, L. (2024). Weakly-supervised learning-based pathology detection and localization in 3D chest CT scans. *Medical Physics*, *51*(11), 8272–8282. DOI: 10.1002/mp.17302

Du, Q., Baine, M., Bavitz, K., McAllister, J., Liang, X., Yu, H., Ryckman, J., Yu, L., Jiang, H., Zhou, S., Zhang, C., & Zheng, D. (2019). Radiomic feature stability across 4D respiratory phases and its impact on lung tumor prognosis prediction. *PLoS One*, *14*(5), e0216480. DOI: 10.1371/journal.pone.0216480

Esteva, A., Chou, K., Yeung, S., Naik, N., Madani, A., Mottaghi, A., Liu, Y., Topol, E., Dean, J., & Socher, R. (2021). Deep learning-enabled medical computer vision. *NPJ Digital Medicine*, *4*(1), 5. DOI: 10.1038/s41746-020-00376-2

Felder, R. M. (2021). Coming to terms with the black box problem: How to justify AI systems in health care. *The Hastings Center Report*, *51*(4), 38–45. DOI: 10.1002/hast.1248

Feng, X., Yang, J., Laine, A. F., & Angelini, E. D. (2017). Discriminative localization in CNNs for weakly-supervised segmentation of pulmonary nodules. In Medical Image Computing and Computer Assisted Intervention – *MICCAI 2017: 20th International Conference,* Quebec City, QC, Canada, September 11–13, 2017, *Proceedings, Part III* (pp. 568–576). Springer. DOI: 10.1007/978-3-319-66179-7_65

Feng, Y., Hao, P., Zhang, P., Liu, X., Wu, F., & Wang, H. (2023). Supervoxel based weakly-supervised multi-level 3D CNNs for lung nodule detection and segmentation. *Journal of Ambient Intelligence and Humanized Computing*, *14*(11), 1–11. DOI: 10.1007/s12652-018-01170-5

Ferlay, J., Ervik, M., Lam, F., Laversanne, M., Colombet, M., Mery, L., Piñeros, M., Znaor, A., Soerjomataram, I., & Bray, F. (2024). *Global Cancer Observatory: Cancer Today.* International Agency for Research on Cancer. https://gco.iarc.who.int/today

Fernandes, M. G. O., Dias, M., Santos, R., Ravara, S., Fernandes, P., Firmino-Machado, J., Antunes, J. P., Fernandes, O., Madureira, A., Hespanhol, V., Rodrigues, C., Vicente, C. A., Alves, S., Mendes, G., Ilgenfritz, R., Pinto, B. S., Alves, J., Saraiva, I., Bárbara, C., & Morais, A. (2024). Recommendations for the implementation of a national lung cancer screening program in Portugal: A consensus statement. *Pulmonology*, *30*(6), 625–635. Advance online publication. DOI: 10.1016/j.pulmoe.2024.04.003

Fletcher, J. W., Djulbegovic, B., Soares, H. P., Siegel, B. A., Lowe, V. J., Lyman, G. H., Coleman, R. E., Wahl, R., Paschold, J. C., Avril, N., Einhorn, L. H., Suh, W. W., Samson, D., Delbeke, D., Gorman, M., & Shields, A. F. (2008). Recommendations on the use of ^{18}F-FDG PET in oncology. *Journal of Nuclear Medicine*, *49*(3), 480–508. DOI: 10.2967/jnumed.107.047787

Gierada, D. S., Black, W. C., Chiles, C., Pinsky, P. F., & Yankelevitz, D. F. (2020). Low-dose CT screening for lung cancer: Evidence from 2 decades of study. *Radiology. Imaging Cancer*, *2*(2), e190058. DOI: 10.1148/rycan.2020190058

Gierlinger, M., Brandner, D., & Zagar, B. G. (2020). Multi-seed region growing algorithm for medical image segmentation. In Heizmann, M., & Längle, T. (Eds.), *Proceedings* (p. 267)., DOI: 10.58895/ksp/1000124383-21

Gillies, R. J., Kinahan, P. E., & Hricak, H. (2016). Radiomics: Images are more than pictures, they are data. *Radiology*, *278*(2), 563–577. DOI: 10.1148/radiol.2015151169

Girvin, F., & Ko, J. P. (2008). Pulmonary nodules: Detection, assessment, and CAD. *AJR. American Journal of Roentgenology*, *191*(4), 1057–1069. DOI: 10.2214/AJR.07.3472

Goldstraw, P., Chansky, K., Crowley, J., Rami-Porta, R., Asamura, H., Eberhardt, W. E. E., Nicholson, A. G., Groome, P., Mitchell, A., Bolejack, V., Goldstraw, P., Rami-Porta, R., Asamura, H., Ball, D., Beer, D. G., Beyruti, R., Bolejack, V., Chansky, K., Crowley, J., & Yokoi, K. (2016). The IASLC lung cancer staging project: Proposals for revision of the TNM stage groupings in the forthcoming (eighth) edition of the TNM classification for lung cancer. *Journal of Thoracic Oncology, 11*(1), 39–51. DOI: 10.1016/j.jtho.2015.09.009

Gonzalez, R. C. (2009). *Digital image processing*. Pearson Education India.

Gould, M. K., Donington, J., Lynch, W. R., Mazzone, P. J., Midthun, D. E., Naidich, D. P., & Wiener, R. S. (2013). Evaluation of individuals with pulmonary nodules: When is it lung cancer? Diagnosis and management of lung cancer: American College of Chest Physicians evidence-based clinical practice guidelines. *Chest, 143*(5), e93S–e120S. DOI: 10.1378/chest.12-2351

Hardavella, G., Frille, A., Sreter, K. B., Atrafi, F., Yousaf-Khan, U., Beyaz, F., Kyriakou, F., Bellou, E., Mullin, M. L., & Janes, S. M. (2024). Lung cancer screening: Where do we stand? *Breathe (Sheffield, England), 20*(2), 230190. Advance online publication. DOI: 10.1183/20734735.0190-2023

. Hasan, M. A., Haque, F., Sabuj, S. R., Sarker, H., Goni, M. O. F., Rahman, F., & Rashid, M. M. (2024). An end-to-end lightweight multi-scale CNN for the classification of lung and colon cancer with XAI integration. *Technologies, 12*(4), 56. MDPI. DOI: 10.3390/technologies12040056

Herbst, R. S., Morgensztern, D., & Boshoff, C. (2018). The biology and management of non-small cell lung cancer. *Nature, 553*(7689), 446–454. DOI: 10.1038/nature25183

Hernández-Vázquez, N., Santos-Arce, S. R., Salido-Ruiz, R. A., Torres-Ramos, S., & Román-Godínez, I. (2024). Automatic cluster selection in K-means lung segmentation. In Flores Cuautle, J. d. J. A. (Eds.), *XLVI Mexican Conference on Biomedical Engineering (CNIB 2023)* (IFMBE Proceedings, Vol. 96). Springer, Cham. DOI: 10.1007/978-3-031-46933-6_17

Hesso, I., Kayyali, R., Dolton, D. R., Joo, K., Zacharias, L., Charalambous, A., Lavdaniti, M., Stalika, E., Ajami, T., Acampa, W., Boban, J., & Nabhani-Gebara, S. (2023). Cancer care at the time of the fourth industrial revolution: An insight into healthcare professionals' perspectives on cancer care and artificial intelligence. *Radiation Oncology (London, England), 18*(1), 167. DOI: 10.1186/s13014-023-02351-z

. Hesso, I., Kayyali, R., Zacharias, L., Charalambous, A., Lavdaniti, M., Stalika, E., Ajami, T., Acampa, W., Boban, J., & Gebara, S. N. (2024). Cancer care pathways across seven countries in Europe: What are the current obstacles? And how can artificial intelligence help? *Journal of Cancer Policy, 39*, 100457. Elsevier. DOI: 10.1016/j.jcpo.2023.100457

Hofmanninger, J., Prayer, F., Pan, J., Röhrich, S., Prosch, H., & Langs, G. (2020). Automatic lung segmentation in routine imaging is primarily a data diversity problem, not a methodology problem. *European Radiology Experimental, 4*(1), 1–13. DOI: 10.1186/s41747-020-00173-2

Holzinger, A., Langs, G., Denk, H., Zatloukal, K., & Müller, H. (2019). Causability and explainability of artificial intelligence in medicine. *Wiley Interdisciplinary Reviews. Data Mining and Knowledge Discovery, 9*(4), e1312. DOI: 10.1002/widm.1312

Hosny, A., Parmar, C., Quackenbush, J., Schwartz, L. H., & Aerts, H. J. W. L. (2018). Artificial intelligence in radiology. *Nature Reviews. Cancer, 18*(8), 500–510. DOI: 10.1038/s41568-018-0016-5

Huang, D., Li, Z., Jiang, T., Yang, C., & Li, N. (2024). Artificial intelligence in lung cancer: Current applications, future perspectives, and challenges. *Frontiers in Oncology, 14*, 1486310. DOI: 10.3389/fonc.2024.1486310

Huang, T.-C., Chou, K.-T., Wang, Y.-C., & Zhang, G. (2014). Motion freeze for respiration motion correction in PET/CT: A preliminary investigation with lung cancer patient data. *BioMed Research International, 2014*(1), 167491. DOI: 10.1155/2014/167491

Hyman, D. M., Taylor, B. S., & Baselga, J. (2017). Implementing genome-driven oncology. *Cell, 168*(4), 584–599. DOI: 10.1016/j.cell.2016.12.015

Itai, Y., Kim, H., Ishikawa, S., Katsuragawa, S., Ishida, T., Nakamura, K., & Yamamoto, A. (2005). Automatic segmentation of lung areas based on SNAKES and extraction of abnormal areas. In *Proceedings of the 17th IEEE International Conference on Tools with Artificial Intelligence (ICTAI 2005)* (pp. 5–10). DOI: 10.1109/ICTAI.2005.44

Jadwaa, S. K. (2022). X-ray lung image classification using a Canny edge detector. *Journal of Electrical and Computer Engineering, 2022*(1), 3081584. Advance online publication. DOI: 10.1155/2022/3081584

Jamal-Hanjani, M., Wilson, G. A., McGranahan, N., Birkbak, N. J., Watkins, T. B. K., Veeriah, S., Shafi, S., Johnson, D. H., Mitter, R., Rosenthal, R., Salm, M., Horswell, S., Escudero, M., Matthews, N., Rowan, A., Chambers, T., Moore, D. A., Turajlic, S., Xu, H., & Swanton, C. (2017). Tracking the evolution of non–small-cell lung cancer. *The New England Journal of Medicine*, *376*(22), 2109–2121. DOI: 10.1056/NEJMoa1616288

Jiang, P., Sinha, S., Aldape, K., Hannenhalli, S., Sahinalp, C., & Ruppin, E. (2022). Big data in basic and translational cancer research. *Nature Reviews. Cancer*, *22*(11), 625–639. DOI: 10.1038/s41568-022-00502-0

Kakeda, S., Moriya, J., Sato, H., Aoki, T., Watanabe, H., Nakata, H., Oda, N., Katsuragawa, S., Yamamoto, K., & Doi, K. (2004). Improved detection of lung nodules on chest radiographs using a commercial computer-aided diagnosis system. *AJR. American Journal of Roentgenology*, *182*(2), 505–510. DOI: 10.2214/ajr.182.2.1820505

Kavitha, M. S., Shanthini, J., & Sabitha, R. (2019). ECM-CSD: An efficient classification model for cancer stage diagnosis in CT lung images using FCM and SVM techniques. *Journal of Medical Systems*, *43*(3), 73. Advance online publication. DOI: 10.1007/s10916-019-1190-z

Kido, S., Kidera, S., Hirano, Y., Mabu, S., Kamiya, T., Tanaka, N., Suzuki, Y., Yanagawa, M., & Tomiyama, N. (2022). Segmentation of lung nodules on CT images using a nested three-dimensional fully connected convolutional network. *Frontiers in Artificial Intelligence*, *5*, 782225. DOI: 10.3389/frai.2022.782225

Kodete, C. S., Saradhi, D. V., Suri, V. K., Varma, P. B. S., Tirumanadham, N. S. K. M. K., & Shariff, V. (2024). Boosting lung cancer prediction accuracy through advanced data processing and machine learning models. In *Proceedings of the 2024 4th International Conference on Sustainable Expert Systems (ICSES)* (pp. 1107–1114). IEEE. DOI: 10.1109/ICSES63445.2024.10763338

Krishnamurthy, S., Narasimhan, G., & Rengasamy, U. (2016). A level set evolution morphology-based segmentation of lung nodules and false nodule elimination by 3D centroid shift and frequency domain DC constant analysis. *International Journal of u- and e-Service. Science and Technology*, *9*(1), 187–198. DOI: 10.14257/ijunesst.2016.9.10.18

Kumar, V., Gu, Y., Basu, S., Berglund, A., Eschrich, S. A., Schabath, M. B., Forster, K., Aerts, H. J. W. L., Dekker, A., Fenstermacher, D., Goldgof, D. B., Hall, L. O., Lambin, P., Balagurunathan, Y., Gatenby, R. A., & Gillies, R. J. (2012). Radiomics: The process and the challenges. *Magnetic Resonance Imaging*, *30*(9), 1234–1248. DOI: 10.1016/j.mri.2012.06.010

Lamare, F., Fayad, H., Fernandez, P., & Visvikis, D. (2015). Local respiratory motion correction for PET/CT imaging: Application to lung cancer. *Medical Physics*, *42*(10), 5903–5912. DOI: 10.1118/1.4930251

Lambin, P., Leijenaar, R. T. H., Deist, T. M., Peerlings, J., de Jong, E. E. C., van Timmeren, J., Sanduleanu, S., Larue, R. T. H. M., Even, A. J. G., Jochems, A., van Wijk, Y., Woodruff, H., van Soest, J., Lustberg, T., Roelofs, E., van Elmpt, W., Dekker, A., Mottaghy, F. M., Wildberger, J. E., & Walsh, S. (2017). Radiomics: The bridge between medical imaging and personalized medicine. *Nature Reviews. Clinical Oncology*, *14*(12), 749–762. DOI: 10.1038/nrclinonc.2017.141

Lavanya, M., Arivalagan, M., Princye, P. H., Sivasubramanian, S., & Madhu, S. (2020). A review on lung nodule segmentation techniques for nodule detection. In *2020 4th International Conference on Electronics, Communication and Aerospace Technology (ICECA)* (pp. 1423–1428). IEEE. DOI: 10.1109/ICECA49313.2020.9297387

LeCun, Y., Bengio, Y., & Hinton, G. (2015). Deep learning. *Nature*, *521*(7553), 436–444. DOI: 10.1038/nature14539

Lee, S.-H., Cho, H., Lee, H. Y., & Park, H. (2019). Clinical impact of variability on CT radiomics and suggestions for suitable feature selection: A focus on lung cancer. *Cancer Imaging; the Official Publication of the International Cancer Imaging Society*, *19*(1), 1–12. DOI: 10.1186/s40644-019-0239-z

Lei, M., Varghese, B., Hwang, D., Cen, S., Lei, X., Desai, B., Azadikhah, A., Oberai, A., & Duddalwar, V. (2021). Benchmarking various radiomic toolkit features while applying the Image Biomarker Standardization Initiative toward clinical translation of radiomic analysis. *Journal of Digital Imaging*, *34*(5), 1156–1170. DOI: 10.1007/s10278-021-00506-6

Li, B., Chen, Q., Peng, G., Guo, Y., Chen, K., Tian, L. F., Ou, S., & Wang, L. (2016). Segmentation of pulmonary nodules using adaptive local region energy with probability density function-based similarity distance and multi-features clustering. *Biomedical Engineering Online*, *15*(1), 49. DOI: 10.1186/s12938-016-0164-3

Li, S., & Zhou, B. (2022). A review of radiomics and genomics applications in cancers: The way towards precision medicine. *Radiation Oncology (London, England)*, *17*(1), 217. DOI: 10.1186/s13014-022-02192-2

Li, X., Li, B., Liu, F., Yin, H., & Zhou, F. (2020). Segmentation of pulmonary nodules using a GMM fuzzy C-means algorithm. *IEEE Access : Practical Innovations, Open Solutions*, *8*, 37541–37556. DOI: 10.1109/ACCESS.2020.2968936

Li, Y., Sadée, C. Y., Carrillo-Perez, F., Selby, H. M., Thieme, A. H., & Gevaert, O. (2024). A 3D lung lesion variational autoencoder. *Cell Reports Methods*, *4*(2), 100695. DOI: 10.1016/j.crmeth.2024.100695

Liu, H., Geng, F., Guo, Q., Zhang, C., & Zhang, C. (2018). A fast weakly-supervised pulmonary nodule segmentation method based on modified self-adaptive FCM algorithm. *Soft Computing*, *22*(12), 3983–3995. DOI: 10.1007/s00500-017-2608-5

Liu, H., Zhang, C. M., Su, Z. Y., Wang, K., & Deng, K. (2015). Research on a pulmonary nodule segmentation method combining fast self-adaptive FCM and classification. *Computational and Mathematical Methods in Medicine*, *2015*(1), 185726. DOI: 10.1155/2015/185726

Liu, S., Sun, Q., & Ren, X. (2023). Novel strategies for cancer immunotherapy: Counter-immunoediting therapy. *Journal of Hematology & Oncology*, *16*(1), 38. DOI: 10.1186/s13045-023-01430-8

Liu, Y., Bai, P., Li, C., & Zhao, Y. (2018). A novel level set model originated from fuzzy connectedness guided initial contours. In *Proceedings of the 2018 IEEE 3rd International Conference on Image, Vision and Computing (ICIVC)* (pp. 288–293). IEEE. DOI: 10.1109/ICIVC.2018.8492772

Liu, Z., Zhang, X.-Y., Shi, Y.-J., Wang, L., Zhu, H.-T., Tang, Z., Wang, S., Li, X.-T., Tian, J., & Sun, Y.-S. (2017). Radiomics analysis for evaluation of pathological complete response to neoadjuvant chemoradiotherapy in locally advanced rectal cancer. *Clinical Cancer Research*, *23*(23), 7253–7262. DOI: 10.1158/1078-0432.CCR-17-1038

Lu, L., Tan, Y., Schwartz, L. H., & Zhao, B. (2015). Hybrid detection of lung nodules on CT scan images. *Medical Physics*, *42*(9), 5042–5505. DOI: 10.1118/1.4927573

Mackin, D., Fave, X., Zhang, L., Yang, J., Jones, A. K., Ng, C. S., & Court, L. (2018). Correction: Harmonizing the pixel size in retrospective computed tomography radiomics studies. *PLoS One*, *13*(1), e0191597. DOI: 10.1371/journal.pone.0191597

MacMahon, H., Naidich, D. P., Goo, J. M., Lee, K. S., Leung, A. N. C., Mayo, J. R., Mehta, A. C., Ohno, Y., Powell, C. A., Prokop, M., Rubin, G. D., Schaefer-Prokop, C. M., Travis, W. D., Van Schil, P. E., & Bankier, A. A. (2017). Guidelines for management of incidental pulmonary nodules detected on CT images: From the Fleischner Society 2017. *Radiology*, *284*(1), 228–243. DOI: 10.1148/radiol.2017161659

Manikandan, T., & Bharathi, N. (2011). Lung cancer diagnosis from CT images using fuzzy inference system. In V. V. Das & N. Thankachan (Eds.), *Computational Intelligence and Information Technology* (CCIS, Vol. 250). Springer, Berlin, Heidelberg. DOI: 10.1007/978-3-642-25734-6_110

Martell, M. B., Linton-Reid, K., Chen, M., & Aboagye, E. O. (2025). Radiomics for lung cancer diagnosis, management, and future prospects. *Clinical Radiology, 106926*, 106926. Advance online publication. DOI: 10.1016/j.crad.2025.106926

Mayerhoefer, M. E., Materka, A., Langs, G., Häggström, I., Szczypiński, P., Gibbs, P., & Cook, G. (2020). Introduction to radiomics. *Journal of Nuclear Medicine, 61*(4), 488–495. DOI: 10.2967/jnumed.118.222893

Mayuri, A. V. R., Rashmi, V., Das, B., Mandal, A., & Neelakandan, S. (2023). Artificial neural network (ANN) with Chan–Vese (CV) algorithm-based plant disease detection and classification. In *Proceedings of the 2023 International Conference on Applied Intelligence and Sustainable Computing (ICAISC)* (pp. 1–6). IEEE. DOI: 10.1109/ICAISC58445.2023.10199472

McIlhagga, W. (2011). The Canny edge detector revisited. *International Journal of Computer Vision, 91*(3), 251–261. DOI: 10.1007/s11263-010-0392-0

Meier-Schroers, M., Homsi, R., Skowasch, D., Buermann, J., Zipfel, M., Schild, H. H., & Thomas, D. (2018). Lung cancer screening with MRI: Results of the first screening round. *Journal of Cancer Research and Clinical Oncology, 144*(1), 117–125. DOI: 10.1007/s00432-017-2521-4

National Comprehensive Cancer Network. (2024). *NCCN Clinical Practice Guidelines in Oncology (NCCN Guidelines): Lung cancer screening* (Version 1.2024) https://www.nccn.org/professionals/physician_gls/pdf/lung_screening.pdf *(Accessed July 10, 2025)*

National Lung Screening Trial Research Team. (2011). Reduced lung-cancer mortality with low-dose computed tomographic screening. *The New England Journal of Medicine, 365*(5), 395–409. DOI: 10.1056/NEJMoa1102873

National Lung Screening Trial Research Team. (2011). The National Lung Screening Trial: Overview and study design. *Radiology, 258*(1), 243–253. DOI: 10.1148/radiol.10091808

Niu, C., Lyu, Q., Carothers, C. D., Kaviani, P., Tan, J., Yan, P., Kalra, M. K., Whitlow, C. T., & Wang, G. (2025). Medical multimodal multitask foundation model for lung cancer screening. *Nature Communications, 16*(1), 1523. DOI: 10.1038/s41467-025-56822-w

O'Shea, R., Manickavasagar, T., Horst, C., Hughes, D., Cusack, J., Tsoka, S., Cook, G., & Goh, V. (2023). Weakly supervised segmentation models as explainable radiological classifiers for lung tumour detection on CT images. *Insights Into Imaging*, *14*(195), 195. Advance online publication. DOI: 10.1186/s13244-023-01542-2

Oneda, E., Abu Hilal, M., & Zaniboni, A. (2020). Biliary tract cancer: Current medical treatment strategies. *Cancers (Basel)*, *12*(5), 1237. DOI: 10.3390/cancers12051237

. Otsu, N. (1975). A threshold selection method from gray-level histograms. *Automatica, 11*(285–296), 23–27.

Oudkerk, M., Devaraj, A., Vliegenthart, R., Henzler, T., Prosch, H., Heussel, C. P., Bastarrika, G., Sverzellati, N., Mascalchi, M., Delorme, S., Baldwin, D. R., Callister, M. E., Becker, N., Heuvelmans, M. A., Rzyman, W., Infante, M. V., Pastorino, U., Pedersen, J. H., Paci, E., & Field, J. K. (2017). European position statement on lung cancer screening. *The Lancet. Oncology*, *18*(12), e754–e766. DOI: 10.1016/S1470-2045(17)30861-6

Parmar, C., Grossmann, P., Bussink, J., Lambin, P., & Aerts, H. J. W. L. (2015). Machine learning methods for quantitative radiomic biomarkers. *Scientific Reports*, *5*(1), 13087. DOI: 10.1038/srep13087

Parmar, C., Leijenaar, R. T. H., Grossmann, P., Rios Velazquez, E., Bussink, J., Rietveld, D., Rietbergen, M. M., Haibe-Kains, B., Lambin, P., & Aerts, H. J. W. L. (2015). Radiomic feature clusters and prognostic signatures specific for lung and head & neck cancer. *Scientific Reports*, *5*(1), 11044. DOI: 10.1038/srep11044

Pei, Q., Luo, Y., Chen, Y., Li, J., Xie, D., & Ye, T. (2022). Artificial intelligence in clinical applications for lung cancer: Diagnosis, treatment and prognosis. [CCLM]. *Clinical Chemistry and Laboratory Medicine*, *60*(12), 1974–1983. DOI: 10.1515/cclm-2022-0291

Prasad, V. (2016). Perspective: The precision-oncology illusion. *Nature*, *537*(7619), S63. DOI: 10.1038/537S63a

Prencipe, B., Delprete, C., Garolla, E., Corallo, F., Gravina, M., Natalicchio, M. I., Buongiorno, D., Bevilacqua, V., Altini, N., & Brunetti, A. (2023). An explainable radiogenomic framework to predict mutational status of KRAS and EGFR in lung adenocarcinoma patients. *Bioengineering (Basel, Switzerland)*, *10*(7), 747. DOI: 10.3390/bioengineering10070747

Ren, H., Zhou, L., Liu, G., Peng, X., Shi, W., Xu, H., Shan, F., & Liu, L. (2020). An unsupervised semi-automated pulmonary nodule segmentation method based on enhanced region growing. *Quantitative Imaging in Medicine and Surgery*, *10*(1), 233–242. DOI: 10.21037/qims.2019.12.02

Rizzo, S., Botta, F., Raimondi, S., Origgi, D., Fanciullo, C., Morganti, A. G., & Bellomi, M. (2018). Radiomics: The facts and the challenges of image analysis. *European Radiology Experimental*, *2*(1), 1–8. DOI: 10.1186/s41747-018-0068-z

Rocha, J., Cunha, A., & Mendonça, A. M. (2020). Conventional filtering versus U-Net based models for pulmonary nodule segmentation in CT images. *Journal of Medical Systems*, *44*(4), 81. DOI: 10.1007/s10916-020-1541-9

Roy, R., Banerjee, P., & Chowdhury, A. S. (2020). A level set based unified framework for pulmonary nodule segmentation. *IEEE Signal Processing Letters*, *27*, 1465–1469. DOI: 10.1109/LSP.2020.3016563

Rudin, C. (2019). Stop explaining black box machine learning models for high stakes decisions and use interpretable models instead. *Nature Machine Intelligence*, *1*(5), 206–215. DOI: 10.1038/s42256-019-0048-x

Samek, W., Wiegand, T., & Müller, K.-R. (2017). Explainable artificial intelligence: Understanding, visualizing and interpreting deep learning models. *arXiv Preprint*, arXiv:1708.08296. https://doi.org//arXiv.1708.08296DOI: 10.48550

Schaefer-Prokop, C., Neitzel, U., Venema, H. W., Uffmann, M., & Prokop, M. (2008). Digital chest radiography: An update on modern technology, dose containment and control of image quality. *European Radiology*, *18*(9), 1818–1830. DOI: 10.1007/s00330-008-0948-3

Seeram, E. (2015). *Computed tomography: Physical principles, clinical applications, and quality control* (4th ed.). Elsevier.

. Silva, F., Pereira, T., Neves, I., Morgado, J., Freitas, C., Malafaia, M., Sousa, J., Fonseca, J., Negrão, E., Flor de Lima, B., et al. (2022). Towards machine learning-aided lung cancer clinical routines: Approaches and open challenges. *Journal of Personalized Medicine, 12*(3), 480. MDPI. DOI: 10.3390/jpm12030480

Song, F., Song, X., Feng, Y., Fan, G., Sun, Y., Zhang, P., Li, J., Liu, F., & Zhang, G. (2023). Radiomics feature analysis and model research for predicting histopathological subtypes of non-small cell lung cancer on CT images: A multi-dataset study. *Medical Physics*, *50*(7), 4351–4365. DOI: 10.1002/mp.16233

Sung, H., Ferlay, J., Siegel, R. L., Laversanne, M., Soerjomataram, I., Jemal, A., & Bray, F. (2021). Global cancer statistics 2020: GLOBOCAN estimates of incidence and mortality worldwide for 36 cancers in 185 countries. *CA: a Cancer Journal for Clinicians*, *71*(3), 209–249. DOI: 10.3322/caac.21660

Suzuki, K. (2017). Computer-aided detection of lung cancer. In Arimura, H. (Ed.), *Image-based computer-assisted radiation therapy* (pp. 9–40). Springer., DOI: 10.1007/978-981-10-2945-5_2

Taha, A. A., & Hanbury, A. (2015). Metrics for evaluating 3D medical image segmentation: Analysis, selection, and tool. *BMC Medical Imaging*, *15*(1), 1–28. DOI: 10.1186/s12880-015-0068-x

Theriault-Lauzier, P., Cobin, D., Tastet, O., Langlais, E. L., Taji, B., Kang, G., Chong, A.-Y., So, D., Tang, A., & Gichoya, J. W.. (2024). A responsible framework for applying artificial intelligence on medical images and signals at the point-of-care: The PACSAI platform. *The Canadian Journal of Cardiology*, *40*(10), 1828–1840. Advance online publication. DOI: 10.1016/j.cjca.2024.05.025

Topol, E. J. (2019). High-performance medicine: The convergence of human and artificial intelligence. *Nature Medicine*, *25*(1), 44–56. DOI: 10.1038/s41591-018-0300-7

Travis, W. D., Asamura, H., Bankier, A. A., Beasley, M. B., Detterbeck, F., Flieder, D. B., Goo, J. M., MacMahon, H., Naidich, D., Nicholson, A. G., ... (2016). The IASLC lung cancer staging project: Proposals for coding T categories for subsolid nodules and assessment of tumor size in part-solid tumors in the forthcoming eighth edition of the TNM classification of lung cancer. *Journal of Thoracic Oncology, 11*(8), 1204–1223. DOI: 10.1016/j.jtho.2016.03.025

Travis, W. D., Brambilla, E., Nicholson, A. G., Yatabe, Y., Austin, J. H. M., Beasley, M. B., Chirieac, L. R., Dacic, S., Duhig, E., Flieder, D. B., Geisinger, K., Hirsch, F. R., Ishikawa, Y., Kerr, K. M., Noguchi, M., Pelosi, G., Powell, C. A., Tsao, M. S., & Wistuba, I. (2015). The 2015 World Health Organization classification of lung tumors: Impact of genetic, clinical, and radiologic advances since the 2004 classification. *Journal of Thoracic Oncology*, *10*(9), 1243–1260. DOI: 10.1097/JTO.0000000000000630

Trebeschi, S., Drago, S. G., Birkbak, N. J., Kurilova, I., Călin, A. M., Delli Pizzi, A., Lalezari, F., Lambregts, D. M. J., Rohaan, M. W., Parmar, C., Rozeman, E. A., Hartemink, K. J., Swanton, C., Haanen, J. B A G., Blank, C. U., Smit, E. F., Beets-Tan, R. G. H., & Aerts, H. J. W. L. (2019). Predicting response to cancer immunotherapy using noninvasive radiomic biomarkers. *Annals of Oncology : Official Journal of the European Society for Medical Oncology*, *30*(6), 998–1004. DOI: 10.1093/annonc/mdz108

Tsimberidou, A. M., Fountzilas, E., Nikanjam, M., & Kurzrock, R. (2020). Review of precision cancer medicine: Evolution of the treatment paradigm. *Cancer Treatment Reviews*, *86*, 102019. DOI: 10.1016/j.ctrv.2020.102019

Tunali, I., Gillies, R. J., & Schabath, M. B. (2021). Application of radiomics and artificial intelligence for lung cancer precision medicine. *Cold Spring Harbor Perspectives in Medicine*, *11*(8), a039537. DOI: 10.1101/cshperspect.a039537

Unterrainer, M., Eze, C., Ilhan, H., Marschner, S., Roengvoraphoj, O., Schmidt-Hegemann, N.-S., Walter, F., Kunz, W. G., af Rosenschöld, P. M., & Jeraj, R.. (2020). Recent advances of PET imaging in clinical radiation oncology. *Radiation Oncology (London, England)*, *15*(1), 1–15. DOI: 10.1186/s13014-020-01519-1

Van der Velden, B. H., Kuijf, H. J., Gilhuijs, K. G., & Viergever, M. A. (2022). Explainable artificial intelligence (XAI) in deep learning-based medical image analysis. *Medical Image Analysis*, *79*, 102470. DOI: 10.1016/j.media.2022.102470

Vellido, A. (2020). The importance of interpretability and visualization in machine learning for applications in medicine and health care. *Neural Computing & Applications*, *32*(24), 18069–18083. DOI: 10.1007/s00521-019-04051-w

Wahl, R. L., Jacene, H., Kasamon, Y., & Lodge, M. A. (2009). From RECIST to PERCIST: Evolving considerations for PET response criteria in solid tumors. *Journal of Nuclear Medicine*, *50*(Suppl. 1), 122S–150S. DOI: 10.2967/jnumed.108.057307

Wang, J., Cheng, Y., Guo, C., & Tamura, S. (2015). A new pulmonary nodules detection scheme utilizing region grow and adaptive fuzzy c-means clustering. *Journal of Medical Imaging and Health Informatics*, *5*(8), 1941–1946. DOI: 10.1166/jmihi.2015.1674

. Wani, N. A., Kumar, R., & Bedi, J. (2024). DeepXplainer: An interpretable deep learning-based approach for lung cancer detection using explainable artificial intelligence. *Computer Methods and Programs in Biomedicine, 243*, 107879. Elsevier. DOI: 10.1016/j.cmpb.2023.107879

Willemink, M. J., Koszek, W. A., Hardell, C., Wu, J., Fleischmann, D., Harvey, H., Folio, L. R., Summers, R. M., Rubin, D. L., & Lungren, M. P. (2020). Preparing medical imaging data for machine learning. *Radiology*, *295*(1), 4–15. DOI: 10.1148/radiol.2020192224

Wilson, R., & Devaraj, A. (2017). Radiomics of pulmonary nodules and lung cancer. *Translational Lung Cancer Research*, *6*(1), 86–91. DOI: 10.21037/tlcr.2017.01.04

Xie, Q., Li, Y., He, N., Ning, M., Ma, K., Wang, G., Lian, Y., & Zheng, Y. (2022). Unsupervised domain adaptation for medical image segmentation by disentanglement learning and self-training. *IEEE Transactions on Medical Imaging*, *43*(1), 4–14. DOI: 10.1109/TMI.2022.3192303

Yadav, M., Lee, J., Kim, H., Lee, S., Um, T., Lee, S., Djunadi, T. A., Chung, L. I.-Y., Yu, J., Rodrigues, D., Gennaro, N., Kim, L., Nam, M., Kim, Y., Hong, I., Jang, J., Kang, G., Cho, A., Velichko, Y., & Chae, Y. K. (2024). Pre-treatment CT radiomics for predicting immunotherapy response in non-small cell lung cancer (NSCLC): RECIST vs. irRECIST criteria. *Journal of Clinical Oncology*, *42*(16, Suppl), e20613. DOI: 10.1200/JCO.2024.42.16_suppl.e20613

Yang, F., Zhang, J., Zhou, L., Xia, W., Zhang, R., Wei, H., Feng, J., Zhao, X., Jian, J., Gao, X., & Yuan, S. (2022). CT-based radiomics signatures can predict the tumor response of non-small cell lung cancer patients treated with first-line chemotherapy and targeted therapy. *European Radiology*, *32*(3), 1538–1547. DOI: 10.1007/s00330-021-08277-y

Yang, H.-H., Wang, F.-E., Sun, C., Huang, K.-C., Chen, H.-W., Chen, Y., Chen, H.-C., Liao, C.-Y., Kao, S.-H., & Wang, Y.-C. F.. (2021). Leveraging auxiliary information from EMR for weakly supervised pulmonary nodule detection. In Medical Image Computing and Computer Assisted Intervention – *MICCAI 2021: 24th International Conference,* Strasbourg, France, September 27–October 1, 2021, *Proceedings, Part VII* (pp. 251–261). Springer. DOI: 10.1007/978-3-030-87234-2_24

Yang, M., Shi, L., Huang, T., Li, G., Shao, H., Shen, Y., Zhu, J., & Ni, B. (2023). Value of contrast-enhanced magnetic resonance imaging-T2WI-based radiomic features in distinguishing lung adenocarcinoma from lung squamous cell carcinoma with solid components ≥ 8 mm. *Journal of Thoracic Disease*, *15*(2), 635–648. DOI: 10.21037/jtd-23-142

Yeghiazaryan, V., & Voiculescu, I. (2015). *An overview of current evaluation methods used in medical image segmentation* (Tech. Rep. RR-15-08, pp. 22). Department of Computer Science, Oxford, UK.

Ying, W., Cunxi, C., Tong, J., & Xinhe, X. (2009). Segmentation of regions of interest in lung CT images based on 2-D Otsu optimized by genetic algorithm. In *2009 Chinese Control and Decision Conference* (pp. 5185–5189). IEEE. DOI: 10.1109/CCDC.2009.5195024

Yousefi, B., Jahani, N., LaRiviere, M. J., Cohen, E., Hsieh, M.-K., Luna, J. M., Chitalia, R. D., Thompson, J. C., Carpenter, E. L., Katz, S. I., ... (2019). Correlative hierarchical clustering-based low-rank dimensionality reduction of radiomics-driven phenotype in non-small cell lung cancer. In *Medical Imaging 2019: Imaging Informatics for Healthcare, Research, and Applications* (Vol. 10954, pp. 278–285). SPIE. DOI: 10.1117/12.2515609

Zarei, M., Sotoudeh Paima, S., McCabe, C., Abadi, E., & Samei, E. (2024). A physics-informed deep neural network for harmonization of CT images. *IEEE Transactions on Biomedical Engineering*, *71*(12), 3494–3504. Advance online publication. DOI: 10.1109/TBME.2024.3428399

Zhang, L., Gopalakrishnan, V., Lu, L., Summers, R. M., Moss, J., & Yao, J. (2018). Self-learning to detect and segment cysts in lung CT images without manual annotation. In *Proceedings of the 2018 IEEE 15th International Symposium on Biomedical Imaging (ISBI 2018)* (pp. 1100–1103). DOI: 10.1109/ISBI.2018.8363763

Zhang, R., Hong, M., Cai, H., Liang, Y., Chen, X., Liu, Z., Wu, M., Zhou, C., Bao, C., Wang, H., Yang, S., & Hu, Q. (2023). Predicting the pathological invasiveness in patients with a solitary pulmonary nodule via Shapley additive explanations interpretation of a tree-based machine learning radiomics model: A multicenter study. *Quantitative Imaging in Medicine and Surgery*, *13*(12), 7828–7845. DOI: 10.21037/qims-23-615

Zhang, W., Zhang, X., Zhao, J., Qiang, Y., Tian, Q., & Tang, X. (2017). A segmentation method for lung nodule image sequences based on superpixels and density-based spatial clustering of applications with noise. *PLoS One*, *12*(9), e0184290. DOI: 10.1371/journal.pone.0184290

Zhang, Y., Oikonomou, A., Wong, A., Haider, M. A., & Khalvati, F. (2017). Radiomics-based prognosis analysis for non-small cell lung cancer. *Scientific Reports*, *7*(1), 46349. DOI: 10.1038/srep46349

Zhong, J., Liu, X., Hu, Y., Xing, Y., Ding, D., Ge, X., Song, Y., Wang, S., Chen, L., Zhu, Y., Lu, W., Zhang, H., & Yao, W. (2024). Robustness of quantitative diffusion metrics from four models: A prospective study on the influence of scan-rescans, voxel size, coils, and observers. *Journal of Magnetic Resonance Imaging*, *60*(4), 1470–1483. DOI: 10.1002/jmri.29192

Zhou, J., Wen, Y., Ding, R., Liu, J., Fang, H., Li, X., Zhao, K., & Wan, Q. (2024). Radiomics signature based on robust features derived from diffusion data for differentiation between benign and malignant solitary pulmonary lesions. *Cancer Imaging; the Official Publication of the International Cancer Imaging Society, 24*(1), 14. DOI: 10.1186/s40644-024-00660-4

. Zhu, E., Muneer, A., Zhang, J., Xia, Y., Li, X., Zhou, C., Heymach, J. V., Wu, J., & Le, X. (2025). Progress and challenges of artificial intelligence in lung cancer clinical translation. *npj Precision Oncology, 9*(1), 210. DOI: 10.1038/s41698-025-00986-7

Zuo, Y., Liu, Q., Li, N., Li, P., Fang, Y., Bian, L., Zhang, J., & Song, S. (2024). Explainable 18F-FDG PET/CT radiomics model for predicting EGFR mutation status in lung adenocarcinoma: A two-center study. *Journal of Cancer Research and Clinical Oncology, 150*(10), 469. DOI: 10.1007/s00432-024-05998-7

Zwanenburg, A., Vallières, M., Abdalah, M. A., Aerts, H. J. W. L., Andrearczyk, V., Apte, A., Ashrafinia, S., Bakas, S., Beukinga, R. J., Boellaard, R., Bogowicz, M., Boldrini, L., Buvat, I., Cook, G. J. R., Davatzikos, C., Depeursinge, A., Desseroit, M.-C., Dinapoli, N., Dinh, C. V., & Löck, S. (2020). The image biomarker standardization initiative: Standardized quantitative radiomics for high-throughput image-based phenotyping. *Radiology, 295*(2), 328–338. DOI: 10.1148/radiol.2020191145

Chapter 8
Machine Learning in Radiation Oncology

Tariq S. Mian
https://orcid.org/0000-0003-2666-9223
Taibah University, Saudi Arabia

Hisham F. Saeed
Fatima Medical and Saleem Surgical Hospital, Sheikhupura, Pakistan

Eman M. Alatawi
Taibah University, Saudi Arabia

ABSTRACT

Machine learning (ML) is transforming radiation oncology by enhancing precision, efficiency, and personalization. Key applications include: (1) Treatment planning—U-Net and nnU-Net achieve >85% Dice scores for tumor segmentation, while GANs optimize dose distribution; (2) Predictive modeling—Radiomics and genomics predict treatment response/toxicity, though data heterogeneity challenges reproducibility; (3) Personalized therapy—Biomarker-driven adaptation and digital twins enable dynamic adjustments. Challenges include data scarcity, model validation, and interdisciplinary collaboration, with federated learning proposed for privacy-preserving data sharing. ML automates workflows, improves outcomes, and addresses resource disparities, but requires standardized protocols, robust validation, and ethical frameworks for equitable adoption. Future directions include federated learning advances, multi-center trials, and prospective studies to translate research into practice.

DOI: 10.4018/979-8-3373-4312-9.ch008

BACKGROUND AND LITERATURE REVIEW

The rising cancer burden, estimated to hit 28.4 million fresh cases every year by 2040 (Grahovac, 2023), has further increased the need to find more accurate, effective, and tailored treatment options. Radiation oncology, which is one of the pillars of cancer treatment, is especially pressed to move beyond the conventional protocols. The major issue is to get the best possible control over tumours and least possible toxicity to the neighbouring healthy tissues, which is naturally complex and differs positively in individual patients.

The artificial intelligence (AI) and clinical medicine have joined forces creating an opportunity to tackle this challenge. Initial computational work in radiation oncology was on the rule-based systems and simple statistical models of processes such as dose calculation. Nevertheless, with the development of machine learning (ML) and deep learning in particular, the shift in approach to automation to intelligent assistance has become possible. It was shown that convolutional neural networks (CNNs), including U-Net, can be used to automate the labour-intensive task of tumour and organ-at-risk segmentation, with Dice coefficients comparable to human experts (Seminal work by (Giraud et al., 2019) and others). At the same time, the so-called radiomics appeared, to which researchers, including (Dercle et al., 2021), attributed quantitative characteristics of medical images as a potential predictor of treatment response and toxicity.

Irrespective of this positive trend, there are some gaps evident in the literature. To start with, the reproducibility crisis affects most ML applications, particularly in the field of radiomics, frequently because of the absence of standardised protocols of image acquisition, preprocessing, and validation (Zhovannik, 2022; Dercle et al., 2021). Second, it has a high level of translational disparity; many of the models are highly accurate in retrospective research, but a minimal number are subject to rigorous prospective clinical verification [Citation: Dercle et al., 2021]. Third, there exist problems of data scarcity and heterogeneity, which restrict the possibility of the generalizability of models to new patient groups and clinical settings (Vuong, 2021). Lastly, the concept of multi-modal data (imaging, genomics, clinical records) integration into unified predictive models is a significant technical and operational challenge (Khansari, 2024).

The objective of the review is to synthesise these advances and issues, critically reviewing the adoption of ML in the main fields of radiation oncology treatment planning, predictive modelling, and therapy personalisation. This work will attempt to bring a clear roadmap on how responsible and effective adoption of ML in clinical practice can be done by consolidating the current state of the art and by clearly solving the identified gaps.

1. INTRODUCTION

The implementation of machine learning (ML) in radiation oncology can be regarded as a major breakthrough in the modern healthcare sector, as it proposes new measures to enhance the precision and efficiency of cancer care delivery. Given the global cancer rates are expected to exceed 28.4 million new cancer cases per year by 2040 [Citation], there is an instant need to find more patient-centred and innovative therapeutic solutions. Radiation oncology as one of the pillars of cancer care has now been challenged to transform its methods to accommodate more complicated clinical demands. The key research question that is critically reviewed in this review paper is as follows: How can ML methods, especially in the processes of treatment planning and delivery, predictive modelling and personalisation, be optimally combined to improve accuracy and efficiency in radiation oncology? We explore this query by conducting a literature review, particularly regarding the transformative opportunities, as well as the ethical, technical, and practical issues that arise due to the implementation of ML.

This review is intended to examine the scientific role of ML in the facilitation of precision and efficiency in radiation oncology with reference to three major domains, namely treatment planning and delivery, predictive modelling, and therapy personalisation. The synthesis of our analysis incorporates established and new applications in literature, but in parallel, we highlight general issues of methodology and implementation. Special attention is paid to such issues as interpretability, data scarcity, validation of algorithms, and ethics. Through the assessment of current research status, determination of major gaps, and recommendation of the avenue of responsible integration, this review will be utilized to offer a way forward in the future of AI in clinical oncology.

In the field of Machine Learning in Radiation Oncology, the connection between artificial intelligence and clinical oncology practice is discussed in the current paper. Even though radiation therapy (RT) has long been considered one of the key treatment modalities used to manage cancer, its effectiveness depends on the delicate process of balancing the need to cause minimal damage to normal tissues and the ability to manage the tumour. This need has become the demand of the advancement of decent treatment planning, therapy individualization and predictive measures of its consequences and adverse effects. Comprising of the algorithms that learn through data so as to make predictions or automate processes, ML presents useful opportunities to respond to such needs. ML can transform clinical processes and clinical outcomes in radiation oncology by automating labour intensive tasks such as tumour segmentation, enhancing the accuracy of dose delivery, and supporting adaptive planning based on patient specific information.

It is based on a literature-based research methodology, in which comparative analysis and critical analysis of the literature were applied in the key domains: automated segmentation algorithms (e.g., U-Net, nnU-Net, SAM, EAV-UNet), AI-assisted dose optimisation (including GANs), and adaptive radiotherapy that could be supported by an advanced imaging device such as MRI-Linac and cone-beam CT. The paper also looks at the integration of radiomics, radiogenomics, and biomarker analysis into predictive modelling and strategies to personalize approaches like Bayesian network-based dose adaptation and digital twins. Special attention is paid to ML model validation, technical and ethics barriers, the role of federated learning and data sharing. This approach will help to clear up the current situation in the field as well as the future perspectives of the ML development in radiation oncology.

The paper design is crafted in such a way that it facilitates an in-depth discussion of the topic. After the introduction, Chapter 2 presents the ML applications in treatment planning among which there is automated segmentation and dose optimisation. Chapter 3 is an analysis of predictive modelling that includes radiomics integration and treatment response assessment methods. Chapter 4 deals with the Personalisation strategies, which involve biomarker-based adaptations and patient-specific planning. Chapter 5 addresses issues such as implementation, such as ethical issues, clinical validation, and technical requirements. Chapter 6 brings the paper to an end with the summarization of the findings and a discussion on future directions of the integration of ML in radiation oncology.

2. MACHINE LEARNING IN TREATMENT PLANNING

Radiation oncology is becoming increasingly personalised, accurate and efficient due to the application of machine learning-based treatment planning. Field workflow can be enhanced through automation in dose change and segmentation. Machine learning promotes planning of treatment, so the knowledge of its use, issues, and future needs is essential in contemporary radiotherapy.

The following table (Table 1) summarises the major variations between traditional models and modern machine learning models, and their effects on clinical workflow and clinical outcomes.

Table 1. Comparison of The Traditional and ML-Based Approaches to Radiation Oncology Treatment Planning.

Feature	Traditional Methods	ML-Based Methods	Key Evidence & Impact
Speed	Manual contouring can take hours to days per case. Plan optimisation is iterative and time-consuming.	Automated contouring in minutes. AI-driven dose optimisation can generate plans in seconds to minutes.	High throughput by reducing planning time significantly. (Fiorentino et al., 2023).
Accuracy	Highly dependent on clinician expertise. Prone to manual errors in complex anatomies.	High quantitative accuracy (e.g., Dice coefficients >85% for many OARs and tumours). Can match or exceed expert-level consistency in defined tasks.	U-Net variants show Dice >85%; EAV-UNet reported F1 score of 96.1% (AbdelAziz et al., 2024).
Inter-Observer Variability	High. Different experts may produce significantly different contours, affecting plan quality and multi-centre trial consistency.	Low. Provides standardised, reproducible contours that minimise variability between and within observers.	Eliminates inter-observer variability, crucial for standardising multi-centre studies (AbdelAziz et al., 2024).
Resource Requirements	High demand for skilled human resources (oncologists, dosimetrists). Lower computational costs.	High upfront computational cost (GPU clusters, data storage). Reduces long-term human labour. Can streamline work in resource-limited settings.	Enables centres with limited expert staff to deliver state-of-the-art care by automating labour-intensive tasks (Fiorentino et al., 2023).

2.1 Automated Segmentation Methods

Machine learning-based radiation oncology benefits from automatic segmentation. Automation minimizes work, improves accuracy, and standardizes treatment. Models can detect cancer and organs-at-risk. Deep learning models U-Net, nnU-Net, SAM, and EAV-UNet segment OARs and tumours. Some U-Nets have 85% Dice coefficients in primary segmentation (AbdelAziz et al., 2024, p. 4). Automatic segmentations are nearly as accurate as expert segmentations and can be utilized clinically. EAV-UNet had 96.1% F1 in the binary segmentation BraTS-Africa dataset (AbdelAziz et al., 2024, p. 4), while SAM had 86.6 Dice. Multiclass segmentations for complex tissues like abdominal or pelvic cancer are lacking, however automated segmentation may improve therapy. SAM's multiclass segmentation Dice was 60.4 (AbdelAziz et al., 2024, p. 4).

The models standardize clinical care and eliminate inter-observer variation by segmenting objects from different patients or centers with identical outlines. For consistency, multi-center research must be uniform. Protocol and process changes can hinder multi-center research due to observer variability. Without this ambiguity, multi-center research could give larger, more consistent datasets (AbdelAziz et al., 2024, p. 4). Deep learning must segment uncommon malignancies or low-quality pictures for therapy. Before implementing these algorithms in clinics, a diverse clinical dataset must assess model resilience (AbdelAziz et al., 2024, p. 4).

Research indicates that Dice-Sørensen coefficients > 90% for OARs such parotid glands align with expert recommendations (Giraud et al., 2019, p. 5). Most patients have unique OARs. This would improve treatment planning speed and quality.

Low-value little OARs lack the appropriate lens or brainstem (Giraud et al., 2019, p. 5). Increasing radiation therapy dosages may make these small cases clinically important but harder to differentiate.

Automated segmentation reduces OAR and tumour target contouring time (Giraud et al., 2019, p. 5; Fiorentino, 2023, p. 1). High-volume treatment centers may automate workflows for faster planning. High-incidence radiation centers may lack resources. Combining these models to streamline workflow will help centers treat more patients and minimize wait times. This may work in breast, prostate, lung, and colorectal cancer-prone areas (Giraud et al., 2019, p. 5; Fiorentino, 2023, p. 1). These tools enable centers swiftly provide excellent cancer care and improve outcomes.

New imaging approaches are employed in adaptive radiotherapy. For adaptive re-planning, 3D/4D volumetric imaging systems and EPIDs use daily or weekly volumetric images (Tunçel, 2021, p. 3). Clinical ART involves weekly plan re-optimisation and per-fraction beam weight modifications (Tunçel, 2021, p. 3). Imaging helps ART systems discover cancers and organs-at-risk, improving dosage compliance and efficacy (Tunçel, 2021, p. 3). Medical imaging is used in every treatment plan, enabling doctors and scientists to have vast labelled datasets for machine learning segmentation and dosimetry algorithms (Tunçel, 2021, p. 3).

Unannotated medical imaging data inhibits automatic segmentation. Teaching model tasks requires enough, well-annotated data (Deist, 2019, p. 17). Automation can contour clinical departments and institutions faster and more consistently, improving treatment delivery in regions with clinical manpower and equipment shortages (Fiorentino et al., 2023, p. 1).

2.2 Dose Optimisation Techniques

From historical planning, AI-driven dose optimisation develops clinically appropriate radiation dose distributions. Treatment planning is faster and more consistent, reducing subjective variability and time waste. For better treatment outcomes, generative adversarial networks (GAN) can optimise clinical goals such dosage to at-risk organs (Archambault et al., 2020, p. 9). Federated learning may allow many institutions to train ML models without exposing patient data to address data quantity and quality challenges (Archambault et al., 2020, p. 9). This may make dose optimisation more generalizable but may face legal and institutional obstacles.

Probabilistic contour uncertainty protects head and neck structures better than isotropic contour expansion in adaptive proton treatment (Bengtsson et al., 2024, p. 3). Planning takes ten times longer than isotropic expansion since this optimisation method requires 200 contour samples (Bengtsson et al., 2024, p. 3). This approach provides clinically acceptable dose distributions with adequate coverage and structural sparing, but routine clinical processes require significant planning time reduction.

IMRT improves moderate and severe xerostomia and submucous fibrosis in head and neck cancer patients compared to 3D conformal radiation therapy, but long-term tumour control is the same (Adhikarimayum, 2023, p. 2). Volumetric-modulated arc therapy (VMAT) has better dosimetric efficiency and beam-on time than IMRT and 3DCRT, reducing treatment planning and beam delivery delays (Adhikarimayum, 2023, p. 2).

Stereotactic body radiation (SBRT) may outperform surgery for 3-year overall survival and decreased toxicity in early-stage non-small cell lung cancer (Adhikarimayum, 2023, p. 2). Modern dose-optimized treatment planning may improve survival and reduce side effects and toxicity. Radiogenomics, electronic medical records, and imaging features can personalize medicines and improve clinical outcomes. Radiogenomic data has linked thousands of genes and radiomic features to tumour morphologies and treatment response (Xia, 2023, pp. 50-56).

According to gene ontology and radiomic region analysis, treatment outcome concepts like local control are more common, supporting individualized dosage planning. Xia (2023, pp. 54-56) linked distant metastases to unique radiomic area sets. Data limitations may make radiation oncology precision treatment problematic, especially in poorer nations with rising cancer incidence. Scalable medicines are needed to lower developing country cancer incidence by 95% by 2040 (Grahovac, 2023, p. 17).

For practical use, ML dosage optimisation must account for inter-patient anatomical variances and heterogeneity. Due to high anatomical heterogeneity and variability in organs at risk contours, head and neck segmentation and dose calculations are problematic and require robust uncertainty quantification (Bengtsson et al., 2024, p. 2). Federated learning can address insufficient training data volume and ensure patient anonymity through data-sharing to provide tailored radiation oncology treatment for a heterogeneous, vast population (Grahovac, 2023, p. 17).

Overall, ML dose optimisation has enhanced radiation therapy planning by improving dose prescription alternatives and clinical outcomes. Overcoming application hurdles requires overcoming major clinical translation constraints.

2.3 Overview of Machine Learning Models in Treatment Planning

Machine learning has changed treatment planning with automatic segmentation and dose optimisation. These advances are motivated by the diversity of ML architectural communities' capabilities and methods. To bring this chapter's ML models into coherence and provide a concise comparison view, Table 2 summarizes their key applications, the best performance measurements in the literature, and some of their drawbacks.

Table 2. Summary of Key Machine Learning Models Discussed in Radiation Oncology

ML Model	Primary Application(s) in Radiation Oncology	Reported Performance (Examples)	Key Limitations
U-Net & Variants (nnU-Net)	**Automated Segmentation** of tumours and Organs-at-Risk (OARs).	Dice coefficients **>85%** for many structures; ~90% for parotid glands (Giraud et al., 2019).	Performance drops for small or complex structures (e.g., multiclass Dice of 60.4 for SAM). Requires large, annotated datasets.
Generative Adversarial Networks (GANs)	**Dose Optimisation & Prediction**, synthetic data generation, plan quality assurance.	Can generate clinically acceptable dose distributions rapidly, mimicking prior high-quality plans (Archambault et al., 2020).	Reliability is highly dependent on the quality and diversity of the training data. It can be unstable during training.
Random Forests / Hard Voting Classifier	**Predictive Modeling**, e.g., stratification based on genetic markers (MGMT) or treatment outcomes.	~86% accuracy for predicting MGMT methylation status in glioblastoma (Miteva, 2025).	Performance is moderate for complex clinical decisions (e.g., AUC ~0.7). It may not capture complex non-linear relationships as well as deep learning.
Convolutional Neural Networks (CNNs)	**Image Classification & Feature Extraction**, e.g., lesion detection, radiomic feature analysis.	Up to **97.2% accuracy** in lung cancer image classification (Chehade et al., 2022).	Act as "black boxes"; lack interpretability. Performance can be biased if training data is not diverse (e.g., lower accuracy on darker skin tones).
Vision Transformers	**Advanced Image Analysis**, e.g., non-invasive biomarker prediction from 3D scans.	**99.13%** accuracy in predicting MGMT status from MRI scans (AbdelAziz et al., 2024).	Extremely computationally intensive to train and run. Requires very large datasets to perform effectively.
Bayesian Networks	**Personalised Therapy**, integrating clinical, genomic, and imaging data to predict radiosensitivity and toxicity risk probabilistically.	Enables uncertainty quantification for safer adaptive planning (Khansari, 2024).	Complex to build and validate. Requires high-quality, harmonized multi-modal data from various sources.

3. PREDICTIVE MODELING APPLICATIONS

Predictive modeling using radiomics, genetics, and multimodal data is improving treatment response and personalizing radiation. Machine learning applications on complicated biology and imaging biomarkers will improve radiation oncology clinical decision-making and treatment response consistency. Predictive modeling, which improves treatment planning and customized medicine, requires validation and interdisciplinary collaboration to increase clinical application.

3.1 Integration of Radiomics

Radiomics uses quantitative imaging biomarkers to characterise malignancies and surrounding tissues, improving radiation oncology precision. Imaging scanner SNR, image preprocessing, and segmentation methodology affect radiomic analysis reliability. Under scanner SNR variation, 62 of 92 radiomic parameters are significantly variable (Zhovannik, 2022, p. 60). Additive correction methods improve feature stability by reducing standard deviation by more than two in 47 features (Zhovannik, 2022, p. 60). These methods show radiomics preprocessing's value. Only 17% of radiomics research notes every methodological step, from scanner to feature extraction. Without documentation, replication and translation are constrained (Dercle et al., 2021, p. 7). Lack of procedure reduces inter-study comparisons and encourages overfitting and weak feature attribution. This misrepresents biomarker prediction and performance (Dercle et al., 2021, p. 7). Reproducibility and clinical validity require harmonised multi-institutional pipelines and quality assurance.

Radiomics must be adaptable to diverse technological and biological settings to improve clinical outcome prediction. High-risk tumours near the mediastinum have worse NSCLC survival rates (Vuong, 2021, p. 5). Histology is better predicted by tumour-adjacent rim features than intratumoural features (Vuong, 2021, p. 6). This shows modeling outside the tumour core may be advantageous. Only 10% of NSCLC radiomic features were consistent across segmentation, patient movements, and protocol modifications. Transferability is limited and unknown (Vuong, 2021, p. 6). Validation sets for prediction had AUCs of 0.72-0.79. To improve radiomic feature repeatability in NSCLC, multi-region and multi-modal features must have rigorous validation and avoid using unstable features (Vuong, 2021, p. 6).

Radioomics can predict patient survival when combined with genetics or clinical data. Multi-omics data can be used to simulate patient-specific radiosensitivity, response, and adverse events. These combined predictive models beat anatomical imaging. Machine learning algorithms can uncover novel therapy targets by using multi-omics data as model features to predict and find non-linear correlations between cancer and tissue responses to treatment (Khansari, 2024, pp. 2-4). Radiomics and molecular data can identify individuals for adaptive dose escalation (in resistant cancers) or dose de-escalation (in sensitive tumours) to optimise treatment (Khansari, 2024, p. 4).

Data availability and heterogeneity are radiomics' main challenges. The field is growing, but high-quality, large-scale, well-annotated imaging datasets are limited. Imaging parameters, techniques, and scanner vendors differ. Thus, most studies recruit fewer than 50 patients and even fewer undertake prospective external validation in retrospectively validated trials with an independent patient group (Dercle et al., 2021, p. 13; p. 11). Radiomics feature transferability is limited, aggravating this. Federated learning addresses limited datasets and data protection. Several institutions train machine learning algorithms in situ to secure and share data (Zhovannik, 2022, p. 11). It benefits but raises regulatory and compliance concerns, especially between countries. Federated learning requires a strict, moral, and transparent framework.

Clinical workflow and oncology disparities are best improved via radiomics. This lets radiomics-based triage and high-throughput patient analysis plan treatment and quickly assess clinic risk (Morgado, 2024, p. 23). Europe's cancer rate would rise 21% by 2040 and 77% globally by 2050 (Morgado, 2024, p. 23). Machine learning-based radiomics reduces manual radiomics personnel and speeds clinical results. Large hospitals/healthcare facilities with many patients can postpone time-sensitive treatment (Morgado, 2024, p. 23).

3.2 Treatment Response Assessment

Radiomics uses quantitative imaging biomarkers to characterise malignancies and surrounding tissues, thereby improving the precision of radiation oncology. Imaging scanner SNR, image preprocessing, and segmentation methodology affect radiomic analysis reliability. Under scanner SNR variation, 62 of 92 radiomic parameters are significantly variable (Zhovannik, 2022, p. 60). Additive correction methods improve feature stability by reducing standard deviation by more than two in 47 features (Zhovannik, 2022, p. 60). These methods show radiomics preprocessing's value. Only 17% of radiomics research notes every methodological step, from scanner to feature extraction. Without documentation, replication and translation are constrained (Dercle et al., 2021, p. 7). Lack of procedure reduces inter-study comparisons and encourages overfitting and weak feature attribution. This misrepresents biomarker prediction and performance (Dercle et al., 2021, p. 7). Reproducibility and clinical validity require harmonised multi-institutional pipelines and quality assurance.

Radiomics must be adaptable to diverse technological and biological settings to improve clinical outcome prediction. High-risk tumours near the mediastinum have worse NSCLC survival rates (Vuong, 2021, p. 5). Histology is better predicted by tumour-adjacent rim features than intratumoural features (Vuong, 2021, p. 6). This shows modeling outside the tumour core may be advantageous. Only 10% of NSCLC radiomic features were consistent across segmentation, patient movements, and protocol modifications. Transferability is limited and unknown (Vuong, 2021, p. 6). Validation sets for prediction had AUCs of 0.72-0.79. To improve radiomic feature repeatability in NSCLC, multi-region and multi-modal features must undergo rigorous validation and not use unstable features (Vuong, 2021, p. 6).

Radioomics can predict patient survival when combined with genetics or clinical data. Multi-omics data can simulate patient-specific radiosensitivity, response, and adverse events. These combined predictive models beat anatomical imaging. Machine learning algorithms can uncover novel therapy targets by using multi-omics data as model features to predict and find non-linear correlations between cancer and tissue responses to treatment (Khansari, 2024, pp. 2-4). Radiomics and molecular data can identify individuals for adaptive dose escalation (resistant cancers) or dose de-escalation (sensitive tumours) to optimise treatment (Khansari, 2024, p. 4).

Data availability and heterogeneity are radiomics' main challenges. The field is growing, but high-quality, large-scale, well-annotated imaging datasets are limited. Imaging parameters, techniques, and scanner vendors differ. Thus, most studies recruit fewer than 50 patients and even fewer undertake prospective external validation in retrospectively validated trials with an independent patient group (Dercle et al., 2021, p. 13; p. 11). Radiomics feature transferability is limited, aggravating this. Federated learning addresses limited datasets and data protection. Several institutions train machine learning algorithms in situ to secure and share data (Zhovannik, 2022, p. 11). It benefits but raises regulatory and compliance concerns, especially between countries. Federated learning requires a strict, moral, and transparent framework.

Clinical workflow and oncology disparities are best improved via radiomics. This lets radiomics-based triage and high-throughput patient analysis plan treatment and quickly assess clinic risk (Morgado, 2024, p. 23). Europe's cancer rate would rise 21% by 2040 and 77% globally by 2050 (Morgado, 2024, p. 23). Machine learning-based radiomics reduces manual radiomics personnel and speeds clinical results. Large hospitals/healthcare facilities with many patients can postpone time-sensitive treatment (Morgado, 2024, p. 23).

4. PERSONALISATION STRATEGIES

Personalisation is changing radiation therapy. A biomarker-guided adaptation strategy and a patient-specific program can improve radiotherapy effectiveness, minimize dose-effect ratios, and provide a more tailored treatment. Nowadays, machine learning and other technologies can provide more precise and effective radiation treatments to many clinical scenarios.

4.1 Biomarker-Based Adaptation

Dynamic customised radiation dose is possible using biomarker-based machine learning models. Bayesian network-based models can probabilistically predict radiosensitivity, treatment response, and toxicity risk using clinical, genetic, and imaging biomarkers. This knowledge helps analyse uncertainty for safer and more effective adaptive planning. Harmonising data across clinical sites and integrating real-time biomarker testing into clinical workflows are needed to construct such models (Khansari, 2024, pp. 2-3).

Machine learning models that incorporate biomarkers like gene mutations, gene expression, and imaging features enable individualised radiation dose by moving from population-based prescription regimens to tumour adaptations. The ability to tailor each fraction to biomarker measurement in real time allows dose distribution and treatment fields to be adjusted to account for tumour heterogeneity. However, the practical implementation of these technologies still faces operational problems. Quick biomarker quantification and analysis are problems. Beyond this, integration of multi-input data streams requires interoperability (Khansari, 2024, pp. 2-4).

Radiogenomics studies found rs28419191 and rs448138 to be related to decreased mucositis rates. Both genes had the T minor allele (Barnett, 2016, p. 2). Personalised medicine can benefit patients by adjusting plans based on risk-modifying genes as biomarkers. Future studies may examine chromosomal diversity in different populations and use machine learning to customise treatment.

Genome-wide association studies reveal risk-modifying polymorphisms in radiation poisoning patients using genomic markers. These studies require many cohorts and genome-sequencing data to get meaningful results. Because they vary across studies, such relationships must be properly checked and integrated using well-constructed prediction work that efficiently uses multi-dimensional inputs (Barnett, 2016, pp. 1-2).

Individual radiation-induced adverse effect risks can be predicted using radiogenomic systems. Such algorithms can recommend personalised schedules and therapies based on risk estimations. For instance, radiogenomics can help biologists adjust radiation dosages using patients' imaging and molecular data (Khansari, 2024, p. 4). Radiogenomics is still limited in cancer treatment despite its predictive power. Complex radiogenomics datasets impede prospective validation and generalizability. Infrastructure for collecting huge patient datasets should be funded by policymakers to fill resource gaps.

In recent investigations, deep learning predicted MGMT methylation status in glioblastoma patients non-invasively. Deep learning methods categorized 99.13% of 3D vision transformer models for MGMT methylation detection (AbdelAziz et al., 2024, p. 10). These deep learning advancements also increase image segmentation and treatment efficiency. F1 scores show that EAV-UNet and SAM are accurate image segmentation models: 96.1% for EAV-UNet and 86.6 for Dice for binary segmentation using deep learning (AbdelAziz et al., 2024, p. 4).

Deep learning improves tumour margin and treatment area detection in automated cancer segmentation. Deep learning helps clinicians create treatment domains for tailored patient care by precisely defining tumours. This will improve risk grouping of patients for plan modification. Automated treatment plan tactics have improved, but repeatability in various clinical settings remains a challenge (Zhovannik, 2022, p. 60).

Machine learning in imaging is sensitive to tissue molecular changes, enabling sensitive plan adaption in glioblastoma. Quantitative imaging biomarker repeatability is a problem. Cierniack found that 62/92 radiomic characteristics had a greater signal-to-noise ratio. An additive correction model reduces variability for nearly all radiomic characteristics by two-fold and improves reliability. This strategy should be validated and implemented at other clinical sites (Zhovannik, 2022, p. 60).

Technical variances from vendors, pulse sequences, scanning equipment, and lack of standardization make imaging biomarkers disadvantageous. The lack of consistent research methodologies prevents radiogenomics from being widely used in machine learning. Research pipelines must be integrated to reduce biases across clinical sites. Federated learning lets clinical sites share patient datasets in a local system through multicenter collaboration. However, ethical issues including data sharing laws in different nations should be considered (Zhovannik, 2022, pp. 11, 13).

A germline biomarker is widely used in adaptive planning for breast cancer treatment to reduce long-term morbidity. The rate of coronary artery disease 20 years following left-sided breast cancer treatment is directly related to heart dose (Cirolla & Lora, 2024, p. 6). Clinicians can use genetic risk factors like BRCA1/2 status to alter treatment plans to avoid cardiac dosage restrictions and lessen these risks. Mean cardiac dosage is less than 5 Gy, and V20Gy is less than 10%. Long-term dangers will be reduced, and as a result, patient care will be improved with such techniques.

Genetic variation can be exploited to plan adaptation in other malignancies and use biomarker-predictive radiation. Example: BRCA1/2 evaluation is used in risk prediction and dose escalation and constraint (Cirolla & Lora, 2024, p. 2). Applying these inherited biomarkers requires infrastructure, training, and genomics education for doctors. Biomarker-derived individualised dosage restriction makes personalised radiotherapy useful.

Artificial intelligence adaptive workflows have shown that they can develop tumour contours in less than a minute and give a plan in 10 minutes for rectal cancer therapy. Machine learning can be used to alter plans to provide high-quality treatments quickly without affecting plan robustness and complexity (Briggs et al., 2021, pp. 12, 14). Further clinical studies of automated working processes are needed (Briggs et al., 2021, p. 2).

4.2 Patient-Specific Planning

AI-based digital twins use multi-level biology. In tissue-scale simulations, digital twins use artificial intelligence-driven partial differential equations to understand tissue radiation-response estimates. Radiobiological impacts are better understood by simulating DNA damage mechanisms at the molecular level. Digital twins reduce risk and improve therapy by in silico iterative treatment (Liu, 2024, p. 18). Digital twins with physiological and immunological data are accurate and promising for precision radiation oncology (Liu, 2024, p. 2).

Due to its ability to recognize trends in large multimodal datasets, machine learning has enabled treatment-planning optimisations that reduce toxicity (Luo et al., 2020, p. 2). Nonlinear techniques like artificial neural networks and support vector machines predict symptomatic lung injury and radiation pneumonitis better than linear statistical methods (Luo et al., 2020, p. 2). Artificial neural networks classify radiation results. For radiotherapy-induced symptomatic lung injury prediction, feed-forward artificial neural networks are trained on pre-radiotherapy biological and physical parameters (Luo et al., 2020, p. 2). Many layers of artificial neural networks learn patterns and predict outputs using different techniques, updating themselves from past mistakes (Driscoll, n.d.). Support vector machines are trained with kernel-based learning of high-dimensional interactions and non-kernel methods to learn any treatment regime pattern while minimizing failure, resulting in personalised treatment plans (Luo et al., 2020, p. 2). Machine learning can stratify patients at high or low risk for toxicity and local failure with biological and physical parameters before radiotherapy and learn a relationship between patient features, treatment dose distributions, and toxicity grades. Multi-deep neural networks using CT simulation scans and clinical variables predict local control for head and neck squamous cell carcinomas more accurately than logistic regression and random forest (Luo et al., 2020, p. 4).

Bayesian networks use clinical, genetic, and imaging information to predict radiosensitivity, toxicity, and other outcomes. These networks can stratify patients to recommend clinical treatments, such as increasing radiotherapy doses for aggressive phenotypes to improve local control or lowering doses for radio-sensitive patients to improve tolerance (Khansari, 2024, p. 2). Machine learning models further analyse the predictive powers of imaging biomarkers by learning from histopathological image patterns and spatial transcriptomics, which map gene activity within the specific spatial context of a tissue sample to analyse immune cell infiltration and vascular heterogeneity (Khansari, 2024, p. 3).

Breast cancer is an example of AI and machine learning in radiotherapy patient-specific planning. It improves risk categorisation and personalises adjuvant therapy, according to various studies (Khansari, 2024, p. 4). It refines risk categorisation in elderly patients. Patients with aggressive cancer characteristics and high risk for major side effects may safely forgo radiation treatment (Khansari, 2024, p. 4). According to clinical trial results, patients at high risk of disease recurrence had a 50% reduction in recurrence after radiotherapy, while those at low risk had no benefit due to their low relapse rate. These benefits have been extended to all cancer therapy stages as imaging and clinical biomarker data increase.

Adaptive radiotherapy is transforming patient-specific planning alongside machine learning and AI. Real-time, automated planning drives this radiation oncology intervention (Tunçel, 2021, p. 3). MRI navigation signals and electronic portal imaging equipment can identify inter- or intrafractional anatomical or tumour motions with great temporal and spatial resolution (Tunçel, 2021, p. 3). This allows clinicians to adjust beam weights to optimize radiation delivery while adjusting treatment plans based on factors like organ shrinkage or repositioning, normal tissue changes, and toxicity. The incorporation of a plan optimisation method during weekly conventionally fractionated radiation sessions is an example. This may improve therapeutic margin without much change or clinical resources compared to intensity modulation for treatment plans and dose escalation (Tunçel, 2021, p. 3). Adaptive methods also reduce toxicities, spare normal tissues from excessive doses, and improve quality of life during and after therapy. Computing power, planning time, and staffing limit real-time, automated adaptation (Tunçel, 2021, p. 3). The future of adaptive radiotherapy may depend on new imaging techniques, algorithmic efficiency, and computer capacity.

Machine learning's major advantage in radiation oncology is detecting interpatient heterogeneity for patient-specific planning, unlike generic patient cohorts or clinical trials (Khansari, 2024, p. 3). Machine learning platforms and non-invasive imaging can uncover radiomic biomarkers such radiogenomic characteristics, which describe radiotherapy response and radiation-induced immune infiltration (Khansari, 2024, p. 3).

Patient-specific planning for rectal cancer treatment has been automated using adaptive radiotherapy platforms. These modern radiotherapy devices can auto-segment patient images to develop tumour contours in under a minute and communicate the best treatment plan for radiation delivery in under ten minutes. Daily adaptive updates are feasible and time-efficient, easing concerns about individualized radiotherapy (Tunçel, 2021, pp. 1, 3).

5. IMPLEMENTATION CHALLENGES AND FUTURE DIRECTIONS

Machine learning in radiology is not merely an improvement of the technique, but a change in the workflow. The treatment planning and customisation based on the use of ML have to cross numerous technological, clinical, ethical, and practical obstacles. This chapter summarizes these concerns into critical areas and recommends the further development.

5.1 Technical Requirements

Any advanced MLs depend on high-quality and rich data and computing capabilities. Heterogeneity and data scarcity are severe technological challenges. It requires large datasets with notes in order to build perfect, challenging models such as dose optimisation or unusual tumour types. The accessibility of the data is constrained by patient privacy issues and institutional silos (Chu, 2021). The heterogeneity of data obtained during imaging, vendor of scanners, and anatomy of a patient lowers the general predictability of the models and may impair their performance in new clinical settings (Bengtsson et al., 2024).

The data scarcity and privacy issue may be addressed by federation learning (FL). FL allows the various institutions to train ML models without accessing patient information, enhancing privacy and security and producing stronger and more generalized models [Citation: Olawade et al., 2025]. FL presupposes the presence of homogeneous data formats and legal frameworks of cross-institutional interaction, among other technological and legal issues.

Advanced ML applications like adaptive proton therapy and digital twins require lots of compute. Computing that would have taken minutes outside of an HPC can now take hours, requiring infrastructure and high-performance computing that may not be available in some clinical settings (Bengtsson et al., 2024; Liu, 2024).

5.2 Clinical Validation

Clinical translation of ML is hampered by the lack of rigorous and transparent validation. Most radiomics works lack a methodological explanation, and only 17% describe picture capture and feature extraction (Dercle et al., 2021). Lack of openness makes reproducibility difficult.

Additionally, most ML models are assessed retroactively. Fewer than 6% of radiomics studies have external validation, and even fewer are tested in prospective clinical trials (Dercle et al., 2021). Models may overfit and fail in varied clinical workflows without prospective validation. Ethos, which received regulatory approval for its efficient adaptive workflows in a conventional treatment slot, shows the need to validate the model's accuracy, clinical feasibility, and workflow integration (Archambault et al., 2020).

5.3 Ethical and Regulatory Concerns

Training data should be representative of the population to avoid algorithmic bias and healthcare disparity. With less representation in training sets, AI-based skin cancer detection systems are less accurate with darker skin (Kumar, 2024).

FDA and other agencies regulate ML-based clinical tools called Software as a Medical Device. This necessitates extensive pre- and post-market testing for safety and efficacy (Kumar, 2024).

Ethos platform received market approval, CE mark, and FDA 510(k) clearance after one prospective clinical validation (Archambault et al., 2020, p. 9). Ethos overcomes the clinical application problem and proves its operational practicality by completing a patient-specific adaptive radiation cycle in 15 minutes. Clinical application is required for ML validation, which typically assesses predictive accuracy.

Some ML models are the most accurate, but accuracy does not guarantee therapeutic efficacy. CNNs can detect lung cancer with 97.2% accuracy, while XGBoost has an F1-score of 99 (Chehade et al., 2022, p. 3). Clinical validation should ensure that the algorithm performs well in different patient groups as certain algorithms function in all. As most AI datasets are based on lighter skin color, AI models for skin cancer diagnosis are less accurate in darker skin patients (Kumar, 2024, p. 12).

MC model validation addresses ethics and regulation. Healthcare-based ML systems must meet regulatory quality norms like post-market follow-ups, bias evaluation, and transparency reporting as SaMDs (Kumar, 2024, pp. 1213).

5.4 Workforce Integration and Workflow Adaptation

Human factors determine implementation success. ML tools require radiation oncologists, medical physicists, dosimetrists, and IT specialists to reinvent clinical processes and collaborate. In adaptive radiotherapy, pre-treatment planning becomes real-time, on-table decision-making (Tunçel, 2021).

6. CONCLUSION

This chapter aimed to explore the possibility of machine learning in radiation oncology and enhance precision, efficiency in treatment planning, predictive modelling, and therapy Personalisation . In my opinion, the review and assessment of the existing machine learning approaches in significant fields of radiation oncology was successfully done in this paper, as it proved that these methods are not only facilitating the process but also promoting the paradigm of personalised patient care in this domain. Machine learning methodologies have been applied to automated segmentation, dose optimisation and predictive modelling via radiomics, and biomarker-driven adaptation, have demonstrated better accuracy and reproducibility of modern radiotherapy practice, as well as identified outstanding challenges in existing operation and methodology.

This literature review has reviewed evidence showing that machine learning has a vast potential to enhance accuracy, precision, efficiency, and personalisation of radiation oncology. ML approaches will transform the standards of care, as the methods that can be utilized to perform automated segmentation evolve into those that can be adapted using biomarkers.

Nevertheless, the key to transferring these technologies between research and practice is the ability to overcome the obstacles critical to the process. Issues of lack of reproducibility, paucity of prospective validation, and heterogeneity of data are still pertinent problems. In this regard, the future should be working on the following:

1. **Advancing Federated Learning:** Promoting multi-institutional collaborations to build robust, generalizable models while preserving data privacy.
2. **Prioritizing Prospective Validation:** Conducting rigorous clinical trials that move beyond retrospective accuracy to demonstrate improvements in patient outcomes, such as survival and toxicity reduction.
3. **Developing Explainable AI (XAI):** Creating models that are not only accurate but also interpretable to clinicians, thereby fostering trust and facilitating human-AI collaboration.
4. **Establishing Ethical Frameworks:** Implementing guidelines to ensure equity, transparency, and accountability in all clinical AI applications.

To conclude, the future of ML in radiation oncology is bright but needs a well-related, interdisciplinary strategy aimed at creating powerful, generalizable, and ethically viable algorithms. With this set of priorities, the field can realise the full potential of ML with respect to developing a new paradigm of personalised and accessible cancer care.

The summary of the findings of this review is as follows. Even though most of these applications are in active development, automated segmentation models make it clear that algorithms can be equally accurate as manual segmentations made by physicians. The AI-assisted optimisation of radiation doses can be applied quicker and deliver distributions comparable to those of the traditional optimisation planning. Radiomics or genomics Applications of predictive modelling processes enhance response assessment and toxicity intolerance assessment, but the predictive accuracy of the process relies on validation. Multimodality imaging data and biomarkers can be integrated into treatment working processes in order to support personalised treatment. Radiation oncology clinical platforms are also able to use machine learning and adaptive treatment workflows to provide more patient-specific treatment and care in a wide variety of environments.

This work has helped fill the fast-paced revolution in the field of radiation oncology in the context of the current revolution of individualized medicine because it evaluates both the current and potential future uses of machine learning methodologies. It is my hope that the findings of this review will spur additional studies in the direction of using big data and algorithms to enhance patient outcome and utilization of health resources in cancer management. Reproducibility of machine learning research and the absence of external validity are major issues that should be resolved to ensure generalizability. The absence of publicly available datasets that have proper annotation is a drawback to machine learning because the existing datasets are not able to reflect on inter-patient and inter-site variances, which in turn influences performance. The computational platforms, data, standards and tools employed in various cancer centres are heterogeneous, which impacts on data pooling. These barriers are problematic to the adoption of machine learning applications to clinical settings. On top of this, machine learning validation is not a popular practice. No accepted benchmarking and assessment criteria exist regarding clinical outcome and safety and quality of life measures.

The future trends in machine learning that would overcome these constraints would not only benefit the radiation oncology field but also the rest of the medical fields. The most important step towards addressing the inherent interpretability issues of complex systems and techniques like deep neural networks is to increase their clinical utility. Moreover, future studies ought to be concerned with ways of addressing small datasets that have low generalizability. One of the potential technologies is federated learning where multiple local models are trained together without sharing patient data. In addition, multi-centre joint research should be developed and encouraged to increase the dissemination of data without causing inequality in the advantages and disadvantages of improving the algorithms among different health care organizations. More comprehensive evaluation must be done by conducting prospective clinical trials. This will demand the presence of interdisciplinary teams that include specialists in the fields of cancer biology, clinical oncology, imaging, computer science, and statistics. The development and adoption of machine learning algorithms and platforms can also be accelerated by future enhancements in the computational resources and informatics infrastructure. The growing trend in applying machine learning methodologies to clinical workflow to adaptively treat or personalize processes is increasing, but issues like computational resources, workforce training, and regulations should be considered to guarantee scalability and sustainability of clinical applications. It could include the integration of AI into the cloud computing infrastructure, thus will entail the aspect of data privacy and protection.

Ethical issues should be considered when developing and applying machine learning. As it was mentioned in the foregoing section, algorithms can be prejudiced against the training data, which they are trained on. Other considerations that should be made include data security, data privacy, and cost of developing an algorithm. My interpersonal communication with other members of the department has shown that they are not only critical considerations to researchers in the field but also to clinical oncologists.

Summing up, machine learning can enhance accuracy, efficiency, and precision of radiation oncology and Personalisation . The creation of strong and transferable algorithms should be sought and ethical analysis carried out regularly to enhance and increase clinical application in cancer treatment.

REFERENCES

AbdelAziz, N. M., Dawood, E. A., Hassan, M. M., & Tantawy, A. A. (2024). *Brain tumour radiogenomic classification and prediction of glioblastoma status using MRI scans with deep learning algorithms. Research Square.* DOI: 10.21203/rs.3.rs-3968021/v1

Adhikarimayum, A. D. (2023). Recent treatment advancements in radiation therapy. Jawaharlal Nehru Institute of Medical Sciences. https://iipseries.org/assets/submission/iip2023BE657E8C33F78BE.pdf

Archambault, Y., Boylan, C., Bullock, D., Morgas, T., Peltola, J., Ruokokoski, E., Genghi, A., Haas, B., Suhonen, P., & Thompson, S. (2020). Making on-line adaptive radiotherapy possible using artificial intelligence and machine learning for efficient daily re-planning. Medical Physics International Journal, 8(2), 77–86. http://mpijournal.org/pdf/2020-02/MPI-2020-02-p077.pdf

Barnett, G. (2016). GWAS in radiogenomics [Dissertation, Cambridge University Hospitals NHS Trust, Department of Oncology, Cambridge, United Kingdom]. Cancer Letters. https://figshare.le.ac.uk/articles/conference_contribution/The_REQUITE_project_integrating_biomarkers_and_clinical_predictors_of_radiotherapy_side_effects/10214567/1/files/18418739.pdf

Bengtsson, I., Smolders, A., Forsgren, A., Lomax, A., Weber, D. C., Fredriksson, A., & Albertini, F. (2024). Robust optimisation for contouring uncertainties in adaptive radiation therapy. 20th International Conference on the Use of Computers in Radiation Therapy, 1–4. https://www.iccr2024.org/papers/524476.pdf

Briggs, A., Fent, I., Brown, R., Hruby, G., Kneebone, A., & Booth, J. (2021). Individual disease site white paper (2.0 (Version 02.00.10) & Ethos Treatment Planning 1.0 (Version 01.00.10)). Adaptive Intelligence™ Consortium. https://filecache.mediaroom.com/mr5mr_varianmedicalaffairs/178507/download/AICBest%20Practices_Rectum.pdf

Chehade, A. H., Abdallah, N., Marion, J.-M., Oueidat, M., & Chauvet, P. (2022). Lung and colon cancer classification using medical imaging: A feature engineering approach. *Research Square.* DOI: 10.21203/rs.3.rs-1211832/v1

Chu, J. C. H. (2021). The role of artificial intelligence in radiation oncology. *International Journal of Radiation Oncology, Biology, Physics*, *110*(3), 674–686.

Cirolla, V. A., & Lora, O. (2024). Breast cancer between radiomics and adaptive radiotherapy. *International Journal of Contemporary Research in Multidisciplinary*, *3*(4), 121–128. https://multiarticlesjournal.com/counter/d/3-4-34/IJCRM-2024-3-4-34.pdf

Deist, T. M. (2019). Distributed learning and prediction modelling in radiation oncology [Doctoral dissertation, Maastricht University]. Proefschrift Maken Maastricht. DOI: 10.26481/dis.20190405td

Dercle, L., Henry, T., Carré, A., Paragios, N., Deutsch, E., & Robert, C. (2021). Reinventing radiation therapy with machine learning and imaging bio-markers (radiomics): State-of-the-art, challenges and perspectives. Methods, 188, 44-60. https://hal.science/hal-04525175/file/S1046202319303184.pdf

Fiorentino, G., Veniero, M., & Romano, C. (2023). AI powered cancer prediction, diagnosis and treatmeNt. *CEUR Workshop Proceedings*, *3486*, 1–6. https://ceur-ws.org/Vol-3486/153.pdf

Giraud, P., Gasnier, A., El Ayachy, R., Kreps, S., Foy, J.-P., Durdux, C., Huguet, F., Burgun, A., & Bibault, J.-E. (2019). Radiomics and machine learning for radiotherapy in head and neck cancers. *Frontiers in Oncology*, *9*, 174. Advance online publication. DOI: 10.3389/fonc.2019.00174 PMID: 30972291

Grahovac, M. (2023). Performance evaluation of in vivo predictive models built on conventional and probabilistic delineation-driven radiomic approaches in tumour patients [Doctoral thesis, Medical University of Vienna]. https://repositorium.meduniwien.ac.at/obvumwhs/content/titleinfo/11491791/full.pdf

Khansari, N. (2024). AI machine learning improves personalised cancer therapies. *The Australasian Medical Journal*, *17*(2), 1166–1173. DOI: 10.21767/AMJ.2024.4019

Kumar, A. (2024). AI driven precision oncology: Predictive biomarker discovery and personalised treatment optimisation using genomic data. *International Journal of Advance Research Publication and Reviews*, *1*(3), 21–39. https://ijarpr.com/uploads/V1ISSUE3/IJARPR0104.pdf. DOI: 10.55248/gengpi.5.0224.0421

Liu, R. (2024). Towards developing an AI-powered digital twin modeling framework for personalised radiotherapy. Midwest Radiation Oncology Symposium, University of Nebraska Medical Center. https://www.unmc.edu/cce/_archived/2024/live/radonc/attendee-info/sat13_liu.pdf

Luo, Y., Chen, S., & Valdes, G. (2020). Machine learning for radiation outcome modeling and prediction. *Medical Physics*, *47*(5), e178–e184. DOI: 10.1002/mp.13570 PMID: 32418338

Miteva, M. D. (2025). Artificial intelligence in radiogenomics: Innovations for supporting diagnosis, treatment decisions, and prognostication in oncology [Doctoral dissertation, Sofia University St. Kliment Ohridski]. https://www.uni-sofia.bg/index.php/eng/layout/set/print/content/download/333402/2148902/version/2/file/Abstract_Mariya_Miteva_EN.pdf

Morgado, R. L. M. (2024). Robust automatic planning for stereotactic body radiation therapy [Doctoral dissertation, Faculty of Sciences and Technology of the University of Coimbra]. https://estudogeral.uc.pt/retrieve/275228/Dissertacao_MIEF_RitaMorgado_vPosDefesa_30_07_2024.pdf

Olawade, D. B., Clement David-Olawade, A., Adereni, T., Egbon, E., Teke, J., & Boussios, S. (2025). Integrating AI into cancer immunotherapy—A narrative review of current applications and future directions. *Diseases (Basel, Switzerland)*, *13*(1), 24. DOI: 10.3390/diseases13010024 PMID: 39851488

Tunçel, N. (2021). Adaptive radiotherapy from past to future frontiers. *International Journal of Radiology & Radiation Therapy*, *8*(2), 81–84. https://avesis.akdeniz.edu.tr/yayin/1be4388d-be5d-477b-a818-97d75a92f181/adaptive-radiotherapy-from-past-to-future-frontiers/document.pdf. DOI: 10.15406/ijrrt.2021.08.00298

Vuong, D. (2021). Radiomics as biomarker in multi-modality treatment of locally advanced non-small cell lung cancer [Doctoral dissertation, Universität Zürich]. https://www.zora.uzh.ch/id/eprint/211927/1/Dissertation_Vuong_2021.pdf

Xia, T. (2023). Radiogenomics framework for associating medical image features with tumour genetic characteristics [Doctoral dissertation, The University of Sydney]. https://core.ac.uk/download/pdf/590715623.pdf

Zhovannik, I. (2022). Pitfalls of image biomarker analysis in radiation oncology [Doctoral dissertation, Radboud University Nijmegen]. https://repository.ubn.ru.nl/bitstream/handle/2066/289611/289611.pdf?sequence=1#page=133

Chapter 9
Machine Learning and Emerging Technologies in Cancer Care

Muhammad Aasim Rafique
https://orcid.org/0000-0002-2896-3162
Department of Information Systems, College of Computer Sciences and Information Technology, King Faisal University, Al Ahsa, Saudi Arabia

Qazi Mudassar Ilyas
https://orcid.org/0000-0003-4238-8093
Universiti Islam Sultan Sharif Ali, Brunei

ABSTRACT

Cancer is the second-leading global cause of death (>10M/year), posing complex economic and social burdens. Current treatments—conventional (chemo, radio) and advanced (targeted, immuno)—are limited by high cost, toxicity, lack of precision, and unpredictable patient response . An urgent paradigm shift requires leveraging Artificial Intelligence (AI) and Machine Learning (ML). AI/ML drives breakthroughs in the entire oncological care pathway: enabling precise diagnosis, robust prognosis, and individualized prediction of therapeutic response via multi-omics analysis. The future of oncology must be defined by AI-powered precision to solve the problem of variable efficacy and achieve universal access to effective care.

1. INTRODUCTION

Cancer remains one of the biggest health challenges for humanity, affecting millions of individuals and families annually. The World Health Organization and

DOI: 10.4018/979-8-3373-4312-9.ch009

the International Agency for Research on Cancer estimates suggest that cancer is responsible for over 10 million deaths annually, making it the second-highest cause of death, behind only cardiovascular diseases, with about 18 million mortalities every year (Sung et al., 2021). These numbers indicate the impact of cancer on the economy and human health, not merely through loss of lives, but also through long periods of patient treatment, health systems, and psychological impact on patients and caregivers. Furthermore, cancer is not a single disease but comprises hundreds of types and subtypes, each having different symptoms and treatments. These challenges make cancer a major risk factor for humanity, requiring serious efforts from all stakeholders, including healthcare professionals, researchers, local governments, and international organizations.

Traditional cancer treatment approaches, such as chemotherapy, radiotherapy, and surgery, have helped countless individuals overcome cancer and live healthy lives. Although these approaches remain focused on current oncology, they suffer from several limitations, including high costs, toxicity, limited precision, variable patient responses to the same treatments, and, in some cases, ineffectiveness for certain patients. Some more recent approaches include targeted therapy and immunotherapy. However, these approaches also have their own limitations, including high cost, inaccessibility for poor and underdeveloped communities, and variable efficacy across patients. To this end, there is a high need for innovative approaches for cancer diagnosis, prognosis, therapeutic interventions, and post-surgery care.

1.1. Artificial Intelligence in Oncology

Recent advancements in algorithms, hardware, and the increasing availability of large datasets have led to unprecedented growth in artificial intelligence, particularly in its subdomains of machine learning and deep learning (DL), over the past decade. Researchers have applied AI to nearly every domain and solved problems that were previously considered unsolvable. The healthcare community has also reaped significant benefits from the use of AI. Some major applications of AI in healthcare include medical imaging (Esteva et al., 2017), drug discovery (Vamathevan et al., 2019), personalized medicine (Kourou et al., 2015), clinical decision support (Sutton et al., 2020), and robotic surgery (Hashimoto et al., 2018). While statistical methods of prediction require predefined assumptions as a prerequisite, machine learning algorithms can directly learn complex nonlinear functions from the underlying data to make accurate predictions on unseen data. This learning and prediction ability is particularly useful in oncology, where clinical decision-making often involves scouring large amounts of medical imaging data, pathology knowledge bases, genome sequences, and patient electronic health records.

AI algorithms are already showing promising results in supporting cancer diagnostics. For example, researchers have achieved similar or higher diagnostic performance compared to human radiologists using DL methods (Ilyas & Ahmad, 2021; Mehmood et al., 2023). While these results require validation through clinical trials, they offer a glimpse into the potential of AI support for clinicians in cancer diagnosis and treatment in the future.

Beyond diagnosis, AI systems are being developed for early detection, medical imaging analysis, histopathology classification, genomic data interpretation, personalized treatment planning, drug discovery, prognosis prediction, clinical decision support, radiotherapy optimization, and remote patient monitoring (Figure 1). Future AI systems have the potential to develop highly personalized cancer treatments tailored to individual patients based on diverse biological data streams. These systems will be able to customize therapeutic interventions based not only on the tumor's profile but also on patient conditions and requirements. The ultimate goal of such a system is to develop and deliver precision medicine tailored to each patient's exact needs.

Figure 1. AI applications in oncology

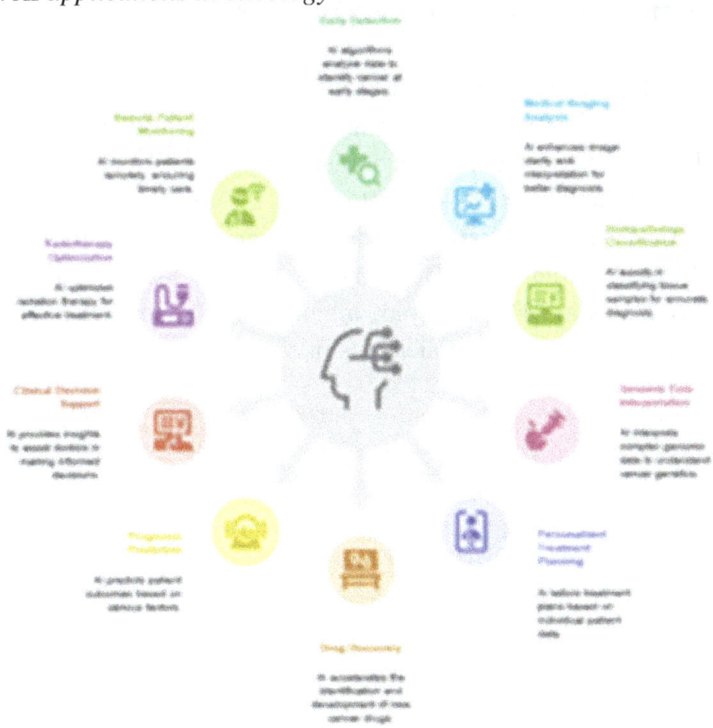

1.2. Convergence with Emerging Technologies

While AI technologies alone have made significant contributions across all domains of life, including healthcare, integrating them with advances in supporting technologies can yield synergistic effects in cancer care. For instance, nanotechnology is being used to develop nanoscale drug carriers that target cancer cells with high precision and minimal or no adverse effects on healthy cells, thereby reducing undesired side effects for cancer patients. AI can accelerate the development of nanoscale drug carriers by supporting nanoparticle design and predicting their interactions with human cells. Similarly, in immune-oncology, AI can help identify biomarkers of the immune response and accelerate the development of personalized immune therapies.

Other emerging technologies in healthcare include wearable sensors and mobile health applications. These technologies can complement AI solutions in oncology by collecting real-time patient data for remote monitoring and personalized care. These solutions are especially useful for cancer survivors, who require long-term care and management of late treatment effects. The integration of AI with these emerging technologies makes the long-term goal of personalized, comprehensive, and patient-centered cancer care realizable in the near future.

1.3. Scope and Objectives of the Chapter

The goal of this chapter is to examine the role of machine learning and emerging technologies in cancer care and to identify their strengths and limitations. The study is not limited to technical aspects of the domain alone; it also offers insights into oncology workflows in real-world settings. A discussion on technical aspects is followed by data availability issues, model explainability, regulatory, and ethical concerns, providing a comprehensive overview of the domain. Figure 2 presents the chapter's scope as a SWOT analysis, highlighting the strengths, weaknesses, opportunities, and threats of AI applications in cancer care.

Figure 2. SWOT analysis of AI in cancer care

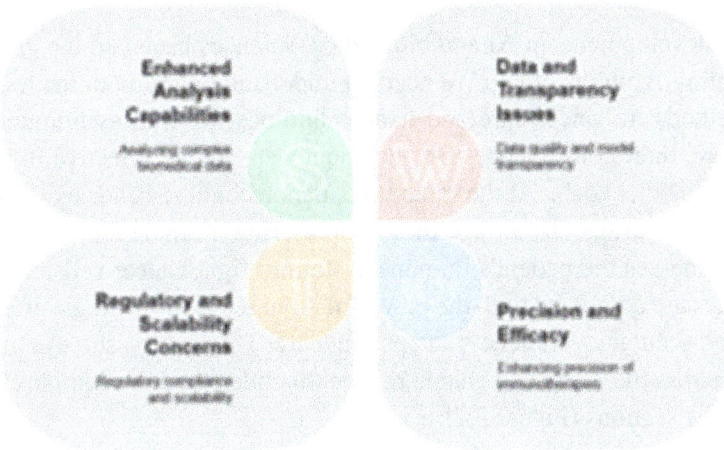

The chapter is organized into the following sections:

- **Background**: This section provides a context for the subsequent sections by reviewing key developments in AI for healthcare in general, and in oncology in particular. This contextual background information lays the groundwork for the subsequent sections.
- **Deep Learning in Cancer Diagnostics and Treatment**: The application of DL techniques in cancer prognosis, diagnosis, pathology, and patient care forms the focus of this section.
- **AI for Patient-Centered Care and Survivorship**: This section examines the role of AI in patient care and follow-up care after cancer treatment, extending beyond the treatment itself.
- **AI in Immunotherapy and Drug Discovery**: This section examines how AI can facilitate the development of immunotherapy and the creation of novel, more effective drugs in oncology.
- **Challenges, Ethics, and Implementation Considerations**: This section addresses the challenges, ethical considerations, and implementation concerns associated with AI applications in cancer care. Issues of bias, transparency, explainability, privacy, and regulatory challenges are highlighted as barriers to the clinical adoption of AI.
- **Future Directions and Conclusions**: The chapter concludes with a discussion on how AI and emerging technologies discussed in this chapter may define the future of oncology in the coming years.

2. BACKGROUND

Recent developments in AI and biomedical sciences have laid the groundwork for integrating AI in oncology. We need an understanding of both the foundations of DL methods in cancer care and nanotechnology, as well as immunotherapy, to appreciate their convergence. DL techniques are highly effective in analyzing complex biomedical data. At the same time, nanotechnology endeavors to develop tools for precise drug delivery and tumor monitoring. Immunotherapy, on the other hand, harnesses the patient's immune system to fight cancer cells. When these technologies are combined with the powerful AI models, the synergic effect results in improved accuracy, efficiency, and patient care. This section surveys the current literature across these areas to enable readers to understand the complex details in the following sections (Figure 3).

Figure 3. AI integration in cancer care

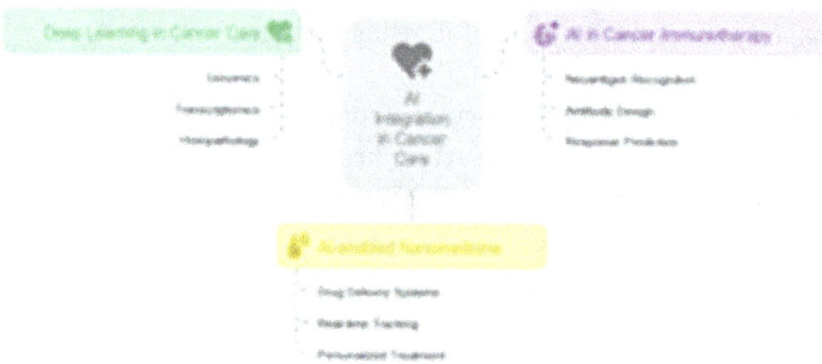

2.1. Deep Learning in Cancer Care

Tran et al. present a comprehensive review of deep learning (DL) applications across several areas in cancer care (Tran et al., 2021). The study highlights the potential of DL methods in oncology while also highlighting potential challenges, such as limited phenotypic diversity and the lack of explainability of these algorithms.

Another recent review by Yao et al. elaborates how DL methods are transforming cancer detection with improved accuracy and speed (Yao et al., 2025). The study also highlights key challenges faced by these techniques, including quality of training data, transparency and trust in the model outputs, standardization by governments, and regulatory compliance of AI models. The study also identifies several potential solutions to these challenges, including federated learning, explainable AI, and the generation of synthetic data.

In addition to cancer detection, DL methods are also being explored for personalized treatment and prognosis. Shao et al. elaborate how radiomics and DL can be used to predict various genetic mutations, such as estimated glomerular filtration rate (EGFR), anaplastic lymphoma kinase (ALK), and programmed death-ligand 1(PD-L1), directly from medical imaging (Shao et al., 2023). The authors also highlight the role of DL in predicting treatment response and survival outcomes of cancer patients.

DL techniques have been applied to address several challenges in oncology. For instance, Boldrini et al. review DL-based autosegmentation in oncology (Boldrini et al., 2019). Wulczyn et al. propose a DL method to predict multiple cancer types from histopathology images (Wulczyn et al., 2020). Waqas et al. review the integration of multimodal cancer data for cancer prevention, prediction, early detection, and treatment (Waqas et al., 2024). Similarly, Partin et al. discuss emerging trends in the prediction of cancer drug response (Partin et al., 2022).

2.2. AI in Cancer Immunotherapy

The recent innovations in cancer immunotherapy include immune checkpoint inhibitors and CAR-T cell therapies. AI researchers have developed various techniques to enhance the precision and efficacy of immunotherapies. Xu et al. present an excellent review on the applications of AI in immunotherapy, including the prediction of drug response using patient immune signatures, as well as imaging and histology (Xu et al., 2021). The authors also highlight future directions to clinical deployment of the proposed techniques in personalized treatments and drug response monitoring.

Another recent review by Li et al. covers a broad range of immunotherapy topics, including neoantigen recognition, antibody design, and response prediction (Li et al., 2023). AI application in neoantigen recognition analyzes massive molecular datasets to identify the most effective tumor-specific antigens. Similarly, AI and machine learning techniques support the creation of antibodies with significantly enhanced effectiveness for cancer patients. The study highlights how AI models can identify patients who are more likely to benefit from specific immunotherapies, thereby customizing and optimizing treatment plans.

Other applications of AI in immunotherapy include diagnosis, biomarker discovery, and trial matching (Huang et al., 2025). However, the proposed AI techniques in these application areas are still in their infancy and struggle with several challenges, including data quality, data access, model transparency, and limited generalization. Researchers are addressing these challenges by adopting better data practices, utilizing explainable AI, developing robust models, and conducting clinical validation through trials.

2.3. AI-Enabled Nanomedicine

The integration of nanomedicine technologies with the power of AI holds immense potential to revolutionize cancer care. AI-enabled nanomedicine can be used to develop precise drug delivery systems that offer several advantages over traditional methods, including targeted therapy, real-time tracking, and personalized treatment strategies (Samathoti et al., 2025). Noury et al. review smart, multifunctional nanocarriers and demonstrate how they facilitate drug loading, enhance drug release mechanisms, ensure biocompatibility, and overcome biological barriers (Noury et al., 2025). Abdullah et al. identify a lack of understanding of drug-delivery dynamics as the primary reason for the failure of most nanoformulations (Abdullah et al., 2025).

Several studies have focused on a specific type of cancer for in-depth research on nanomedicines. For instance, Bhange and Telange explore how AI techniques can be applied to the design of nanomedicine and to the real-time monitoring of its effectiveness in liver cancer patients (Bhange & Telange, 2025). The study emphasizes that AI techniques must be used to enhance patient satisfaction by tailoring treatment to individual needs. They highlight regulatory challenges and poor explainability as key issues in AI for nanomedicine.

Similarly, Shirzad et al. studied the application of AI in nanocarriers for breast cancer (Shirzad et al., 2025). The study underscores the role of AI in improved drug discovery, theranostics, and diagnostic precision. The authors identify data access, interpretability, and scalability as the main challenges in the domain. Furthermore, Dipankar et al. identify several AI applications in brain cancer, including gliomas, biomarker discovery, prognosis, and personalized therapeutic design (Dipankar et al., 2025).

3. DEEP LEARNING IN CANCER DIAGNOSIS AND TREATMENT

This section dives deeper into the applications of DL in diagnosis and treatment. The section focuses on advanced DL techniques in oncology, such as multi-omics, attention, transformers, radiomics, image-driven decision support, autoencoding, transfer learning, interpretability, and biomarker innovations. The section presents the latest breakthroughs, novel modeling strategies, and the future outlook of DL applications in cancer care.

Figure 4. Deep learning applications in oncology

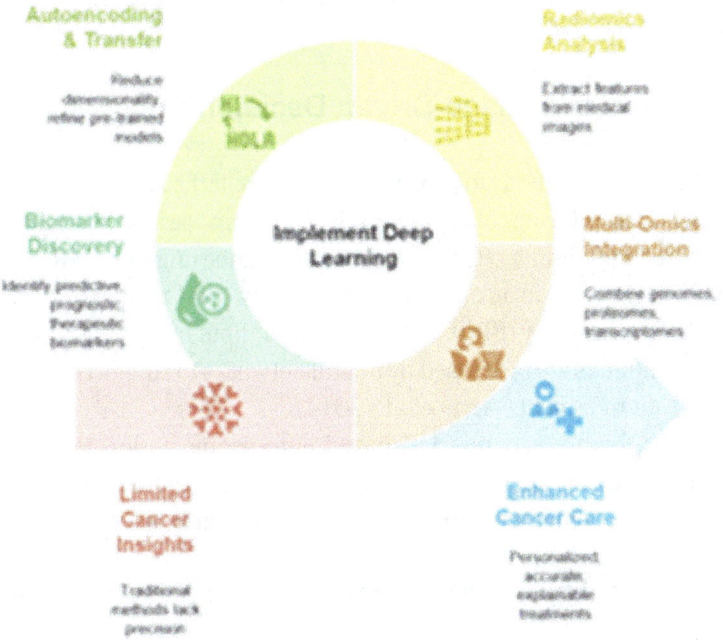

3.1. Adaptive Treatment Response Prediction through Multi-Omics and Attention

The latest trend in DL research for oncology involves using multi-omics (genomes, epigenomes, transcriptomes, and proteomes, etc.) to predict cancer treatment responses for individual patients. Wang et al. employed this approach in a graph-embedded neural network, integrating genome data, copy number variations, mutations, and protein data to predict drug response in cancer patients (Wang et al., 2022). The study employed an attention mechanism to dynamically adjust the weights of various omics. The authors achieved 90% accuracy in the Cancer Cell Line Encyclopedia (CCLE) and Genomics of Drug Sensitivity in Cancer (GDSC) datasets. Another study by Zhang et al. proposed consDeepSignaling, a DL model based on biological signaling pathways (Zhang et al., 2021). The proposed architecture utilizes the Kyoto Encyclopedia of Genes and Genomes (KEGG) pathways to make highly accurate predictions. Using KEGG also improves the interpretability of predictions compared to conventional DL methods. These novel techniques not only improve the overall performance of cancer treatment response prediction but also represent a shift from black-box DL models to more transparent, explainable architectures with greater interpretability. These innovations are crucial for the translational adoption of these techniques in the healthcare domain, which demands high user trust in model outcomes.

3.2. Radiomics and Image-Driven Decision Support

The ability of DL methods to process and analyze large amounts of imaging data makes them suitable for oncology imaging data from various modalities, such as X-ray, computed tomography (CT), magnetic resonance imaging (MRI), ultrasound, and nuclear imaging (positron emission tomography (PET) and single photon emission computed tomography (SPECT)). High-throughput image features extracted by quantitative radiomics are processed by neural networks to support cancer prognosis and personalized treatment (Aerts et al., 2014).

Furthermore, highly accurate DL-based auto-segmentation models are being employed to delineate organs-at-risk and tumor volumes (Erdur et al., 2025). It enables physicians to plan oncology treatments more effectively.

3.3. Autoencoding, Transfer Learning, and Interpretability

Due to the presence of multiple distinct cancer types, diverse modalities with unique characteristics, and data concerns in healthcare, such as privacy, availability, and physician time constraints, researchers face challenges of limited sample sizes and high-dimensional data. Researchers have used various intelligent strategies to overcome these challenges. Autoencoders are one such technique used by researchers for dimensionality reduction and pretraining in oncology. Partin et al. discuss emerging trends in cancer treatment prediction and elaborate on how variational autoencoders are used to compress gene expression profiles, thereby reducing the overfitting risk of treatment prediction models (Partin et al., 2023).

Transfer learning is another emerging trend in oncology, where the weights of a pre-trained model are refined for a cancer type on which the model was not originally trained. This results in significant performance, efficiency, and economic gains due to reduced resource and data requirements. DeepDR is one such model, developed by Jiang and Li, which is trained on a large oncology dataset, The Cancer Genome Atlas Program (TCGA) (Jiang & Li, 2024). The model provides pretrained weights that can be further refined for smaller drug screening datasets at significantly lower training costs and times.

A major roadblock to the widespread adoption of AI in healthcare applications is the black-box nature of AI model outputs. To this end, an emerging trend in DL research in oncology is to use interpretability-based architectures. Samal et al. developed HiDRA, which utilizes hierarchical attention across gene- and pathway-level representations (Samal et al., 2022). These representations allow the model to trace their "thought" process and explain the inference drawn. This work builds a foundation for explainable AI in oncology.

3.4. DL and Biomarkers in Oncology

The human body has several biomarkers that reflect various biological states and can provide significant clues for disease diagnosis, progression, and response to drugs and other treatments. Carlomagno et al. identify three types of biomarkers in oncology: predictive, prognostic, and therapeutic biomarkers (Carlomagno et al., 2017). The integration of DL models in biomarker discovery and interpretation has significantly enhanced their role in cancer care. For example, Coudray et al. developed a convolutional neural network model to identify biomarkers of mutational status, such as EGFR and KRAS, from histopathology slides of lung cancer (Coudray et al., 2018). Similarly, Wei et al. trained a DL model to detect prognosis biomarkers from colorectal cancer tissue images (Wei et al., 2024). Table 2 gives a summary of DL innovations in biomarkers in oncology.

Table 2. Traditional vs DL-enabled biomarker approaches in oncology

Biomarker Type	Traditional Approach	DL-Enabled Innovation	Representative Study
Diagnostic Biomarkers (early detection)	Genetic testing and immunohistochemistry for mutation detection (e.g., EGFR, KRAS).	CNNs applied to histopathology slides can directly infer mutational status from tissue images, thereby bypassing some molecular assays.	(Coudray et al., 2018)
Prognostic Biomarkers (disease outcomes)	Manual histological grading of tissue morphology by pathologists.	DL models trained on colorectal cancer tissue images predict patient survival more accurately than standard grading.	(Wei et al., 2024)
Predictive Biomarkers (treatment response)	Radiologist assessment of tumor shrinkage via RECIST criteria in imaging studies.	Radiomics features combined with DL predict immunotherapy response in NSCLC from CT scans.	(Prelaj et al., 2024)

continued on following page

Table 2. Continued

Biomarker Type	Traditional Approach	DL-Enabled Innovation	Representative Study
Immunological Biomarkers (tumor–immune microenvironment)	Manual quantification of tumor-infiltrating lymphocytes (TILs) in histopathology.	DL-based automated quantification of TILs from digital slides offers scalable and reproducible prognostic indicators.	(Lopez-Beltran et al., 2018)
Surrogate Phenotypic Biomarkers (non-traditional indicators)	Clinical risk factors (age, BMI, performance status) assessed manually.	Exploratory DL approaches use facial imaging or phenotypic features to estimate biological age or treatment outcomes.	(Aronson, 2005)

4. AI FOR PATIENT-CENTERED CARE AND SURVIVORSHIP

Cancer has been among the leading causes of death in the United States for the last seventy years, and its diagnosis affects not only the patient but also close family members. In such anxious circumstances, special attention is needed, and the same level of care should extend to survivors. Trained healthcare staff should adopt a patient-centered approach and evaluate all related aspects of care.

It is important to note that patient-centered care is distinct from personalized care. The latter focuses on using a patient's biological data or specimens to devise a treatment plan, whereas the former is a holistic philosophy that respects patients' preferences, accommodates their needs, and honors their values.

Patient-centered care emphasizes partnering with patients and their families in the delivery of healthcare. It includes strategies such as empowering patients through education, counseling, and shared decision-making, while fostering the confidence needed to manage their health throughout the process.

Healthcare services do not end when patients step out of the facility. Particularly after cancer treatment, survivors need post-recovery support. Survivorship is an additional phase of care that focuses on the long-term and late effects of treatment, lifestyle management, and psychosocial support for survivors.

Digital health services support both patient-centered care and survivorship, with advances in AI making care more convenient and scalable. Figure 5 gives an overview of AI's role in patient-centered care and survivorship.

Figure 5. AI's role in patient-centered care and survivorship

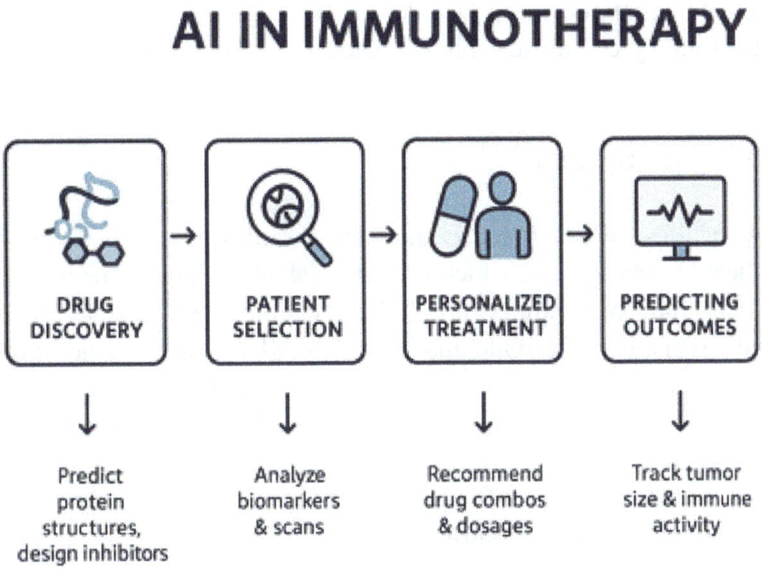

4.1 AI in Patient-Centered Care

A challenge for the healthcare system in adopting patient-centered care is the diversity of patients' needs. AI—particularly machine learning (ML) and deep learning—leverages vast datasets (genomic, clinical, behavioral) to create Personalized Patient Care Plans (PPCPs) (Baig, M.M et al., 2024)

4.2 AI in Cancer Survivorship

Cancer survivors go through an excruciating physical and mental experience during treatment. It can drastically alter their lives, and they need support on all fronts. Fortunately, advances in AI technology span a wide range of supportive areas, particularly lifestyle adaptation and stress-coping counseling. Both were expensive, placed a heavy financial burden on patients, and were not readily available. AI provides inexpensive, personalized, and timely survivorship support. AI-empowered Digital Health Technologies (DHTs) are being applied to cancer survivorship care, with positive outcomes including improved patient-reported outcomes (PROs), reduced fatigue and pain, and better quality of life and physical function. Globally, a significant number of cancer survivors report long-term or late physical, cognitive, and psychological effects (Schmidt et al., 2022). A Norwegian study of cancer survivors reported that 83% respondents experienced one or more long-term effects of treatment, including fatigue, sleep disorder, or nerve damage (Kristoffersen et al., 2022). These findings call for scalable AI-enabled survivor support systems for cancer patients.

4.2.1 Mobile Health Systems

An example of lifestyle adaptation is monitoring cardiovascular (CV) health using mobile health technologies, which provide scalable solutions for tracking risk-reducing behaviors and guiding lifestyle interventions (Benzo et al., 2025.). Another example is the use of mobile apps like iCANSleep—an evidence-based Cognitive Behavioral Therapy for Insomnia (CBT-I)—which provide accessible interventions for cancer survivors with minimal barriers related to cost or geography (Etli, D., et al., 2024).

4.2.2 Generative AI–Based Chatbots

Generative AI–based chatbots serve as counselors and provide assistive support that mimics healthcare settings (Kurniawan, M.H., 2024). Agentic AI is advancing, with large language models (LLMs) as the underlying technology for conversational agents; these systems offer accessible healthcare information and support. They aim to ensure that patients receive validated information for self-management (Najar N., et al. 2025). Moreover, agents can benefit from mining consumer-generated data, such as program reviews and blogs detailing self-management needs and the experiences of cancer survivors, particularly during periods of reduced clinical oversight (Wang, L., et al. 2025).

4.3 Challenges of AI in Patient-Centered Care and Survivorship

A persistent challenge for AI in care is the lack of human confidence in machines. For instance, patient and caregiver attitudes toward AI in cancer care are split, with roughly 50% positive and 50% negative (Najar N., et al. 2025). A primary concern is that AI could reduce crucial in-person time and the personal connection with clinicians. Patients and advocates stress the importance of transparency, seeking to understand AI's role, capabilities, and limitations in their care and decision-making (Moy, S., et al., 2024). An ever-growing concern reappears here: privacy and data security. These are significant issues across all healthcare applications of AI, requiring established controls to protect sensitive medical information. More on this appears in the next section.

Individuals feel vulnerable when left alone during difficult times, and AI has not yet replaced the warmth of another person. This suggests that patients are generally comfortable with AI when human involvement remains central (Moy, S., et. Al. 2024). Therefore, AI in an assistant role is viewed as a valuable tool for information gathering, but not as a source of definitive health advice.

5. AI IN IMMUNOTHERAPY AND DRUG DISCOVERY

Cancer cells can evade the body's immune defenses, and patients may need immunotherapy or other interventions. The immune system resists foreign cells and agents, including harmful bacteria, viruses, and damaged cells. White blood cells in our bodies are tasked with identifying and attacking dangerous cells. However, cancer cells, although harmful, can deceive the immune system by producing signals that prevent white blood cells from attacking.

Immunotherapy helps train the immune system to recognize cancer cells as threats and fight them. It strengthens the body's immune system, and scientists have discovered ways to train our natural defenses using various types of immunotherapy. These techniques include immune checkpoint inhibitors, T-cell therapy, monoclonal antibodies, vaccines, and immune system boosters. If immunotherapy alone cannot contain the cancer cells, scientists develop supporting drugs that can fight these harmful cells. However, a common challenge for both approaches is the adaptability of cancer cells; even a minuscule change in the cell or the patient's immune response can create numerous control groups. Another humanitarian concern involves the hazardous effects of drugs on test subjects.

These two challenges can be summarized as insufficient resources to carry out safe experiments in a timely manner. Although medical and pharmaceutical technological advancements are fast-paced, progress is impeded by human factors. Contemporary advances in computing and the rise of successful ventures in artificial intelligence mitigate these challenges: first, AI spares human scientists the drudgery by exploring vast avenues of drug discovery. Second, patients can be relieved from early, excruciating experiences by having AI perform tests in simulated environments.

5.1 Immunotherapy Process and AI Opportunities

Cancer cells trick our immune system, evading the hunter cells by using immune checkpoints, e.g., PD-L1. These checkpoints bind to the PD-1 receptor on immune cells (T cells), causing the T cells to stop attacking cancer cells. Therefore, T-cell receptors can be modified to avoid being deceived, and immunotherapy drugs block the receptors from receiving these stop signals, thus exploiting the camouflage of harmful cancer cells. Cancer cells are then targeted by T cells, and the reinvigorated immune system destroys harmful cells. The whole process can be summarized in four steps: recognize, block, attack, and follow-up. However, each of these steps involves numerous choices—from drug discovery for receptor modification to predicting immunotherapy outcomes—which creates opportunities to use AI at different stages, as shown in Figure 6.

Figure 6. Various opportunities of AI to be used in immunotherapy

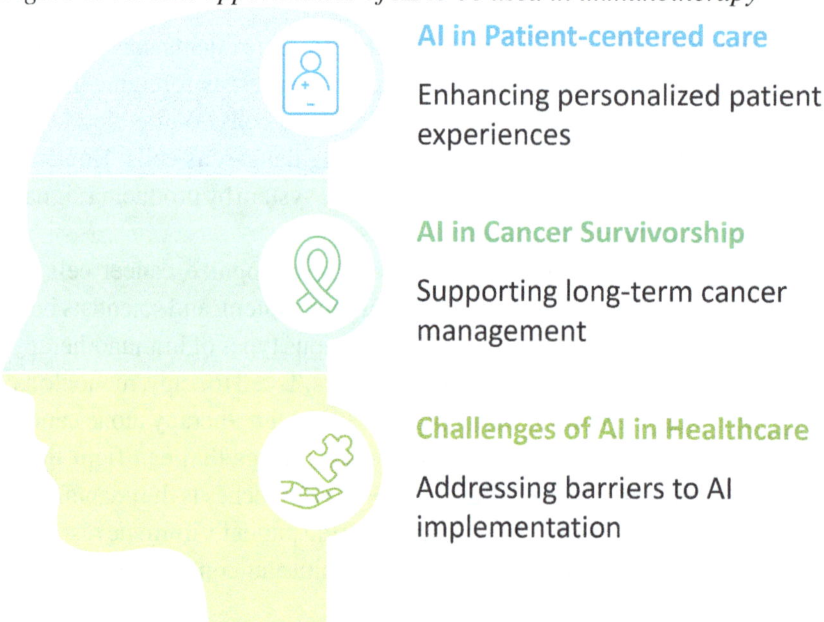

5.1.1 AI Opportunities

5.1.1.1 Drug Discovery for Immunotherapy

AlphaFold (Jumper, J., et al., 2021), an AI model, wins its developers (AI researchers) an unprecedented Nobel Prize in Chemistry, shared with a biochemist. It predicts protein structures, which are the building blocks for checkpoint inhibitors. Previously, protein structure prediction involved mostly drudgery and could take hundreds of hours in the laboratory to identify a viable protein structure that could act as a PD-1/PD-L1 inhibitor for T cells. Tech companies like Insilico Medicine have used their AI platforms to identify novel inhibitors for targets relevant to tumor immune evasion, such as QPCTL, advancing these molecules into the oncology pipeline.

Beyond protein-structure prediction, modern drug-discovery platforms such as Exscientia and Insilico Medicine have developed first-in-class small molecules for immune-oncology treatment. These platforms employed reinforcement learning, multi-objective optimization, and automated lab validation to develop these solutions.

5.1.1.2 Patient Biomarker Discovery

A prior examination of a patient's test results may prevent unnecessary treatments, and timely evaluation is crucial. However, resource limitations and the need to assess numerous data types—genomics, proteomics, pathology, and radiomics—pose challenges. AI can assist clinicians by automating tasks such as predicting hot or cold tumors and timely identifying patients with hot (immune-active) tumors. For example, image analysis of histopathology slides can predict whether a patient has high PD-L1 expression; these patients often respond better to pembrolizumab.

This process extends to personalized immunotherapy plans that include genomic data, medical history, and assessments of cancer cells. It is resource-intensive, and AI can help identify a plan that doctors and scientists can verify. AI models are trained on data from thousands of patients and can simulate combinations of drugs to suggest better treatments for new patients. For instance, studies used Machine Learning (ML) to analyze genomic and clinical data from over 78,000 cancer patients to identify genetic changes that directly impacted survival outcomes across 20 cancer types. The team developed a machine learning tool to predict how patients with advanced Non-Small Cell Lung Cancer (NSCLC) might respond to immunotherapy, based on their complex mutational profiles, which helps doctors select the most effective therapies (Liu, R., et al. 2024).

5.1.1.3 Monitoring Treatment Response

Immunotherapy can be demanding for patients and healthcare staff. Patients often undergo frequent examinations during treatment, and healthcare staff must remain vigilant and attentive. AI can ease the burden for both by supporting healthcare staff and improving patient convenience. It can continuously monitor vital signs and symptoms and help detect immune-related adverse events (irAEs). In addition, AI can assist healthcare staff by automating the evaluation of expected immunotherapy responses in pathology labs and medical imaging, as specified by clinicians.

For example, AI-driven monitoring using wearable devices to collect multivariate physiological data can detect the risk of Cytokine Release Syndrome (CRS) in patients undergoing CAR T-cell therapy or T-cell engager therapies, enabling prompt intervention. Another example uses a deep learning model called NeoPred that integrates pre-treatment and pre-surgery dual-phase CT imaging with clinical variables to reliably and non-invasively predict the pathological response (such as major pathological response or pCR) to neoadjuvant chemo-immunotherapy in NS-CLC, significantly outperforming unaided expert assessment (Zheng J, et al. 2025).

6. CHALLENGES OF THE USE OF AI IN CANCER CARE

The challenges of using ML, AI, and emerging technologies stem from the broader issues associated with disruptive innovation and the need to accommodate cultural change. Cheng et al. provide an excellent overview of the challenges that must be overcome to facilitate broader adoption of AI technologies (Cheng et al. 2025). To keep the discussion brief and precise, we categorize the challenges into ethical, legal, implementation, and acceptability (Mohammed & Malhotra, 2025) (Figure 7).

Figure 7. Challenges of the use of AI in cancer care

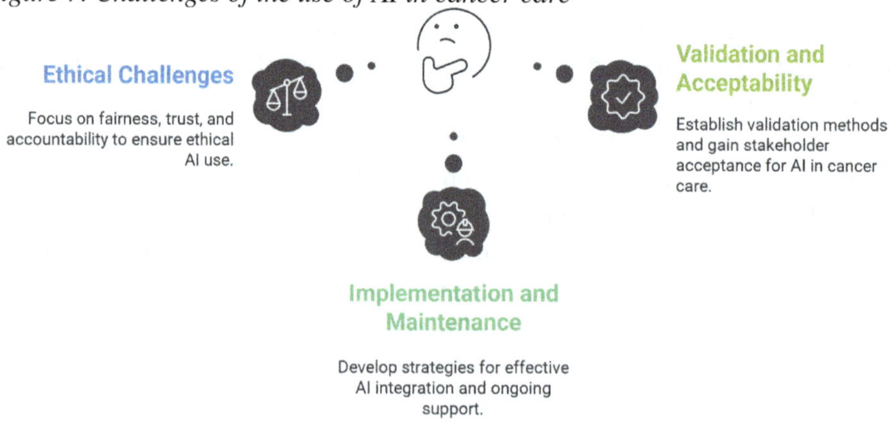

6.1 Ethical Challenges

Ethical challenges concern trust, fairness, and accountability in the technologies being developed. In recent years, ML and AI development has been heavily data-driven, and many challenges arise from data issues such as bias, underrepresentation, and insufficiency. Healthcare contexts are diverse, and outcomes may not generalize when control groups are neglected. Similarly, ML algorithms are often trained on data from limited demographics that represent only a fraction of the population, as well as from specific clinical settings. Bias is particularly pronounced in rapidly evolving technologies like ML and AI. An inherent challenge in cancer care is the shift from generalization to personalization; bias that is harmful in one context may be an intentional feature in another.

6.1.1 Fairness and Equity

From a humanitarian perspective, fairness and equity pose additional challenges. Although basic or experimental functions of new technologies may be available to broad populations, core capabilities and mature products often remain out of reach for many. For instance, studies have shown that over 80% of the genomic data in public oncology datasets (e.g., TCGA) are from individuals of European ancestry (Molina-Aguilar & Robles-Espinoza, 2023), thereby limiting generalizability to underrepresented populations. This creates a dilemma for humanitarian organizations: whether to support beneficial technologies and advocate for accessibility, or to protest against exploitation and inequity. The recent developments in federated learning and light-weight AI models offer solutions to this issue by enabling model training across geographically and ethnically diverse datasets without centralizing sensitive data.

6.1.2 Trust and Transparency Challenges

A valid—though sometimes overstated—criticism of state-of-the-art ML techniques is their "black-box" nature (Lu, S-C., et al.,2023). This fuels debates about explainability, patient autonomy, and trust. Explainability issues arise in both standalone systems and shared decision-making systems. The former requires interpretability of the decisions, plans, and recommendations produced by the system, whereas the latter demands that healthcare practitioners understand the system well enough. A lack of understanding among staff—or vague justifications of recommendations to patients—undermines the autonomy of both clinicians and patients. This exacerbates criticism of AI use in healthcare, particularly in cancer care.

6.1.3 Accountability and Liability

The classic trolley problem is relevant—and perhaps more acute—in cancer care. What constitutes the right decision, and who is responsible for it, is often unclear. Accountability lies at the heart of responsibility, yet when an error occurs, it is often ambiguous who is accountable—the clinician who relied on the recommendation, the hospital that implemented the system, or the developer who created the algorithm. Moreover, there is a substantial gap between technological advancement and regulatory oversight. The regulatory landscape for AI-powered medical care is still evolving and fragmented, which can delay implementation and complicate cross-jurisdictional use. Robust frameworks are required to ensure that stakeholders—from developers to healthcare providers—prioritize ethical conduct and clear accountability.

6.2 Implementation and Maintenance Challenges

AI techniques and ML models often originate in labs, and translating findings into clinical practice for cancer care still faces substantial infrastructure, operational, and human-factor barriers. A key requirement for successful ML models is data—with diverse patient representation and appropriate control groups—which, in reality, reside in fragmented electronic health records (EHRs) (Ardito, V., et al. 2023). Available data are often not interoperable across systems, making aggregation difficult. For instance, in the United States, EHR data are not recorded in a standardized format (Hu, Q., et al., 2024). Another challenge is the lack of infrastructure and computational resources; hosting ML and AI models can consume a significant share of IT budgets. Moreover, technical expertise is often limited, especially in resource-constrained environments, widening the gap between academic centers and community practices and creating further health equity concerns. Unlike traditional software, ML models require continuous monitoring and updates (ModelOps) to account for data drift—changes in patient populations or clinical practice over time—to ensure that accuracy and relevance are maintained.

6.3 Validation and Acceptability

Although AI, ML, and emerging technologies have a strong presence, different disciplines maintain distinct rules and criteria. Most technologies used in medical practice require approval from established regulatory bodies such as the FDA. Cancer-care practitioners must accept ideas developed in research labs into clinical settings, and healthcare professionals may be either reluctant to adopt—or overuse—AI tools in cancer care (Garcia-Saiso, S., et al., 2024). Another major technical barrier to widespread implementation is the need for rigorous external validation. As noted earlier, AI models that perform well on local, internal datasets often fail to generalize when deployed in new clinical settings with different patient populations, equipment, or data characteristics. The lack of standardized protocols for validating AI predictions remains a significant barrier to clinical translation.

7. FUTURE DIRECTIONS

The current research trends in applications of AI in cancer care indicate a future dominated by several technologies working together to improve diagnostics, prediction, and treatment of cancer. Future cancer care systems are expected to integrate and process data from multi-omics, imaging, and wearable devices to achieve personalized care. These systems will not only support cancer diagnostics but also predict treatment response and monitor adverse cases in cancer care. Future developments in AI are also expected to address the current challenges related to hallucinations, transparency, bias, and data privacy. These developments will make AI solutions more reliable and trustworthy for patients and clinicians alike.

In addition to technical advancements, a coherent approach involving various stakeholders, such as researchers, practitioners, policymakers, and standardization bodies, is crucial for the successful application of AI in cancer care in the future. A standardized approach to AI applications in cancer care would ensure equitable access and benefit all populations, rather than just the privileged few. In the future, we might also witness unprecedented progress in drug discovery through breakthroughs in quantum computing, synthetic biology, nanotechnology, and robotics. Additionally, these discoveries may enhance precision surgery and immunotherapy. Furthermore, future digital health ecosystems might deliver personalized, high-quality cancer care to patients at home.

In the long term, research in multimodal intelligence, federated learning, and quantum-enhanced drug discovery will redefine the oncology landscape. These technologies will help develop robust cancer treatments, equitable data representations, and personalized diagnostic and clinical interventions. As these technologies mature and gain widespread adoption at the root level, cancer management might become decentralized, continuous, and patient-centered (Riaz et al., 2025).

Ultimately, we expect AI to adopt a patient-centered paradigm, where these technologies will not only be used as a decision-support mode, but also empower patients, greatly enhance quality of life, and convert cancer from a life-threatening condition into a manageable chronic disease.

8. CONCLUSION

This chapter discusses how AI and emerging technologies are transforming every aspect of cancer care, from early detection to treatment and survivorship. The chapter has demonstrated that integrating AI with immunotherapy, nanotechnology, robotics, and precision surgery can transform the entire landscape of cancer care. These technologies can be used to achieve high accuracy, personalization, and treatment effectiveness. The chapter also highlights several barriers to achieving this vision, including data quality, trustworthiness, transparency, explainability, ethics, and regulatory issues. Future developments in the domain must strive to create equitable, interpretable, and patient-centered AI systems that complement, rather than replace, human experts.

Looking ahead, these developments suggest a highly flexible, continuously learning oncology care paradigm that is well integrated with biological, clinical, and research data streams. These systems will transform cancer care from reactive to proactive disease management and patient care. In this new paradigm, cancer could be prevented and managed through highly personalized interventions to achieve the highest level of survivorship and improve quality of life. As these technologies become more mature, they will not only improve patient care but also change our understanding of how cancer is understood, managed, and ultimately reduced to an ordinary chronic disease.

ACKNOWLEDGEMENT

This work was supported by the Deanship of Scientific Research, Vice Presidency for Graduate Studies and Scientific Research, King Faisal University, Saudi Arabia [Grant No. KFU254239].

REFERENCES

Abdullah, K. M., Sharma, G., Singh, A. P., & Siddiqui, J. A. (2025). Nanomedicine in Cancer Therapeutics: Current Perspectives from Bench to Bedside. *Molecular Cancer, 24*(1), 169. Advance online publication. DOI: 10.1186/s12943-025-02368-w PMID: 40490771

Aerts, H. J. W. L., Velazquez, E. R., Leijenaar, R. T. H., Parmar, C., Grossmann, P., Carvalho, S., Bussink, J., Monshouwer, R., Haibe-Kains, B., Rietveld, D., Hoebers, F., Rietbergen, M. M., Leemans, C. R., Dekker, A., Quackenbush, J., Gillies, R. J., & Lambin, P. (2014). Decoding tumour phenotype by noninvasive imaging using a quantitative radiomics approach. *Nature Communications, 5*(1), 4006. Advance online publication. DOI: 10.1038/ncomms5006 PMID: 24892406

Ardito, V., Golubev, G., Ciani, O., & Tarricone, R. (2023). Evaluating Barriers and Facilitators to the Uptake of mHealth Apps in Cancer Care Using the Consolidated Framework for Implementation Research: Scoping Literature Review. *JMIR Cancer, 9*, e42092. DOI: 10.2196/42092 PMID: 36995750

Aronson, J. K. (2005). Biomarkers and surrogate endpoints. *British Journal of Clinical Pharmacology, 59*(5), 491–494. DOI: 10.1111/j.1365-2125.2005.02435.x PMID: 15842546

Baig, M. M., Hobson, C., GholamHosseini, H., Ullah, E., & Afifi, S. (2024). Generative AI in Improving Personalized Patient Care Plans: Opportunities and Barriers Towards Its Wider Adoption. *Applied Sciences (Basel, Switzerland), 14*(23), 10899. DOI: 10.3390/app142310899

Benzo, R. M., Gogineni, A., Tetrick, M. K., Singh, R., Washington, P., Fernandez, S., Paskett, E. D., Penedo, F. J., Ghazi, S., Osei, A., Clinton, S. K., Krok-Schoen, J., Weyrauch, S., & Addison, D. (2025). mHealth technologies in research studying cardiovascular health in cancer: A systematic review. *PLOS Digital Health, 4*(9), e0001027. DOI: 10.1371/journal.pdig.0001027 PMID: 40996972

Bhange, M., & Telange, D. (2025). Convergence of nanotechnology and artificial intelligence in the fight against liver cancer: A comprehensive review. *Discover. Oncology, 16*(1), 77. Advance online publication. DOI: 10.1007/s12672-025-01821-y PMID: 39841330

Boldrini, L., Bibault, J.-E., Masciocchi, C., Shen, Y., & Bittner, M.-I. (2019). Deep Learning: A Review for the Radiation Oncologist. *Frontiers in Oncology, 9*, 977. DOI: 10.3389/fonc.2019.00977 PMID: 31632910

Carlomagno, N., Incollingo, P., Tammaro, V., Peluso, G., Rupealta, N., Chiacchio, G., Sandoval Sotelo, M. L., Minieri, G., Pisani, A., Riccio, E., Sabbatini, M., Bracale, U. M., Calogero, A., Dodaro, C. A., & Santangelo, M. (2017). Diagnostic, Predictive, Prognostic, and Therapeutic Molecular Biomarkers in Third Millennium: A Breakthrough in Gastric Cancer. *BioMed Research International, 2017*, 1–11. DOI: 10.1155/2017/7869802 PMID: 29094049

Cheng, C. H., & Shi, S. (2025). Artificial intelligence in cancer: Applications, challenges, and future perspectives. *Molecular Cancer, 24*(1), 274. DOI: 10.1186/s12943-025-02450-3 PMID: 41168799

Coudray, N., Ocampo, P. S., Sakellaropoulos, T., Narula, N., Snuderl, M., Fenyö, D., Moreira, A. L., Razavian, N., & Tsirigos, A. (2018). Classification and mutation prediction from non–small cell lung cancer histopathology images using deep learning. *Nature Medicine, 24*(10), 1559–1567. DOI: 10.1038/s41591-018-0177-5 PMID: 30224757

Dipankar, P., Salazar, D., Dennard, E., Mohiyuddin, S., & Nguyen, Q. C. (2025). Artificial intelligence based advancements in nanomedicine for brain disorder management: An updated narrative review. *Frontiers in Medicine, 12*, 1599340. Advance online publication. DOI: 10.3389/fmed.2025.1599340 PMID: 40432717

Erdur, A. C., Rusche, D., Scholz, D., Kiechle, J., Fischer, S., Llorián-Salvador, Ó., Buchner, J. A., Nguyen, M. Q., Etzel, L., Weidner, J., Metz, M.-C., Wiestler, B., Schnabel, J., Rueckert, D., Combs, S. E., & Peeken, J. C. (2025). Deep learning for autosegmentation for radiotherapy treatment planning: State-of-the-art and novel perspectives. *Strahlentherapie und Onkologie, 201*(3), 236–254. DOI: 10.1007/s00066-024-02262-2 PMID: 39105745

Esteva, A., Kuprel, B., Novoa, R. A., Ko, J., Swetter, S. M., Blau, H. M., & Thrun, S. (2017). Dermatologist-level classification of skin cancer with deep neural networks. *Nature, 542*(7639), 115–118. DOI: 10.1038/nature21056 PMID: 28117445

Etli, D.. (2024). Generative AI and Patient Care: A Systematic Review Examining Applications, Limitations, and Future Directions for ChatGPT in Healthcare. *J. Qual. Healthc. Eco.*, *7*(1), 000361. DOI: 10.23880/jqhe-16000361

Garcia-Saiso, S., Marti, M., Pesce, K., Luciani, S., Mujica, O., Hennis, A., & D'Agostino, M. (2024). Artificial Intelligence as a Potential Catalyst to a More Equitable Cancer Care. *JMIR Cancer*, *10*, e57276. DOI: 10.2196/57276 PMID: 39133537

Hashimoto, D. A., Rosman, G., Rus, D., & Meireles, O. R. (2018). Artificial Intelligence in Surgery: Promises and Perils. *Annals of Surgery*, *268*(1), 70–76. DOI: 10.1097/SLA.0000000000002693 PMID: 29389679

Hu, Q., Yao, Y., Han, J., Yang, X., & Parton, J. (2024). Examining the existing usage gap of electronic health records in the United States: A study of National Health Survey. *SSM - Population Health*, *25*, 101577. DOI: 10.1016/j.ssmph.2023.101577 PMID: 38094223

Huang, L., Wu, X., You, J., Jin, Z., He, W., Sun, J., Shen, H., Liu, X., Yue, X., Cai, W., Zhang, S., & Zhang, B. (2025). Artificial Intelligence Can Predict Personalized Immunotherapy Outcomes in Cancer. *Cancer Immunology Research*, *13*(7), 964–977. DOI: 10.1158/2326-6066.CIR-24-1270 PMID: 40499001

Ilyas, Q. M., & Ahmad, M. (2021). An Enhanced Ensemble Diagnosis of Cervical Cancer: A Pursuit of Machine Intelligence Towards Sustainable Health. *IEEE Access : Practical Innovations, Open Solutions*, *9*, 12374–12388. DOI: 10.1109/ACCESS.2021.3049165

Jiang, Z., & Li, P. (2024). DeepDR: A deep learning library for drug response prediction. *Bioinformatics (Oxford, England)*, *40*(12), btae688. Advance online publication. DOI: 10.1093/bioinformatics/btae688 PMID: 39558584

Jumper, J., Evans, R., Pritzel, A., Green, T., Figurnov, M., Ronneberger, O., Tunyasuvunakool, K., Bates, R., Žídek, A., Potapenko, A., Bridgland, A., Meyer, C., Kohl, S. A. A., Ballard, A. J., Cowie, A., Romera-Paredes, B., Nikolov, S., Jain, R., Adler, J., & Hassabis, D. (2021). Highly accurate protein structure prediction with AlphaFold. *Nature*, *596*(7873), 583–589. DOI: 10.1038/s41586-021-03819-2 PMID: 34265844

Kourou, K., Exarchos, T. P., Exarchos, K. P., Karamouzis, M. V., & Fotiadis, D. I. (2015). Machine learning applications in cancer prognosis and prediction. *Computational and Structural Biotechnology Journal*, *13*, 8–17. DOI: 10.1016/j.csbj.2014.11.005 PMID: 25750696

Kristoffersen, A. E., Wider, B., Nilsen, J. V., Bjelland, M., Mora, D. C., Nordberg, J. H., Broderstad, A. R., Nakandi, K., & Stub, T. (2022). Prevalence of late and long-term effects of cancer (treatment) and use of complementary and alternative medicine in Norway. *BMC Complementary Medicine and Therapies*, *22*(1), 322. DOI: 10.1186/s12906-022-03790-z PMID: 36471296

Kurniawan, M. H., Handiyani, H., Nuraini, T., Hariyati, R. T. S., & Sutrisno, S. (2024). A systematic review of artificial intelligence-powered (AI-powered) chatbot intervention for managing chronic illness. *Annals of Medicine*, *56*(1), 2302980. DOI: 10.1080/07853890.2024.2302980 PMID: 38466897

Li, T., Li, Y., Zhu, X., He, Y., Wu, Y., Ying, T., & Xie, Z. (2023). Artificial intelligence in cancer immunotherapy: Applications in neoantigen recognition, antibody design and immunotherapy response prediction. *Seminars in Cancer Biology*, *91*, 50–69. DOI: 10.1016/j.semcancer.2023.02.007 PMID: 36870459

Liu, R., Rizzo, S., Wang, L., Chaudhary, N., Maund, S., Garmhausen, M. R., McGough, S., Copping, R., & Zou, J. (2024). Characterizing mutation-treatment effects using clinico-genomics data of 78,287 patients with 20 types of cancers. *Nature Communications*, *15*(1), 10884. DOI: 10.1038/s41467-024-55251-5 PMID: 39738052

Lopez-Beltran, A., Henriques, V., Cimadamore, A., Santoni, M., Cheng, L., Gevaert, T., Blanca, A., Massari, F., Scarpelli, M., & Montironi, R. (2018). The Identification of Immunological Biomarkers in Kidney Cancers. *Frontiers in Oncology*, *8*, 456. Advance online publication. DOI: 10.3389/fonc.2018.00456 PMID: 30450335

Lu, S.-C., Swisher, C. L., Chung, C., Jaffray, D., & Sidey-Gibbons, C. (2023). On the importance of interpretable machine learning predictions to inform clinical decision making in oncology. *Frontiers in Oncology*, *13*, 1129380. DOI: 10.3389/fonc.2023.1129380 PMID: 36925929

Mehmood, A., Gulzar, Y., Ilyas, Q. M., Jabbari, A., Ahmad, M., & Iqbal, S. (2023). SBXception: A Shallower and Broader Xception Architecture for Efficient Classification of Skin Lesions. *Cancers (Basel)*, *15*(14), 3604. DOI: 10.3390/cancers15143604 PMID: 37509267

Mohammed, S., & Malhotra, N. (2025). Ethical and regulatory challenges in machine learning-based healthcare systems: A review of implementation barriers and future directions. BenchCouncil Transactions on Benchmarks. *Standards and Evaluations*, *5*(1), 100215. DOI: 10.1016/j.tbench.2025.100215

Molina-Aguilar, C., & Robles-Espinoza, C. D. (2023). Tackling the lack of diversity in cancer research. *Disease Models & Mechanisms*, *16*(9), dmm050275. Advance online publication. DOI: 10.1242/dmm.050275 PMID: 37681401

Moy, S., Irannejad, M., Manning, S. J., Farahani, M., Ahmed, Y., Gao, E., Prabhune, R., Lorenz, S., Mirza, R., & Klinger, C. (2024). Patient Perspectives on the Use of Artificial Intelligence in Health Care: A Scoping Review. *Journal of Patient-Centered Research and Reviews, 11*(1), 51–62. DOI: 10.17294/2330-0698.2029 PMID: 38596349

Najar Najafi, N., Hajihassani, H., & Azimzadeh Irani, M. (2025). The Impact of Artificial Intelligence on Cancer Diagnosis and Treatment: A Review. *Cancer Informatics, 24*, 11769351251371273. DOI: 10.1177/11769351251371273 PMID: 40979169

Noury, H., Rahdar, A., Romanholo Ferreira, L. F., & Jamalpoor, Z. (2025). AI-driven innovations in smart multifunctional nanocarriers for drug and gene delivery: A mini-review. *Critical Reviews in Oncology/Hematology, 210*, 104701. DOI: 10.1016/j.critrevonc.2025.104701 PMID: 40086770

Partin, A., Brettin, T. S., Zhu, Y., Narykov, O., Clyde, A., Overbeek, J., & Stevens, R. L. (2022). Deep learning methods for drug response prediction in cancer: Predominant and emerging trends (No. arXiv:2211.10442). arXiv. https://doi.org//arXiv.2211.10442DOI: 10.48550

Partin, A., Brettin, T. S., Zhu, Y., Narykov, O., Clyde, A., Overbeek, J., & Stevens, R. L. (2023). Deep learning methods for drug response prediction in cancer: Predominant and emerging trends. *Frontiers in Medicine, 10*, 1086097. Advance online publication. DOI: 10.3389/fmed.2023.1086097 PMID: 36873878

Prelaj, A., Miskovic, V., Zanitti, M., Trovo, F., Genova, C., Viscardi, G., Rebuzzi, S. E., Mazzeo, L., Provenzano, L., Kosta, S., Favali, M., Spagnoletti, A., Castelo-Branco, L., Dolezal, J., Pearson, A. T., Lo Russo, G., Proto, C., Ganzinelli, M., Giani, C., & Pedrocchi, A. L. G. (2024). Artificial intelligence for predictive biomarker discovery in immuno-oncology: A systematic review. *Annals of Oncology : Official Journal of the European Society for Medical Oncology, 35*(1), 29–65. DOI: 10.1016/j.annonc.2023.10.125 PMID: 37879443

Riaz, I. B., Khan, M. A., & Osterman, T. J. (2025). Artificial intelligence across the cancer care continuum. *Cancer, 131*(16), e70050. DOI: 10.1002/cncr.70050 PMID: 40810209

Samal, B. R., Loers, J. U., Vermeirssen, V., & De Preter, K. (2022). Opportunities and challenges in interpretable deep learning for drug sensitivity prediction of cancer cells. *Frontiers in Bioinformatics, 2*, 1036963. Advance online publication. DOI: 10.3389/fbinf.2022.1036963 PMID: 36466148

Samathoti, P., Kumarachari, R. K., Bukke, S. P. N., Rajasekhar, E. S. K., Jaiswal, A. A., & Eftekhari, Z. (2025). The role of nanomedicine and artificial intelligence in cancer health care: Individual applications and emerging integrations—a narrative review. *Discover. Oncology*, *16*(1), 697. Advance online publication. DOI: 10.1007/s12672-025-02469-4 PMID: 40338421

Schmidt, M. E., Goldschmidt, S., Hermann, S., & Steindorf, K. (2022). Late effects, long-term problems and unmet needs of cancer survivors. *International Journal of Cancer*, *151*(8), 1280–1290. DOI: 10.1002/ijc.34152 PMID: 35657637

Shao, J., Feng, J., Li, J., Liang, S., Li, W., & Wang, C. (2023). Novel tools for early diagnosis and precision treatment based on artificial intelligence. *Chinese Medical Journal Pulmonary and Critical Care Medicine*, *01*(03), 148–160. DOI: 10.1016/j.pccm.2023.05.001 PMID: 39171128

Shirzad, M., Shaban, M., Mohammadzadeh, V., Rahdar, A., Fathi-karkan, S., Hoseini, Z. S., Najafi, M., Kharaba, Z., & Aboudzadeh, M. A. (2025). Artificial Intelligence-Assisted Design of Nanomedicines for Breast Cancer Diagnosis and Therapy: Advances, Challenges, and Future Directions. *BioNanoScience*, *15*(3), 354. Advance online publication. DOI: 10.1007/s12668-025-01980-w

Sung, H., Ferlay, J., Siegel, R. L., Laversanne, M., Soerjomataram, I., Jemal, A., & Bray, F. (2021). Global Cancer Statistics 2020: GLOBOCAN Estimates of Incidence and Mortality Worldwide for 36 Cancers in 185 Countries. *CA: a Cancer Journal for Clinicians*, *71*(3), 209–249. DOI: 10.3322/caac.21660 PMID: 33538338

Sutton, R. T., Pincock, D., Baumgart, D. C., Sadowski, D. C., Fedorak, R. N., & Kroeker, K. I. (2020). An overview of clinical decision support systems: Benefits, risks, and strategies for success. *NPJ Digital Medicine*, *3*(1), 17. DOI: 10.1038/s41746-020-0221-y PMID: 32047862

Tran, K. A., Kondrashova, O., Bradley, A., Williams, E. D., Pearson, J. V., & Waddell, N. (2021). Deep learning in cancer diagnosis, prognosis and treatment selection. *Genome Medicine*, *13*(1), 152. DOI: 10.1186/s13073-021-00968-x PMID: 34579788

Vamathevan, J., Clark, D., Czodrowski, P., Dunham, I., Ferran, E., Lee, G., Li, B., Madabhushi, A., Shah, P., Spitzer, M., & Zhao, S. (2019). Applications of machine learning in drug discovery and development. *Nature Reviews. Drug Discovery*, *18*(6), 463–477. DOI: 10.1038/s41573-019-0024-5 PMID: 30976107

Wang, C., Lye, X., Kaalia, R., Kumar, P., & Rajapakse, J. C. (2022). Deep learning and multi-omics approach to predict drug responses in cancer. *BMC Bioinformatics*, *22*(S10), 632. Advance online publication. DOI: 10.1186/s12859-022-04964-9 PMID: 36443676

Wang, L., Lu, Q., Li, R., Harrison, T. B., Jia, H., Huang, M., Dowst, H., Zhang, R., Badr, H., Fan, J. W., & Liu, H. (2025). Understanding Cancer Survivorship Care Needs Using Amazon Reviews: Content Analysis, Algorithm Development, and Validation Study. *JMIR Cancer*, *11*, e71102. DOI: 10.2196/71102 PMID: 40986859

Waqas, A., Tripathi, A., Ramachandran, R. P., Stewart, P., & Rasool, G. (2024). Multimodal Data Integration for Oncology in the Era of Deep Neural Networks: A Review. *Frontiers in Artificial Intelligence*, *7*, 1408843. DOI: 10.3389/frai.2024.1408843 PMID: 39118787

Wei, B., Li, L., Feng, Y., Liu, S., Fu, P., & Tian, L. (2024). Exploring prognostic biomarkers in pathological images of colorectal cancer patients via deep learning. *The Journal of Pathology. Clinical Research*, *10*(6), e70003. Advance online publication. DOI: 10.1002/2056-4538.70003 PMID: 39343999

Wulczyn, E., Steiner, D. F., Xu, Z., Sadhwani, A., Wang, H., Flament, I., Mermel, C. H., Chen, P.-H. C., Liu, Y., & Stumpe, M. C. (2020). Deep learning-based survival prediction for multiple cancer types using histopathology images. *PLoS One*, *15*(6), e0233678. DOI: 10.1371/journal.pone.0233678 PMID: 32555646

Xu, Z., Wang, X., Zeng, S., Ren, X., Yan, Y., & Gong, Z. (2021). Applying artificial intelligence for cancer immunotherapy. *Acta Pharmaceutica Sinica. B*, *11*(11), 3393–3405. DOI: 10.1016/j.apsb.2021.02.007 PMID: 34900525

Yao, I. Z., Dong, M., & Hwang, W. Y. K. (2025). Deep Learning Applications in Clinical Cancer Detection: A Review of Implementation Challenges and Solutions. *Mayo Clinic Proceedings. Digital Health*, *3*(3), 100253. DOI: 10.1016/j.mcpdig.2025.100253 PMID: 40822144

Zhang, H., Chen, Y., & Li, F. (2021). Predicting Anticancer Drug Response With Deep Learning Constrained by Signaling Pathways. *Frontiers in Bioinformatics*, *1*, 639349. Advance online publication. DOI: 10.3389/fbinf.2021.639349 PMID: 36303766

Zheng, J., Yan, Z., Wang, R., Xiao, H., Chen, Z., Ge, X., Li, Z., Liu, Z., Yu, H., Liu, H., Wang, G., Yu, P., Fu, J., Zhang, G., Zhang, J., Liu, B., Huang, Y., Deng, H., Wang, C., & Liang, H. (2025). NeoPred: Dual-phase CT AI forecasts pathologic response to neoadjuvant chemo-immunotherapy in NSCLC. *Journal for Immunotherapy of Cancer*, *13*(5), e011773. DOI: 10.1136/jitc-2025-011773 PMID: 40449955

Chapter 10
Introduction to Machine Learning in Cancer Care

Tariq S. Mian
https://orcid.org/0000-0003-2666-9223
Taibah University, Saudi Arabia

Hisham F. Saeed
Fatima Medical and Saleem Surgical Hospital, Sheikhupura, Pakistan

Eman M. Alatawi
Taibah University, Saudi Arabia

ABSTRACT

Machine learning (ML) is revolutionizing oncology by enhancing diagnostic accuracy, prognostic predictions, and personalized treatment strategies. This chapter explores the integration of ML into cancer care, focusing on its applications in medical imaging, molecular profiling, and treatment optimization. Advanced algorithms, such as convolutional neural networks (CNNs), have demonstrated diagnostic accuracy comparable to or surpassing human experts, while techniques like radiogenomics bridge imaging and genomic data for non-invasive diagnostics. Despite these advancements, challenges such as data heterogeneity, model interpretability, and ethical concerns—including patient privacy and algorithmic bias—remain significant barriers to clinical implementation.

1. INTRODUCTION

The study of oncology is a fast-growing discipline, with the growing use of machine learning (ML) algorithms in the clinical process. Machine learning (ML)

DOI: 10.4018/979-8-3373-4312-9.ch010

in clinical oncology has diverse clinical implications in terms of enhancing diagnostic and prognostic accuracy and the personalisation of therapeutic decisions. This part is dedicated to the implementation of modern technologies in the clinical field logistics. The question of its primary research is the following: How can ML be applied successfully in the clinical workflow of oncology to enhance clinical outcomes, considering the diversity of data sources, interpretability, and ethics? This question is the stimulus of the current work.

Machine learning is a field of AI and has become a household in most industries. This might be particularly applicable to the healthcare sector, as cancer is a complicated, dynamic condition on the molecular, genetic, and phenotypic levels. Therefore, machine learning has increasingly been applied in oncology because the ability to extract patterns in vast amounts of medical imaging, genomic, and EHR data has established an ability to individualise cancer care to a degree that is more accurate. The section will address the background and early understanding of ML that would be instrumental in explaining its use in healthcare, including a brief history of the history of AI in oncology and some of the applications of machine learning to further cause precision oncology.

2. MACHINE LEARNING FUNDAMENTALS IN HEALTHCARE

It is necessary to learn the fundamental concepts and processes of machine learning to use its revolutionary potential in healthcare, especially in oncology. In this section, I am going to discuss the core algorithms and data processing methods and measures which are the basis of practical AI applications. Creating these basics, the work preconditions the understanding of the sophisticated improvements of machine learning to diagnostics, prognosis, and personalised treatment in cancer care.

2.1 Core Algorithms and Architectures

Machine learning in oncology aims to support diagnostic and prognostic applications, as well as treatment planning and decision-making. Supervised learning uses labelled data, such as histopathological images, to classify input data, malignant or benign tumours. This is used in reproducible oncological diagnoses with measurable performance characteristics (Introduction to Machine Learning in Cancer. The cost, time, and resource requirements to collect labelled data can lead to a need to reduce the required amount through semi-supervised and active learning techniques.

Unsupervised learning utilises unlabelled data to extract hidden patterns relevant to clinical purposes, such as glioblastoma subtype clustering and personalised treatment.

MYCIN used fixed rules for diagnosing infections based on available information. Today, computer programs can improve with the increasing amount of data in modern neural networks. Complex architectures, such as AlexNet, have demonstrated performance comparable to that of radiologists in cancer screening.

Neural networks can learn complex non-linear relationships and extract hierarchical features, which is key to the high complexity of cancer data. Some modern clinical applications include multimodal fusion and medical image analysis. Due to their black box nature, this calls for explainable methods to maintain clinical trust.

The introduction of the AlexNet architecture for medical image analysis popularised the application of deep learning techniques in this area. Several domain-specific algorithms in oncology are now widely utilised in clinical practice. Clinically relevant model design is essential for use in practical settings. The selection of model architectures for practical clinical implementations should also address biases introduced by non-generalizable data.

The application of neural networks in paediatric oncology includes diagnostic and prognostic applications. Gaussian Mixture Models and neural networks are highly effective in distinguishing between therapy-induced leukoencephalopathy and leukaemia. A recall score of 0.9 can be achieved at a precision of 0.81 (accuracy = 0.81, recall = 0.9, F1 = 0.8). High AUROC scores of neural networks (up to 0.904) have shown their predictive power for predicting recurrence (Elsayid et al., 2025, p. 7). The varying patient numbers and datasets of cancer care require additional external validation to confirm the robustness and reliability of different approaches.

Through image segmentation, neural networks can accurately differentiate between pathological and standard conditions for effective intervention strategies. This enables an earlier and more objective approach (Elsayid et al., 2025, p. 7). Monte Carlo-based models can then apply these predictors for recurrence and are an extremely effective prediction strategy (Elsayid et al., 2025, p. 7). In each application, there is a benefit to understanding algorithm design and implementation in the context of the patient's needs. However, inequitable access to machine learning remains an ethical challenge in the field of paediatric cancer (Păcuraru et al., 2025, pp. 1, 5).

With the growing quantities of data that healthcare services must process and the burden on staff due to understaffing, machine learning technologies are becoming increasingly relevant in improving resource utilisation and clinical performance (Păcuraru et al., 2025, p. 4). Algorithms can now commonly find complex connections in biological data. The issue of the uninterpretability and ethical issues of this quickly growing practice should be addressed. This is because these complications of AI in health applications also heighten the concern that disparities between the care of marginalised populations and better-represented populations will be amplified (Farasati Far, 2023, p. 2).

Machine learning algorithms must be designed in a manner that promotes transparency and instils trust and confidence among healthcare professionals and explain the possible error in their decisions, which must be driven by ethics. AccurateAn accurate and transparent algorithm is in the best interest of all parties involved, and the mechanisms that measure the effects of such choices, such as fairness and accountability, should exist (Farasati Far, 2023, p. 2).

2.2 Data Processing Methods

Data cleansing, normalisation, and harmonisation are necessary to provide machine learning model stability and accuracy in complicated cancer datasets. Redundancy, incorrect data, and ambiguous data must be deleted during data pre-processing to improve prediction accuracy and precision and avoid misleading clinical judgments. TThis is shown in the lung cancer survivorship data pre-processing stage, when individuals aged 30 to 79 were selected (Jabin and Rahman, 2021, p. 4). Standardisation protocols are needed to integrate demographic data, clinical and pathology reports, and patient genomics in machine learning in oncology, especially in heterogeneous patient cohorts. These processes decrease systematic disparities between source databases due to data gathering methods or measures. The lung cancer survivorship study filtered patient data to homogenize data for model performance ((Jabin & Rahman, 2021, p. 4).

Feature normalisation and augmentation scale features and generate different samples to improve machine learning models. For analysis and model training, multi-modal data including omics, histology, and EHR clinical reports may contain unbalanced and unstandardized data (Kumar et al., 2024, p. 1). Managing large cancer datasets and collecting clinical information for machine learning models like PCA and autoencoders requires proper feature extraction and dimensionality reduction. Feature extraction and dimensionality reduction have helped identify the most important qualities, reducing the computing cost of machine learning analysis and minimizing the "curse of dimensionality" (Farasati Far, 2023, p. 2; Kumar et al., 2024, p. 2).

Healthcare professionals collaborate to build participatory data processing procedures that meet clinical demands and make machine learning more accessible in clinical settings. A participatory approach was used to construct the INCISIVE toolbox, which included feedback from physicians from seven nations and five clinics in iterative workshops on data integration protocols. Data integration in oncology requires strong de-identification and data handling standards to ensure patient privacy. Data integration from several sources raises the danger of patient re-identification due to the increased number of identifiable data points in every integrated dataset (Farasati Far, 2023, p. 2).

2.3 Model Evaluation Techniques

To evaluate oncology machine learning models in clinical settings, performance measures must be carefully considered. Accuracy, precision, recall, F1 score, and ROC-AUC measure predictive performance. Model accuracy simply measures total correctness. However, it is not always informative, especially when one class is substantially more prevalent than the others, such as in cancer recurrence prediction. Even if accuracy is excellent, it may not show a large rate of false negatives, which can ruin cancer management. Thus, precision and recall are more precise measurements, with precision measuring the percentage of correct true positives and recall measuring the model's sensitivity, which measures whether it recognizes all relevant situations. The F1 score calculates a more balanced weighted average to balance precision and recall. On the other hand, ROC-AUC evaluates model performance across thresholds. This is useful for survival forecasts since sensitivity and specificity must be balanced to make educated treatment decisions. Ahuja et al. (2024) showed that the artificial neural network (ANN) could predict prostate cancer survival rates with 84.14 accuracy, 0.8108 precision, 0.8333 recall, 0.8219 F1 score, and 0.8405 ROC-AUC. The study found that machine learning methods predicted prostate cancer survival with higher value, recall, precision, F1 scores, and ROC-AUC scores than other methods (p. 7). Logistic regression was used as a reference test (p. 7).

ROC-AUC score can be used to compare models and choose the best oncology model. The AUC measures a classifier's likelihood of properly distinguishing two result classes (p. 1). Hamano et al. (2024) found that the KSVM (AUC 0.834) outperformed fractional polynomial regression (AUC: 0.799) and XGBoost models in predicting 30-day survival in advanced cancer patients (p. 1, 4). The ROC-AUC score allows threshold performance comparisons, but it may not capture performance variations due to threshold choice or false positive/negative utility (p. 1, 3). Data size and variety exceeded XGBoost. ROC-AUC scores are used to rank classifiers, although the AUC is insensitive when events are far fewer than non-events.

Benchmarking machine learning algorithms against human skill to assess oncology model applicability and reliability is another important step. CNNs have diagnostic accuracy comparable to dermatologists for some tasks. The CNN found clinical patterns related to some skin cancer kinds at levels comparable to dermatologists (Elhaddad & Hamam, 2024, p. 2). Elhaddad and Hamam (2024, p. 5) quoted research that reported 91% to 98% OCTA imaging accuracy for diabetic retinopathy identification. To be accepted by oncologists, clinicians, and physicians, machine learning techniques must be seen as adjuncts to human performance, not replacements. Thus, benchmarking is essential, especially when the role of human input in model development is uncertain and an erroneous prediction may raise clinical risk.

C-index, or concordance index, is the most frequent classical statistical metric for survival prediction approaches (p. 33). Biccler (2019) states that the C-index is the most commonly used survival prediction metric (p. 33). It measures prognosis by comparing the model's predictions against survival rates. A 0.5 C-index score suggests no prognostic significance (p. 33), as the prediction is random. To justify real-world machine learning applications in research subjects like DLBCL diagnosis, the C-index must be over 0.5. To be considered a proper machine learning system, a machine learning-powered algorithm must perform at or above a C-index of 0.5, regardless of its clinical accuracy.

Generalizing in real-world healthcare contexts is essential for testing model efficacy and showing that machine learning models are robust across patient groups. The uneven, diversified, and limited dataset caused XGBoost to fail in Hamano et al. 's assessment (p. 1). Thus, patient validation of machine learning technologies requires generalizability (p. 5). Interpretability and usability are also important in model evaluation and user confidence in system predictions. It is an emerging field that seeks to explain why some of the most accurate and best machine learning models are worthless. Other issues include that these problems require interdisciplinary discussions with medical, marketing, business, and legal experts.

3. EVOLUTION OF AI IN ONCOLOGY

The evolution of AI in oncology is characterised by a progression from basic rule-based systems to more complex and sophisticated deep learning models. This introduction provides a concise overview of these developments, outlining the plan for the remainder of the section and setting the context for the subsequent discussion on historical milestones, current trends, and future avenues for the application of AI in oncology.

3.1 Historical Development and Milestones

Over the past few decades, oncology has slowly incorporated machine learning, although the number of published studies and novel approaches or applications has expanded. Between 1988 and 2021, 214 documents were indexed, demonstrating the growing importance of AI in oncology. Artificial intelligence and machine learning in cancer have grown in importance and publications from 1988 to 2017. Machine learning in oncology matures after 2017, as publication rates rise (Musa et al.,

2021, p. 3). Between 1988 and 2021, publications averaged 5.32 authors (Musa et al., 2021, p. 4). Complex feature learning and automated feature extraction improve classification accuracy and reduce manual involvement (Singla & Singla, 2020, p. 1).

Allowing the AI model to decide and learn on its own will remove experts' biases when determining data importance in models and allow data to have its own intrinsic value. Deep learning models can process high-dimensional, multi-modal medical data, including imaging and omics data (Singla & Singla, 2020, p. 2). Convolutional neural networks have met or exceeded human radiography and histopathologic image classification accuracy in recent years (Singla & Singla, 2020, p. 1). Oncology facilities now get patient-level tumour behaviour information and better clinical management. Deep learning has been utilized for omics analyses and imaging data classification. Clear cell renal cell carcinoma (ccRCC) showed unique immune microenvironment markers and genetic changes (Singla & Singla, 2020, p. 2).

For ccRCC tumour progression, metastatic behavior, and integrated clinical characteristics, the TRACERx Renal Consortium uses multi-level omics studies using multiregional, targeted genomic analysis (Singla & Singla, 2020, p. 2). Diagnostic accuracy has improved with deep learning systems for imaging-based diagnosis. Deep learning algorithms for imaging-based pneumonia diagnosis have sensitivities of 87% and specificities of 92% (Ankita & Singh, 2024, pp. 2-3). A smartphone-based diagnostic AI technology might detect skin cancer with a 95% early detection rate and accurately define melanoma lesions within 10 seconds (Ankita & Singh, 2024, p. 3).

Deep learning applications are effective in diagnostic laboratories and point-of-care (POC) settings when utilized with EHRs. Most clinical laboratory diagnostic tests have AUROC scores of 0.98 with deep learning (Ankita & Singh, 2024, p. 4). Automating various diagnostic procedures in healthcare, such as laboratory analysis, frees up clinical laboratory workers to focus on patient care. Clinical nurses spend 25% of their time on non-care activities (Ankita & Singh, 2024, p. 4).

Kernel support vector machines (KSVM) have the highest prognostic accuracy, predicting 30-day survival for cancer patients admitted to a hospital's internal medicine department with a mean AUC score of 0.834 (Hamano et al., 2024, p. 4). In addition, this method predicts patient survival better in a training dataset than in a broad testing dataset. A metastatic breast cancer study found that some machine learning algorithms had high sensitivity and specificity in experimental settings but performed poorly in the general cohort (0.6 AUC, 0.65 sensitivity, 0.42 specificity) (Hamano et al., 2024, p. 1). A study employing the same machine learning methods using clinical and CT data from general cancer patients who received surgery, chemotherapy, or radiation supports this. This study used XGBoost with comparable results (Hamano et al., 2024, p. 1).

3.2 Current Applications

AI enhances adaptive radiation workflow (Archambault et al., 2020, p. 1). Varian's Ethos therapy automates real-time radiotherapy planning with machine learning (ML) in every clinical step of adaptive radiation (Archambault et al., 2020, pp. 1-2). Radiotherapy replanning used to be time-consuming and limit treatment (Archambault et al., 2020, pp. 1-2). Ethos therapy uses ML models trained on imaging and ground truth contours to adapt to many new patients' anatomy in real time (Archambault et al., 2020, pp. 1-2). ML improves throughput, reduces cognitive strain, and generalizes because Ethos therapy uses datasets from America, Europe, Australia, and Asia (Archambault et al., 2020, p. 2).

CE marking and FDA 510(k) authorization for automated contouring and planning prove Ethos therapy can adapt safely and efficiently. These regulatory approvals accelerate clinical oncology automated plan adaptation (Archambault et al., 2020, p. 9). Integration with clinical environments allows adaptive plans and physician approval in under 15 minutes, ensuring efficient workflow for high patient volume and comfort (Archambault et al., 2020, p. 9). Ethos' interface lets doctors adjust and monitor automated treatment planning to ensure its proper application in clinical practice and not be used as a standalone decision support system (Archambault et al., 2020, p. 9).

AI-powered tailored therapy suggestion systems give oncologists treatment plans based on malignant tumour genetics (DeFrank & Luiz, 2022, pp. 2, 5). AI-powered technologies give oncologists real-time, tumour-specific treatment recommendations (DeFrank & Luiz, 2022, pp. 2, 5). Treatment recommendation engines anticipate risk and side effects (DeFrank & Luiz, 2022, p. 5). Side effects and risks help doctors and patients decide on therapy, enhancing adherence (DeFrank & Luiz, 2022, p. 5). The treatment suggestion engine will enable oncologists uncover cancer genetic causes to develop therapeutic targets and deliver more targeted molecular therapy options (DeFrank & Luiz, 2022, p. 2). For patient consultation, the AI-powered treatment recommendation engine can provide immediate and consistent advice from a growing dataset of therapeutic treatments (DeFrank & Luiz, 2022, p. 5).

Oncology clinics need AI-powered therapy recommendation engines since 600,000 Americans will die from cancer in 2022 (DeFrank & Luiz, 2022, p. 4). This method is challenging, costly, and underused (DeFrank & Luiz, 2022, p. 4). AI systems are costly and hard to exchange between centers (DeFrank & Luiz, 2022, p. 4). Cancer recurrence is high despite standard chemotherapy (DeFrank & Luiz, 2022, p. 4). Reduce barriers to advanced technology like an AI-powered therapy suggestion engine. Quality and quantity of AI performance are measured. AI-generated treatments are assessed by mean value. ML evolves and must be evaluated for therapeutic value (DeFrank & Luiz, 2022, p. 5).

In CAD and radiomics, ML detects cancer (Bongurala et al., 2025, p. 2). ML-powered CAD tools improve imaging and detect oncological results humans cannot (Bongurala et al., 2025, p. 2). Cancer detection earlier than manually improves patient survival (Bongurala et al., 2025, p. 2). Radiomics allows quantitative texture, morphology, and volumetric imaging (Bongurala et al., 2025, p. 2). Virtual oncology drug screening using ML decreases the time needed to screen hundreds of compounds and find promising new therapeutic molecules (Bongurala et al., 2025, p. 2).

Prevention is possible with early discovery of certain illnesses. Broad and flexible risk stratification algorithms for cancer and patient heterogeneity are constraints of the system (Bongurala et al., 2025, p. 2). AI systems also prevent misdiagnosis and inaccurate treatment regimens, improving patient care (Păcuraru et al., 2025, p. 1). Oncologists and doctors save time, money, and resources (Păcuraru et al., 2025, p. 5). AI enhances cancer diagnosis, treatment, and prevention (Păcuraru et al., 2025, pp. 4-5). These advances are essential to cancer treatment. Though increasing, this field has problems. Many issues hinder large-scale clinical AI use. The lack of cancer care AI regulations, AI's external evaluation, and AI training and education are all difficulties (Păcuraru et al., 2025, p. 7).

AI and ML improve human errors, turnaround times, diagnosis, and workflow in radiology (Bejarano, 2023, pp. 1-2). A study found that automated software cut human chest X-ray and biomarker studies to 10.3 seconds from 30.1 seconds (Bejarano, 2023, p. 2). AI's pattern-recognition and analysis improve diagnosis, but experts should always utilize the applications because medical technology is imperfect (Bejarano, 2023, pp. 1-3). AI in imaging can detect early trends in patients' massive histories and data (Bejarano, 2023, p. 2). AI will extract image-derived features, segment tissues and organs, detect anomalies, and quantify features (Bejarano, 2023, pp. 2-3). Even though lung and breast cancer are more likely to die from late diagnosis, early detection can improve prognosis (Bejarano, 2023, p. 2). Quantitative image analysis (QIA) quantifies longitudinal imaging datasets for therapy and diagnosis picture consistency (Bejarano, 2023, p. 3). AI and automation reduce inter-rater variability and standardise data interpretation (Bejarano, 2023, p. 3). Computational radiology workflow help that manages medical scan images and data using AI and AI-assisted applications has grown in popularity (Bejarano, 2023, p. 2). AI-automated preprocessing and report preparation allow radiologists to focus on clinically relevant decision-making (Bejarano, 2023, p. 2). Reduced human errors and better diagnosis increase patient quality of life (Bejarano, 2023, pp. 1-3).

4. MACHINE LEARNING IN CANCER CARE

4.1 Diagnostic Applications

Medical image analysis and molecular profiling are improving oncology diagnosis and early detection. Using deep learning and genomic data, these breakthroughs can help diagnose and treat cancer.

4.1.1 Medical Image Analysis

CNN models are 98.5%, 97.3%, and 96.1% sensitive, respectively. This makes them excellent at identifying and classifying cancers. They help radiologists reduce misunderstood pictures and diagnostic errors. CNN models can discover patterns on medical images, and U-Net can segment images to detect cancer locations to classify and arrange illness treatment and follow-up (Golden et al., 2025, p. 9). The high Dice coefficient of 0.92 in cancer segmentation shows that AI models are good at localising and quantifying tumours in medical imagery. They also measure visible tumour size to determine cancer spread and growth. AI-based image analysis needs external validation on varied and heterogeneous patient populations (Hesso et al., 2023, p. 6).

Research shows ANNs are 84.14% accurate and logistic regression 76.82. ANNs predict survival more accurately with a ROC-AUC of 0.8405. With a precision rate of 0.8108, recall of 0.8333, and F1 of 0.8219, ANNs can make more accurate clinical predictions (Ahuja et al., 2024, p. 7). Although more expensive, ANNs and other advanced machine learning models are more accurate than conventional models. Many AI applications work in a black-box environment that physicians distrust because of cost, resources, and ability. Thus, these strategies improve interpretability by evolving explanation methods (Hesso et al., 2023, p. 6). Healthcare professionals with the highest mean rank score of 2.25 in diagnosing benign and malignant lesions are interested in machine learning technologies that automatically define several persons. Resource shortages, with a mean rank score of 1.17, may be the main machine learning implementation challenge (Hasso et al., 2023, pp. 3, 6).

Algorithms should also be evaluated routinely to identify and fix AI model biases so they don't affect certain groups (Farasati Far, 2023, p. 2). Healthcare institutions must address patient data privacy to effectively implement artificial intelligence technologies. Transparency and clinical recommendations are crucial. The FDA provides guidelines for responsible machine learning use. Ethicists and regulators should establish systems using these technologies (Farasati Far, 2023, p. 2; Hesso et al., 2023, p. 6). Medical and computer science researchers must collaborate and consider the medical sector perspective to solve the AI technology development and oncologic treatment problem (Hesso et al., 2023, pp. 3, 6).

4.1.2 Molecular Profiling

Cancer molecular profiling using machine learning represents a major leap in processing multi-omic, proteomic, and complex genomic data. This allows actionable insights to improve patient care (Farasati Far, 2023, p. 2). High-quality machine learning-based predictions still face data integrity and dependability issues. Lack of molecular data information or annotation prevents reliable and reproducible predictions (Hesso et al., 2023, p. 6).

Machine-learning based molecular profiling could improve cancer phenotyping and therapy decisions for diagnosis and prognosis. These machine learning-based methods can detect overlapping tumour characteristics, demonstrating its potential to help with diagnosis (Arslan, 2023, p. 4). Complex biological systems like cancer require machine learning models that can adapt to changing molecular data modalities. As more molecular data is obtained, machine learning models must be generalized across populations to maintain predictive accuracy and avoid diagnostic discrepancies (Hesso et al., 2023, p. 6).

Radiogenomics uses deep learning to bridge the gap between imaging features from CT or MRI and genomics to predict patient genotype-phenotype (Arslan, 2023, p. 4). It helps identify quantitative imaging and genetic biomarkers for individual risk stratification. Radiogenomics and multi-omics profiles classify tumour subtypes (Arslan, 2023, p. 4). Radiomics has identified aspects of genetic alterations like EGFR in lung cancer. Quantitative features from radiographic pictures can reveal a tumour's genetic profile, making it promising for non-invasive molecular diagnostics. Current multimodal datasets struggle to reach high model accuracy and generalizability, despite their proven benefits. Interdisciplinary collaboration to collect and understand multimodal imaging and molecular data improves radiogenomic analysis (Hesso et al., 2023, p. 3).

Effective implementation and interpretation of machine learning models require tools that show the reasoning and contributions of sophisticated algorithms that are not totally transparent. Model-agnostic interpretability mechanisms like FI and ALE charts help doctors understand and make therapeutic judgments. FI calculates the impact of each genetic variable on prediction, while ALE helps doctors assess the association between model predictors and predictions, adding accountability (Lu et al., 2023, pp. 6-7). This method has proved successful, but has restricted adoption due to the difficulty in interpreting model predictions with insufficient machine learning knowledge. To improve clinician-machine learning model developer collaboration, visualising model interpretability and iterative feedback are necessary (Hesso et al., 2023, p. 3).

Poor interpretability and data heterogeneity hamper molecular profiling generalizability. Genomic sequencing, proteomics, and clinical factors can affect data quality, annotation, and format. Thus, the integration process hinders the establishment of generalizable, high-performing medical models and institutions (Hesso et al., 2023, p. 6; Lu, p. 1). Generalizable models across data repositories require standardised feature extraction, data normalisation, and harmonisation (Hesso et al., 2023, pp. 3, 6).

Machine learning models perform differently in curated research environments and complex clinical settings, indicating the need for proper validation to make accurate predictions. Thus, multi-institutional research must account for institutional variation across varied populations, healthcare infrastructure, and clinical practice (Hesso et al., 2023, p. 6). Algorithms should be constantly checked for bias throughout development and implementation (Farasati Far, 2023, p. 2). Molecular profiling examines genetic and health data about a customer and their family members. Therefore, patient privacy and molecular data protection should be prioritized (Farasati Far, 2023, p. 2). Working with ethicists, clinicians, data scientists, and patients during model construction can help deploy the technology effectively (Hesso et al., 2023, p. 3). Such algorithms that track bias and produce fair model predictions are required to promote such a practice (Hesso et al., 2023, p. 6).

4.2 Treatment Optimization

Advances in machine learning can be used to treat cancer with more personalized and adaptive approaches.

4.2.1 Personalized Therapy Selection

By using varied clinical and genomic data, machine learning algorithms have transformed cancer treatment choices. Some studies have indicated that customized treatment options based on cancer-specific genetic data improve patient outcomes (Păcuraru et al., 2025, p. 5). Recent research has shown that deep learning models can diagnose HRD with 74% accuracy, helping patients get customized cancer treatment (Ugemuge et al., 2024, p. 3). Personalization also reduced resource and healthcare staff waste (Păcuraru et al., 2025, p. 4). Outlier elimination, imputation for missing information, and feature engineering for trustworthy AI modeling improve AI model repeatability across clinics (Gaur & Jagtap, 2022, p. 3). Oncology care benefits from AI's ability to find patterns and links that statistical approaches cannot. This may reveal novel oncology therapy targets (Farasati Far, 2023, p. 2).

AI-based virtual screening of compounds for drug discovery could improve and personalize oncology treatments quickly (Bongurala et al., 2025, p. 2).

When paired with multi-omic data, AI is more effective than single-type clinical data at identifying patients with personalized therapy (Păcuraru et al., 2025, p. 5). Individualised cancer treatment strategies combined with machine learning have helped healthcare workers with workforce constraints and cancer patients receive timely, personalized treatment (Păcuraru et al., 2025, p. 4). Improved workflow and data standards are essential for real-world cancer applications. Healthcare experts and technicians are trained to provide tailored patient care in clinics. Data sources vary in quality and diversity, hence AI model developers must normalise them to improve clinic repeatability (Gaur & Jagtap, 2022, p. 3). Data harmonisation and rigorous validation across clinics enable real-world deployment and generalization of these therapy regimens (Păcuraru et al., 2025, p. 5). If AI-based algorithms are used in a dataset with incomplete racial profiles or lacking women or other races than whites, they may make biased predictions about patients in real life (Farasati Far, 2023, p. 2). AI-based systems contain high-dimensional and individualized patient data, such as genomic data, which requires compliance with genomics and medicine ethical frameworks to protect patient privacy (Farasati Far, 2023, p. 2).

Patient autonomy and permission procedures, data sharing standards, and data regulations must be followed for regulatory compliance (Farasati Far, 2023, p. 2). Regular ethicist monitoring and auditing could achieve this (Farasati Far, 2023, p. 2). This requires continuous monitoring and model updates with the latest datasets to ensure AI system accountability (Farasati Far, 2023, p. 2). Governance and management must also be explored, including the development of multidisciplinary clinical healthcare teams, to eliminate biases and ethics issues in these AI models to individually treat cancer (Farasati Far, 2023, p. 2).

4.2.2 Response Prediction

Comparative studies show that ML models, which are artificial neural networks (ANNs), predict therapy outcomes and survival rates better. An ANN model for prostate cancer was 84.14% accurate, compared to 76.82% for a logistic regression model (Ahuja et al., 2024, p. 7). ANN model technical performance is shown by improved precision, recall, and F1 scores. ANN had a precision of 0.8108 and a recall of 0.8333, resulting in an F1 score of 0.8219 and ROC-AUC of 0.8405, lower than the logistic regression model, which scored 0.7428 and 0.7222, respectively. ML models can manage huge non-homogenous datasets to uncover non-linear connections between clinical factors and therapy outcomes (Păcuraru et al., 2025, p. 7; Farasati Far, 2023, p. 2). ML algorithms can also improve risk categorization and prognosis by revealing nuances, leading to more appropriate aggressive treatment and less overtreatment. However, these improved forecasts may lose strength when used on other cohorts (Ahuja et al., 2024, p. 7). AI helps quickly stratify patients by therapy benefit and risk. Such systems can swiftly analyze clinical and genetic differences based on medical histories, therapy management, and scans to connect patients to customised treatment or clinical trials (Bongurala et al., 2025, p. 2). These tools should incorporate validation metrics and be presented to patients and clinical personnel for clinical transparency and acceptance. Multi-omic and molecular data must be combined with clinical data to optimize ML prediction and treatment. Combining clinical and genetic variables in early breast cancer patients increased AUC to 0.82. This clinical data-only prediction improvement highlights the importance of multi-modal combination (Kubeyev et al., 2023). ML-based response prediction has great potential to improve treatment decisions, but data annotation, quality, and completeness issues hinder reproducibility and generalizability (Hesso et al., 2023, p. 6). Response prediction systems also use patient privacy, which is often based on massive data repositories (Farasati Far, 2023, p. 2). Diversification of training data and bias monitoring of model training and deployment can reduce these biases and improve model accuracy for underrepresented groups (Farasati Far, 2023, p. 2). When using AI systems to predict responses and treat patients individually, model accountability must be included in addition to regulatory attention to minimize prejudices and other ethical difficulties and encourage clear model usage (Farasati Far, 2023, p. 2). Due to ML systems' increasing predictive powers, responding patients need prompt diagnoses and individualized therapy (Păcuraru et al., 2025, p. 4). ML systems have more modalities than traditional treatment for analysing tumour images, genetic sequences, and other clinical data. They optimise personalised treatment programmes in real time to improve tumour control, patient survival, and treatment side effects (Păcuraru et al., 2025, p. 5). These technologies can change treatment plans in time to achieve desired tumour control outcomes while minimizing overtreatment and the need for subsequent therapies (Bongurala et al., 2025, p. 2). To improve clinical transparency and acceptability in real-world situations, response prediction tasks should incorporate data heterogeneity, model interpretability, and algorithm performance and clinical decision-making (Ahuja et al., 2024, p. 7). Interdisciplinary collaboration between clinicians, data scientists, and data governance boards can improve fairness and bias, accountability, data reliability and robustness, and the need for multiple modal integrations (Bongurala et al., 2025, p. 2).

5. IMPLEMENTATION CHALLENGES AND ETHICS

5.1 Data Privacy and Security

Security breaches increase as cloud storage providers consolidate or integrate patient data into hospitals (Farasati Far, 2023, p. 2). GDPR and HIPAA safeguard patient data. Businesses have data access and storage protocols, but their methods differ. Institutional variability can compromise cancer data and hinder standardization (Farasati Far, 2023, p. 2). Harmonizing privacy laws globally could fix this. Federated learning compiles without sharing patient data by sending its learning algorithm to it (Farasati Far, 2023, p. 2). These methods are time-consuming and complicated to develop without a standard approach, hence they are rarely used. Data curation is needed because many diagnostic algorithms are inaccurate across groups (Harishbhai Tilala et al., 2024, p. 3). Sadly, prediction algorithms often include socioeconomic factors, demonstrating healthcare inequality. Socioeconomic considerations favour patients with healthcare assets or greater social status (Harishbhai Tilala et al., 2024, p. 3). Prejudice reduction is costly. Regular audits, algorithm transparency, and group and patient advocate interaction are essential (Harishbhai Tilala et al., 2024, p. 3).

Varian's Ethos therapy system meets FDA and CE mark criteria and safeguards patient data between clinics, allowing physicians to employ the AI algorithm to improve cancer treatment without compliance or privacy issues (Archambault et al., 2020, p. 9 AI and RPA cut operational costs 22%–30% (Sharma, 2023, p. 5). RPA reduces billing errors and claims processing time by 40-50% (Sharma, 2023, p. 4). To lessen patient autonomy and safety issues when applying machine learning in clinical cancer care, protocols and ethical frameworks must be implemented for patients and personnel. Tighter regulatory oversight is needed to address AI algorithm biases and protect patient privacy (Farasati Far, 2023, p. 2; Harishbhai Tilala et al., 2024, p. 3

5.2 Clinical Integration

Knowledge, technology, and culture affect clinical machine learning. Lack of ML-based technology expertise and training is a major barrier to adoption. Nearly 35% of healthcare companies cite knowledge and training deficiencies as a major hurdle (Preti et al., 2024, p. 1). Another study found that inadequate computing, data storage, and obsolete Electronic Health Records (EHRs) were the initial obstacles (Preti et al., 2024, p. 1). Healthcare machine learning (ML) adoption also depends on organisational culture. New technologies are unpopular in risk-averse, hierarchical companies. For instance, 26% of healthcare institutions cite cultural resistance as a hurdle (Preti et al., 2024, p. 1). A preliminary investigation on the barriers to acceptance and potential benefits of ML applications in oncology imaging found that lesion categorization to benefit patients was highly ranked (Hesso et al., 2023, p. 20). Healthcare workers list insufficient time, technical assistance, and training as impediments to ML-based tool implementation (Hesso et al., 2023, p. 21). Matching ML applications to healthcare workflows requires feedback and iterative design to increase practicality, validity, and confidence (Hesso et al., 2023, pp. 3, 6). A recent study found that imaging, genomics, and mortality data in publicly available oncology datasets have serious completeness issues (Waqas et al., 2024, p. 19). Biased data affects machine learning (ML) systems, according to Harishbhai Tilala et al. (2024). It suggests integrating multiple populations into ML model training sets (p. 3). To achieve trust, explainability, and reproducibility, clinical, IT, data scientist, and biostatistician must collaborate on data curation and governance (Preti et al., 2024, p. 1). ML can automate data entry, billing, appointment reminders, and patient scheduling, reducing workload and optimising resources (Harishbhai Tilala et al., 2024, p. 1). Minorities are less accurate at cancer diagnosis using ML than other groups (Harishbhai Tilala et al., 2024, p. 3).

5.3 Regulatory Compliance

Regulatory frameworks for artificial intelligence (AI) and machine learning (ML) systems in oncology are essential for ensuring their lawful, ethical, and technically robust deployment. Clinical oncology necessitates that AI-assisted clinical decision-making is accurate and trusted by both clinicians and patients. According to the European Union (EU), "regulatory guidelines mandate that AI must be auditable and transparent to ensure patients' health and safety" (Singh & Keche, 2025, p. 4). Additionally, regulations stipulate that ML algorithms in oncology can only be used if they can demonstrate that they meet a safety threshold determined by regulatory authorities to protect patients from harm. One of the major features of ML system training in the field of oncology is the integration of large and heterogeneous data. These data sets should be under good stewardship to ensure their integrity as well as adherence to the privacy norms. The regulatory structures and standards are also applied at the local level, and this sometimes complicates the harmonisation at international levels. Nevertheless, it may be a problem because to achieve its potential application in healthcare, AI would be required to implement universal standards (Farasati Far, 2023, p. 2).

Moreover, as part of reacting to the FDA Total Product Lifecycle (TPLC) strategy, the ML algorithms are to be constantly supervised and revised based on the regulatory guidelines (Singh and Keche, 2025, p. 5). An example is that clinical algorithms might have to be reassessed and retrained with novel evidence in cancer biology arising. The algorithms should also be rerun as the demographics of patients change. These guidelines will help to guarantee that ML models do not worsen with time. The TPLC approach also offers a mechanism of determining the unintended changes in the system amidst constant updating of the system. As per these standards, developers also need to revise their algorithms that are used in AI since they can introduce new information to their training process. This helps in safeguarding the patients since the model predictions might be compromised and the algorithms would then have to be reevaluated to be used in a clinical misuse. Although the TPLC methodology is patient-focused and high-quality, it needs significant resources to guarantee quality. This is an issue, and many healthcare institutions find it difficult to meet the regulations without having to bear a hefty financial cost.

The transparency of the regulation of ML systems is also paramount in order to avoid the formation of the black box tool that would lower ethical standards (Farasati Far, 2023, p. 2). It is therefore controlled that the ML algorithms are sufficiently transparent and should be responsible to ensure patient welfare. Such a regulation is enforced not only to guarantee privacy but also to make sure that oncology practices continue to be unequal due to these algorithms. Patients and doctors should have the opportunity to rely on and interpret the algorithmic procedure of decision-making that can make a drastic change in the health outcomes of a patient. One of the ethical standards that are being exercised as part of the regulatory oversight is the need to have transparent documentation on how decisions are being made. In the case where a patient is not satisfied with the result arrived at using the ML algorithm, then there must be proper records showing how these decisions were made. Although all these requirements are highly helpful in enhancing ethical principles, the intricacy and obscurity of certain AI models can restrain the transparency and clarity of the model. To resolve this problem, regulatory authorities are putting forward the idea of more interpretable machine learning (ML) algorithms in the clinical setting. But in certain clinical scenarios, the trade-off may be having a lower accuracy when applying less complex interpretable algorithms. This raises the question of whether it is putting too much of an emphasis on explainability at the costs of this requirement at the cost of accuracy. To solve this, an emphasis must be put on creating intrinsically interpretable algorithms, with an accompaniment of investment in more opaque model interpretative aids.

The issues of privacy and security are more topical than ever with the growing access to ML tools dealing with personal clinical and genomic data. Hypothetically, medical and genomic data may be disclosed when data is stashed, accessed, and exchanged, without proper cybersecurity measures in place (Farasati Far, 2023, p. 2; Harishbhai Tilala et al., 2024, p. 1). The regulations state that data access should be role-based, which means that only the data required by people accessing and using the algorithms of ML should be available to them. Another regulatory standard to ensure accountability is audits of activity using a system. Medical and genomic data de-identification is a requirement that is common in most jurisdictions, and HIPAA is no exception (Harishbhai Tilala et al., 2024, p. 1). The ML technology of the organisations might lead to a massive loss of privacy in case the organisations do not meet the standards governing the personal information. It has been discovered that sensitive data can sometimes be de-anonymised with the help of publicly available information to identify patients. Although progress in encryption can mitigate the re-identification of anonymised data, their application is rarely used in practice because of the question of computational feasibility. In this regard, regulatory enforcement is justified to avoid security gaps.

The ethical considerations should also be on the forefront in the case of regulations of AI in clinical oncology. Unless patients and/or practitioners trust AI systems, they might never fulfill their potential (Farasati Far, 2023, p. 1). Regulatory bodies should deal with issues like biases which may be involved in coming up with these models and their implementation. Rules and regulations, including the Indian Council of Medical Research (ICMR) policies state that any study involving underrepresented groups is to be included during the modelling of the ML. When certain groups of people are not represented in a training dataset, then the precision of the machine learning (ML) model may decrease significantly. The problem of bias in AI is also increasing, and this is why the rules of transparency and accountability should be established (Singh and Keche, 2025, p. 6; Harishbhai Tilala et al., 2024, p. 3). This is not an exception in healthcare, since bias can arise when medical models are trained using past data about patients and results in unfair or inaccurate patient prognosis of ethnic or racially diverse people. Regulatory boards are to consider the fact that the healthcare setting will be getting more complex as machine learning (ML) technologies are further developed. Regulatory policies must be flexible, therefore, capable of adapting to increasing developments.

Currently, the application of machine learning (ML) in healthcare presents significant challenges in harmonising heterogeneous data, such as molecular and imaging datasets. An example of a rare disease database, ApreciseKUre for alkaptonuria, emphasises the need for quality controls in data sources to meet regulations regarding ethical and clinical use (Visibelli, 2022, p. 20). Regulation over data quality is vital because data must be standardised in a way that enables data interoperability, facilitating the integration of disparate datasets. Many ML algorithms utilise datasets across a combination of data formats, so the datasets must be interoperable to enable integrated analysis. Another issue is data completeness. The more complete the data is, the better results are given by an ML algorithm. Regulations addressing data quality and data completeness will significantly improve ML research. Therefore, this oversight needs to be provided by regulatory agencies. Regulatory agencies must recognise the gaps in the regulation of ML algorithms in oncology so that more standards can be established to benefit all patients. Regulation of ML technologies can only have positive benefits, ensuring that these systems operate ethically and equitably.

Artificial intelligence (AI) and machine learning (ML) in oncology should be regulated to guarantee that these systems work within the law, ethically, and technically. The use of MDSS in oncology clinical decision support entails a lot of clinical decisions that require the right usage of these algorithms by the clinicians. Therefore, the European Union regulatory framework focuses on the transparency and auditing of AI to improve patient safety and allow adherence to the ethical standards (Singh & Keche, 2025, p. 4). Moreover, one must prove that algorithms used in oncological healthcare can reach safety levels prescribed by regulatory agencies. Oncology machine learning systems require the effective integration of massive, non-homogeneous datasets to train their systems and this requires a robust data management regulatory system. International regulatory differences are common because the regulatory standards and guidelines tend to be modified in the local market. Nevertheless, the complete potential of AI to be applied to healthcare ought to be realised with universal standards (Farasati Far, 2023, p. 2).

The FDA requires the Total Product Lifecycle (TPLC) approach (Singh & Keche, 2025, p. 5) involves constant review and revision of algorithms. This will serve to modify the outputs of ML-aided approaches to emerging information in tumour biology and adapt them to changing patient demographic data. The advantages of the algorithm updates are multiplied as the performance of the ML-based oncological systems may be enhanced as well as the patient harm can be reduced. Another advantage of the TPLC approach is that unintended but significant changes in the algorithm can be identified and corrected. Despite this highly effective regulatory intervention in ML-supported decision-making in oncology, there are also disadvantages. The effort required to meet these regulatory demands is considerable and involves significant costs. Additionally, specialised personnel with expertise are needed, which can restrict the development of these applications.

The protection of sensitive patient data is another ethical aspect that requires regulatory measures. ML algorithms must therefore also be developed in compliance with data protection regulations. Ensuring data protection through technical safeguards is necessary to prevent sensitive medical and genomic information from being disclosed to unauthorised third parties (Farasati Far, 2023, p. 2; Harishbhai Tilala et al., 2024, p. 1). This protects patient privacy; however, not all data protection standards are current. Typically, the clinical and genomic data used to train machine learning (ML) algorithms are de-identified beforehand to ensure patient anonymity. Nevertheless, techniques exist that can identify patients by linking anonymised datasets with public information.

For patients and medical professionals to trust the decisions made by ML algorithms, these algorithms should be transparent (Farasati Far, 2023, p. 2). Therefore, if there is uncertainty about an ML algorithm's decision, sufficient documentation should be available showing how the algorithm arrived at that decision. Documenting the data used by the ML system to explain an individual's prognosis provides clarity for patients regarding their health status and the course of their fight against cancer. This clarity comes from understanding the reason for their prognosis, knowing which data were used, how that data was evaluated, and the impact of the results on their therapy and future life.

6. CONCLUSION

The purpose of the present paper is to discuss the use of machine learning in oncology and outline the opportunities of the implemented technology in cancer diagnostics, prognosis, and therapy. First of all, it was determined that AI can contribute greatly to the improvement of precision oncology provided that major technical, organisational, and regulatory issues are mitigated. Resting on the principles of machine learning, basic algorithms, data processing and model evaluation, it was established that the application of this high-tech in the field of oncology has many advantages. The development that has been achieved through the development of rule-based systems to deep neural networks and the present state of the art in AI models over the past years was examined to address the main question about machine learning in the oncological setting and whether it can be used to implement it in the modern context of oncological care.

The section of this paper shows the present state of the art in AI in oncology. Based on these sections, some of the critical conclusions have been drawn. Supervised and unsupervised learning methods have been useful in the advancement of diagnosis, prognostication, and prediction of effective cancer therapies in the application of machine learning techniques. Included are the complex models like the neural network architecture and the innovative feature extraction mechanisms that are all now established in cancer research. Predictive models require effective data processing and workflow, such as data cleaning, normalisation, and harmonisation, and privacy protection and reproducibility considerations, among other steps are required to achieve optimal performance of predictive models. Standard measures like accuracy, ROC-AUC and C-index are used to model performance evaluation, now standard measures of assessing model effectiveness and model validity regularly compared to conventional statistical procedures and human analysis. Machine-learning can be applied in oncology in a wide range, such as diagnostic imaging, molecular profiling, adaptive radiotherapy, and precision cancer therapy. Based on the exploration and the challenges of this technology, it could be inferred that the challenge of privacy and security, regulatory acceptance, data integration and interpretation, and clinical acceptance and system usability are all major obstacles in the translation of AI into oncological practice. It is thus important to consider such implementation challenges and to emphasize an interdisciplinary and collaborative approach among computer science, oncology, and ethics in order to get over these challenges and enable the successful adoption of this technology in oncology.

This paper has several significant contributions to the literature compared to other studies that were conducted in the past. The present results are consistent with the existing literature of the possibilities of machine learning in the oncological field to advance diagnosis, prognosis, and prediction of treatment response as compared to the existing technologies. This is relevant to the current literature as it presents a more detailed overview and discussion of the current state of machine learning within the oncology sector with recent developments, as well as key areas of algorithm development, model deployment, and ethical concerns. Additionally, the study has novel contributions over current review papers about the application of machine learning in oncology, such as the identification of issues in the implementation of the data privacy and security concerns, and the regulation requirement, and a critical analysis of the model development in oncology. The available reviews do not contain these views on the implication of regulatory frameworks and application in the clinical settings. The present results further elaborate on the existing knowledge on the impediments of implementation of machine learning in oncology by also establishing the essentiality of the interdisciplinary engagement between the technical and non-technical staff including computer scientists and oncologists to enhance the standardisation and interpretation of data. Regarding the results provided in the ethics and regulation of AI in oncology, it is possible to make a variety of extensions when compared to the current theoretical literature on ethical AI schemes. The paper introduces tangible issues in the field of healthcare, namely concerning ethics and regulations, where a variety of issues are outlined, which involve fairness and transparency, explainability, patient autonomy and consent, data privacy, regulatory approvals, and governance.

The major shortcoming of this research is that the study is based on the available scientific literature and presented original data is not an experimental study. The machine learning technologies are quite dynamic, and it is impossible to examine all the models and applications in a comprehensive way, and certain models might have changed significantly within the last few years. There also lies the problem of generalizability because the sources and the reporting styles of the various studies used in this paper are heterogeneous and diverse in terms of the type of data and measures that they report. Hence, implementation of strict and standardised data formatting, curation and metric reporting in different laboratories and published reports would be required to enable generalizability in systematic reviews. These limitations are met by rendering these findings straightforward and contextual, hence allowing informed interpretations which will more likely guarantee generalizability and accuracy, and will lead to additional research and development.

The findings that are presently available suggest that several future development directions can be taken to enhance this state-of-the-art technology in the field of oncology. The scalability of model interpretability is required as deep learning approaches are still infiltrating medical practice, which will have positive implications on future development efforts on model training and performance measurement. Data generation, training, and validation of data have to be completed on all patient groups to ensure that data is not biased by algorithmic sub-optimization to enhance equitable cancer diagnosis, prognostication, and treatment strategies. The additional progress may also be directed towards the adaptive regulatory frameworks to evaluate the iterative updates in machine learning, introduce constant monitoring of the model, and strengthen both international standardisations to optimise AI performance and adoption in different organisations. The research and development in the future should be geared towards integrating the models by coming up with clinician-friendly, user-friendly interfaces. The transparency and patient data governance should also be enhanced in the future by applying proper procedures and steps to improve the practice of patient centric data and algorithms and thus providing the patients more autonomy and control over their own personal health data. As machine learning has gained greater significance in the field of oncology, the further developmental goals should be founded on interdisciplinary and multi-stakeholder governance models enhancing the levels of transparency, standardisation, responsibility, data integrity, performance, and accountability of successful and safe integration of artificial intelligence in modern oncological healthcare.

The completion of this work has led to the further understanding that further development of the technological methods in the sphere of healthcare is important. The excitement of working with machine learning technologies dictated my desire to develop the existing technology to be applied to cancer treatment to make it more efficient and successful.

In summary, this chapter suggests that AI can find applications to most existing health problems and can offer significant improvements by enabling more sophisticated treatment.

REFERENCES

Ahuja, G., Priyal, P., Kaur, I., & Virmani, D. (2024). Prostate cancer survival prediction and treatment recommendation: A machine learning perspective. *Indian Journal of Science and Technology*, *17*(11), 1097–1106. DOI: 10.17485/IJST/v17i11.3157

Ankita, & Singh, J. (2024). A review on the integration of artificial intelligence for clinical and laboratory diagnosis. Int. J Med. Pharm. Res., 5(2), 59–64. https://ijmpr.in/article/download/pdf/548/

Archambault, Y., Boylan, C., Bullock, D., Morgas, T., Peltola, J., Ruokokoski, E., Genghi, A., Haas, B., Suhonen, P., & Thompson, S. (2020). Making Online Adaptive Radiotherapy Possible Using Artificial Intelligence and Machine Learning for Efficient Daily Re-Planning. Medical Physics International Journal, 8(2), 77–86. https://cdn0.scrvt.com/7b8dc61d55f0deedb776692474194f7c/8cb0a379b8b6f934/dec7d1475b79/Ethos-Paper-MPI.pdf

Arslan, M. (2023). Improving cancer diagnosis and treatment with deep learning and radiogenomics in precision oncology [Research proposal, Bahauddin Zakariya University Multan]. http://legiit-service.s3.amazonaws.com/f099253bd24292702dc008211e74ce27/0168f1f14104be45c1b441d3ef1cc35a.pdf

Bejarano, A. (2023). The benefits of artificial intelligence in radiology: Transforming healthcare through enhanced diagnostics and workflow efficiency. *The Review of Contemporary Scientific and Academic Studies*, *3*(8), 1–4. DOI: 10.55454/rcsas.3.08.2023.005

Biccler, J. L. (2019). Statistical and machine learning methods for the dynamic prediction of prognosis in haematological malignancies [Doctoral dissertation, Aalborg University]. Aalborg Universitetsforlag. DOI: 10.5278/vbn.phd.med.00127

Bongurala, A. R., Save, D., & Virmani, A. (2025). Progressive role of artificial intelligence in treatment decision-making in the field of medical oncology. *Frontiers in Medicine*, *12*, 1–5. DOI: 10.3389/fmed.2025.1533910 PMID: 40018354

DeFrank, J., & Luiz, A. (2022). AI-based personalised treatment recommendation for cancer patients. *Journal of Carcinogenesis*, *21*(2), 57–63. https://submissions.carcinogenesis.com/index.php/Carcinog/article/download/63/19/184

Elhaddad, M., & Hamam, S. (2024). AI-driven clinical decision support systems: An ongoing pursuit of potential. *Cureus*, *16*(4), 1–9. https://www.cureus.com/articles/244463-ai-driven-clinical-decision-support-systems-an-ongoing-pursuit-of-potential.pdf. DOI: 10.7759/cureus.57728 PMID: 38711724

Elsayid, N. N., Aydaross Adam, E. I., Yousif Mahmoud, S. M., Saadeldeen, H., Nauman, M., Ahmed, T. A. A., & Awad Taha, A. I. (2025). The role of machine learning approaches in pediatric oncology: A systematic review. *Cureus, 17*(1), e77524. DOI: 10.7759/cureus.77524 PMID: 39822251

Farasati Far, B. (2023). Artificial intelligence ethics in precision oncology: Balancing advancements in technology with patient privacy and autonomy. *Exploration of Targeted Anti-tumor Therapy, 4*, 685–689. DOI: 10.37349/etat.2023.00160 PMID: 37720345

Gaur, K., & Jagtap, M. M. (2022). Role of artificial intelligence and machine learning in prediction, diagnosis, and prognosis of cancer. *Cureus, 14*(11), e31008. DOI: 10.7759/cureus.31008 PMID: 36475188

Golden, N., Bhuvaneswari, E., & Venkatesan, R. (2025). A deep learning-driven multi-layer digital twin framework with IoT for precision oncology in cancer diagnosis. *Journal of Intelligent Systems and Internet of Things, 17*(01), 16–26. DOI: 10.54216/JISIoT.170102

Hamano, J., Takeuchi, A., Keyaki, T., Nose, H., & Hayashi, K. (2024). Optimal machine learning models for developing prognostic predictions in patients with advanced cancer. *Cureus, 16*(12), 1–8. DOI: 10.7759/cureus.76227 PMID: 39845249

Harishbhai Tilala, M., Kumar Chenchala, P., Choppadandi, A., Kaur, J., Naguri, S., Saoji, R., & Devaguptapu, B. (2024). Ethical considerations in the use of artificial intelligence and machine learning in health care: A comprehensive review. *Cureus, 16*(6), 1–8. DOI: 10.7759/cureus.62443 PMID: 39011215

Hesso, I., Kayyali, R., Charalambous, A., Lavdaniti, M., Stalika, E., Ajami, T., Nabhani-Gebara, S., Boban, J., & Zacharias, L. (2023). Artificial Intelligence (AI) and Machine learning (ML) for optimising cancer imaging: A User Experience (UX) study. *JMIR Preprints*. DOI: 10.2196/preprints.52639

Jabin, I., & Rahman, M. M. (2021). Predicting lung cancer survivability: A machine learning regression model. Network Biology, 11(2), 68-81. http://www.iaees.org/publications/journals/nb/articles/2021-11(2)/predicting-lung-cancer-survivability.pdf

Kubeyev, A., Giorni, A., Sivasubramaniam, P., Silva, L., Laurie, J., Foster, M., Griffiths, M., & Asghar, U. (2023). A prognostic machine learning model for early breast cancer which combines clinical and genetic data in patients treated with neo/adjuvant chemotherapy. Concr. https://concr.co/ASSETS/files/AACR-OS-Breast-Cancer.pdf

Kumar, D., Pawar, P. P., Gonaygunta, H., Nadella, G. S., Meduri, K., & Singh, S. (2024). Machine learning's role in personalised medicine & treatment optimisation. *World Journal of Advanced Research and Reviews*, *21*(02), 1675–1686. DOI: 10.30574/wjarr.2024.21.2.0641

Lu, S.-C., Swisher, C. L., Chung, C., Jaffray, D., & Sidey-Gibbons, C. (2023). On the importance of interpretable machine learning predictions to inform clinical decision making in oncology. *Frontiers in Oncology*, *13*, 1–11. DOI: 10.3389/fonc.2023.1129380 PMID: 36925929

Musa, I. H., Zamit, I., Okeke, M., Akintunde, T. Y., & Musa, T. H. (2021). Artificial Intelligence and Machine Learning in Oncology: Historical Overview of Documents Indexed in the Web of Science Database. EJMO, 5(3), 239–248. https://www.ejmo.org/pdf/Artificial%20Intelligence%20and%20Machine%20Learning%20in%20Oncology%20Historical%20Overview%20of%20Documents%20Indexed%20in%20the%20Web%20of%20Science%20Database-24856.pdf

Păcuraru, I.-M., Chirvase, C.-S., & Tiriteu, Ş.-I. (2025). The role of artificial intelligence in personalised medicine: Advancements, challenges, and future perspectives. *Business Excellence and Management*, *15*(1), 59–60. DOI: 10.24818/beman/2025.15.1-05

Preti, L. M., Ardito, V., Compagni, A., Petracca, F., & Cappellaro, G. (2024). Implementation of machine learning applications in health care organisations: Systematic review of empirical studies. *Journal of Medical Internet Research*, *26*, e55897. https://www.jmir.org/2024/1/e55897/PDF. DOI: 10.2196/55897 PMID: 39586084

Sharma, V. (2023). Automating complex healthcare workflows with AI and RPA: A new era of efficiency. [IJLRP]. *International Journal of Leading Research Publication*, *4*(2), 1–8. https://www.ijlrp.com/papers/2023/1/1249.pdf

Singh, M. P., & Keche, Y. N. (2025). Ethical integration of artificial intelligence in healthcare: Narrative review of global challenges and strategic solutions. *Cureus*, *17*(5), 1–16. DOI: 10.7759/cureus.84804 PMID: 40568260

Singla, N., & Singla, S. (2020). Harnessing Big Data with Machine Learning in Precision Oncology. *Kidney Cancer Journal : Official Journal of the Kidney Cancer Association*, *18*(3), 83–84. http://www.kidney-cancer-journal.com/pdf/KCJ_nirmish.pdf PMID: 33163139

Ugemuge, P. K., Khandalkar, G. G., & Ingle, R. G. (2024). Artificial intelligence could be the personalised treatment strategy for cancer. *International Journal of Pharmaceutical Quality Assurance*, *15*(2), 1017–1022. https://impactfactor.org/PDF/IJPQA/15/IJPQA,Vol15,Issue2,Article72.pdf. DOI: 10.25258/ijpqa.15.2.72

Visibelli, A. (2022). Machine learning in Bioinformatics: Novel approaches to Precision Medicine, Life Sciences and Healthcare [Doctoral dissertation, University of Siena]. https://tesidottorato.depositolegale.it/bitstream/20.500.14242/87419/1/phd_unisi_085878.pdf

Waqas, A., Tripathi, A., Ramachandran, R. P., Stewart, P., & Rasool, G. (2024). Multimodal data integration for oncology in the era of deep neural networks: A review. https://arxiv.org/pdf/2303.06471

Compilation of References

Abbaoui, W., Retal, S., El Bhiri, B., Kharmoum, N., & Ziti, S. (2024). Towards revolutionizing precision healthcare: A systematic literature review of artificial intelligence methods in precision medicine. *Informatics in Medicine Unlocked*, *46*, 101475.

Abbas, E., Fanni, S. C., Bandini, C., Francischello, R., Febi, M., Aghakhanyan, G., Ambrosini, I., Faggioni, L., Cioni, D., Lencioni, R. A., & Neri, E. (2023). Delta-radiomics in cancer immunotherapy response prediction: A systematic review. *European Journal of Radiology Open*, *11*, 100511. DOI: 10.1016/j.ejro.2023.100511 PMID: 37520768

AbdelAziz, N. M., Dawood, E. A., Hassan, M. M., & Tantawy, A. A. (2024). *Brain tumour radiogenomic classification and prediction of glioblastoma status using MRI scans with deep learning algorithms. Research Square*. DOI: 10.21203/rs.3.rs-3968021/v1

Abdel-Zaher, A. M., & Eldeib, A. M. (2016). Breast cancer classification using deep belief networks. *Expert Systems with Applications*, *46*, 139–144. DOI: 10.1016/j.eswa.2015.10.015

Abdullah, K. M., Sharma, G., Singh, A. P., & Siddiqui, J. A. (2025). Nanomedicine in Cancer Therapeutics: Current Perspectives from Bench to Bedside. *Molecular Cancer*, *24*(1), 169. Advance online publication. DOI: 10.1186/s12943-025-02368-w PMID: 40490771

Abraham, N., & Khan, N. M. (2019, April). A novel focal tversky loss function with improved attention u-net for lesion segmentation. In *2019 IEEE 16th international symposium on biomedical imaging (ISBI 2019)* (pp. 683-687). IEEE. DOI: 10.1109/ISBI.2019.8759329

Acharjee, A., Larkman, J., Xu, Y., Cardoso, V. R., & Gkoutos, G. V. (2020). A random forest-based biomarker discovery and power analysis framework for diagnostics research. *BMC Medical Genomics*, *13*(1), 1–14. DOI: 10.1186/s12920-020-00826-6 PMID: 33228632

Acs, B., Rantalainen, M., & Hartman, J. (2020). Artificial intelligence is the next step towards precision pathology. *Journal of Internal Medicine*, *288*(1), 62–81. DOI: 10.1111/joim.13030 PMID: 32128929

Adachi, T., Nagasawa, R., Nakamura, M., Kakino, R., & Mizowaki, T. (2022). Vulnerabilities of radiomic features to respiratory motion on four-dimensional computed tomography-based average intensity projection images: A phantom study. *Journal of Applied Clinical Medical Physics*, *23*(3), e13498. DOI: 10.1002/acm2.13498

Adams, R., & Bischof, L. (1994). Seeded region growing. *IEEE Transactions on Pattern Analysis and Machine Intelligence*, *16*(6), 641–647. DOI: 10.1109/34.295913

Adhikarimayum, A. D. (2023). Recent treatment advancements in radiation therapy. Jawaharlal Nehru Institute of Medical Sciences. https://iipseries.org/assets/submission/iip2023BE657E8C33F78BE.pdf

Aerts, H. J. W. L., Velazquez, E. R., Leijenaar, R. T. H., Parmar, C., Grossmann, P., Carvalho, S., Bussink, J., Monshouwer, R., Haibe-Kains, B., Rietveld, D., Hoebers, F., Rietbergen, M. M., Leemans, C. R., Dekker, A., Quackenbush, J., Gillies, R. J., & Lambin, P. (2014). Decoding tumour phenotype by noninvasive imaging using a quantitative radiomics approach. *Nature Communications*, *5*(1), 4006. DOI: 10.1038/ncomms5006 PMID: 24892406

Ahmed, H. S. (2025). Navigating ethical dimensions in algorithmic radiology: A call for action to ensure representation of low-resource contexts. *Indian Journal of Medical Ethics*, *10*(2), 138–145. DOI: 10.20529/IJME.2025.001 PMID: 40036128

Ahrari, S., Zaragori, T., Zinsz, A., Oster, J., Imbert, L., & Verger, A. (2024). Application of PET imaging delta radiomics for predicting progression-free survival in rare high-grade glioma. *Scientific Reports*, *14*(1), 3256. DOI: 10.1038/s41598-024-53693-x PMID: 38332004

Ahuja, G., Priyal, P., Kaur, I., & Virmani, D. (2024). Prostate cancer survival prediction and treatment recommendation: A machine learning perspective. *Indian Journal of Science and Technology*, *17*(11), 1097–1106. DOI: 10.17485/IJST/v17i11.3157

Al Mudawi, N., & Alazeb, A. (2022). A model for predicting cervical cancer using machine learning algorithms. *Sensors (Basel)*, *22*(11), 4132. DOI: 10.3390/s22114132 PMID: 35684753

Alawee, W. H., Al-Haddad, L. A., Basem, A., & Al-Haddad, A. A. (2024). A data augmentation approach to enhance breast cancer detection using generative adversarial and artificial neural networks. *Open Engineering*, *14*(1), 20240052.

Alharbi, F., Vakanski, A., Zhang, B., Elbashir, M. K., & Mohammed, M. (2024). Comparative Analysis of Multi-Omics Integration Using Advanced Graph Neural Networks for Cancer Classification. *arXiv preprint arXiv:2410.05325*.

Alharbi, F., Vakanski, A., Zhang, B., Elbashir, M. K., & Mohammed, M. (2025). Comparative Analysis of Multi-Omics Integration Using Graph Neural Networks for Cancer Classification. *IEEE Access : Practical Innovations, Open Solutions*, *13*, 37724–37736. DOI: 10.1109/ACCESS.2025.3540769 PMID: 40123934

Alharbi, W. S., & Rashid, M. (2022). A review of deep learning applications in human genomics using next-generation sequencing data. *Human Genomics*, *16*(1), 26. DOI: 10.1186/s40246-022-00396-x PMID: 35879805

Ali, A. M., & Mohammed, M. A. (2024). Optimized Cancer Subtype Classification and Clustering Using Cat Swarm Optimization and Support Vector Machine Approach for Multi-Omics Data. *Journal of Soft Computing and Data Mining*, *5*(2), 223–244. DOI: 10.30880/jscdm.2024.05.02.017

Ali, H. (2023). Artificial intelligence in multi-omics data integration: Advancing precision medicine, biomarker discovery and genomic-driven disease interventions. *Int J Sci Res Arch*, *8*(1), 1012–1030. DOI: 10.30574/ijsra.2023.8.1.0189

Ali, M. D., Saleem, A., Elahi, H., Khan, M. A., Khan, M. I., Yaqoob, M. M., Khattak, U. F., & Al-Rasheed, A. (2023). Breast cancer classification through meta-learning ensemble technique using convolution neural networks. *Diagnostics (Basel)*, *13*(6), 1021. DOI: 10.3390/diagnostics13132242 PMID: 37443636

Ali, M. M., Ahmed, K., Bui, F. M., Paul, B. K., Ibrahim, S. M., Quinn, J. M., & Moni, M. A. (2021). Machine learning-based statistical analysis for early-stage detection of cervical cancer. *Computers in Biology and Medicine*, *139*, 104985. DOI: 10.1016/j.compbiomed.2021.104985 PMID: 34735942

Alves, M. A., Lamichhane, S., Dickens, A., McGlinchey, A., Ribeiro, H. C., Sen, P., Wei, F., Hyötyläinen, T., & Orešič, M. (2021). Systems biology approaches to study lipidomes in health and disease. *Biochimica et Biophysica Acta (BBA)-. Biochimica et Biophysica Acta. Molecular and Cell Biology of Lipids*, *1866*(2), 158857. DOI: 10.1016/j.bbalip.2020.158857 PMID: 33278596

Alzubaidi, L., Zhang, J., Humaidi, A. J., Al-Dujaili, A., Duan, Y., Al-Shamma, O., Santamaría, J., Fadhel, M. A., Al-Amidie, M., & Farhan, L. (2021). Review of deep learning: Concepts, CNN architectures, challenges, applications, future directions. *Journal of Big Data*, *8*(1), 53. DOI: 10.1186/s40537-021-00444-8 PMID: 33816053

Ankita, & Singh, J. (2024). A review on the integration of artificial intelligence for clinical and laboratory diagnosis. Int. J Med. Pharm. Res., 5(2), 59–64. https://ijmpr.in/article/download/pdf/548/

Archambault, Y., Boylan, C., Bullock, D., Morgas, T., Peltola, J., Ruokokoski, E., Genghi, A., Haas, B., Suhonen, P., & Thompson, S. (2020). Making on-line adaptive radiotherapy possible using artificial intelligence and machine learning for efficient daily re-planning. Medical Physics International Journal, 8(2), 77–86. http://mpijournal.org/pdf/2020-02/MPI-2020-02-p077.pdf

Archambault, Y., Boylan, C., Bullock, D., Morgas, T., Peltola, J., Ruokokoski, E., Genghi, A., Haas, B., Suhonen, P., & Thompson, S. (2020). Making Online Adaptive Radiotherapy Possible Using Artificial Intelligence and Machine Learning for Efficient Daily Re-Planning. Medical Physics International Journal, 8(2), 77–86. https://cdn0.scrvt.com/7b8dc61d55f0deedb776692474194f7c/8cb0a379b8b6f934/dec7d1475b79/Ethos-Paper-MPI.pdf

Ardito, V., Golubev, G., Ciani, O., & Tarricone, R. (2023). Evaluating Barriers and Facilitators to the Uptake of mHealth Apps in Cancer Care Using the Consolidated Framework for Implementation Research: Scoping Literature Review. *JMIR Cancer*, *9*, e42092. DOI: 10.2196/42092 PMID: 36995750

Arevalo, J., González, F. A., Ramos-Pollán, R., Oliveira, J. L., & López, M. A. (2016). Representation learning for mammography mass lesion classification with convolutional neural networks. *Computer Methods and Programs in Biomedicine*, *127*, 248–257. DOI: 10.1016/j.cmpb.2015.12.014 PMID: 26826901

Armato, S. G.III, McLennan, G., Bidaut, L., McNitt-Gray, M. F., Meyer, C. R., Reeves, A. P., Zhao, B., Aberle, D. R., Henschke, C. I., Hoffman, E. A., Kazerooni, E. A., MacMahon, H., van Beek, E. J. R., Yankelevitz, D., Biancardi, A. M., Bland, P. H., Brown, M. S., Engelmann, R. M., Laderach, G. E., & Clarke, L. P. (2011). The lung image database consortium (LIDC) and image database resource initiative (IDRI): A completed reference database of lung nodules on CT scans. *Medical Physics*, *38*(2), 915–931. DOI: 10.1118/1.3528204

Aronson, J. K. (2005). Biomarkers and surrogate endpoints. *British Journal of Clinical Pharmacology*, *59*(5), 491–494. DOI: 10.1111/j.1365-2125.2005.02435.x PMID: 15842546

Arooj, S., Rahman, A.-U., Zubair, M., Khan, M. F., Alissa, K., Khan, M. A., & Mosvi, A. (2022). Breast cancer detection and classification empowered with transfer learning. *Frontiers in Public Health, 10*, 10. DOI: 10.3389/fpubh.2022.924432 PMID: 35859776

Arravalli, T., Chadaga, K., Muralikrishna, H., Sampathila, N., Cenitta, D., Chadaga, R., & Swathi, K. S. (2025). Detection of breast cancer using machine learning and explainable artificial intelligence. *Scientific Reports, 15*(1), 26931.

Arrieta, A. B., Díaz-Rodríguez, N., Del Ser, J., Bennetot, A., Tabik, S., Barbado, A., García, S., Gil-López, S., Molina, D., & Benjamins, R.. (2020). Explainable Artificial Intelligence (XAI): Concepts, taxonomies, opportunities and challenges toward responsible AI. *Information Fusion, 58*, 82–115. DOI: 10.1016/j.inffus.2019.12.012

Arslan, M. (2023). Improving cancer diagnosis and treatment with deep learning and radiogenomics in precision oncology [Research proposal, Bahauddin Zakariya University Multan]. http://legiit-service.s3.amazonaws.com/f099253bd24292702dc008211e74ce27/0168f1f14104be45c1b441d3ef1cc35a.pdf

Arthur, D., & Vassilvitskii, S. (2006). *k-means++: The advantages of careful seeding* (Technical Report). Stanford University. https://dl.acm.org/doi/10.5555/1283383.1283494

Ayad, S., Al-jamimi, H. A., & ElKheir, A. (2025). Integrating advanced techniques RFE SVM feature engineering and Nelder-Mead optimized XGBoost for accurate lung cancer prediction. *IEEE Access : Practical Innovations, Open Solutions.*

Azenkot, T., Rivera, D. R., Stewart, M. D., & Patel, S. P. (n.d.). Artificial intelligence and machine learning innovations to improve design and representativeness in oncology clinical trials. *American Society of Clinical Oncology Educational Book.*

Azuaje, F. (2019). Artificial intelligence for precision oncology: Beyond patient stratification. *NPJ Precision Oncology, 3*(1), 6. DOI: 10.1038/s41698-019-0078-1 PMID: 30820462

Azzarelli, R., Simons, B. D., & Philpott, A. (2018). The developmental origin of brain tumours: A cellular and molecular framework. *Development (Cambridge, England), 145*(10), dev162693. DOI: 10.1242/dev.162693 PMID: 29759978

Bach, P. B., Mirkin, J. N., Oliver, T. K., Azzoli, C. G., Berry, D. A., Brawley, O. W., Byers, T., Colditz, G. A., Gould, M. K., Jett, J. R., Sabichi, A. L., Smith-Bindman, R., Wood, D. E., Qaseem, A., & Detterbeck, F. C. (2012). Benefits and harms of CT screening for lung cancer: A systematic review. *Journal of the American Medical Association, 307*(22), 2418–2429. DOI: 10.1001/jama.2012.5521

Bade, B. C., & Dela Cruz, C. S. (2020). Lung cancer 2020: Epidemiology, etiology, and prevention. *Clinics in Chest Medicine*, *41*(1), 1–24. DOI: 10.1016/j.ccm.2019.10.001

Baig, M. M., Hobson, C., GholamHosseini, H., Ullah, E., & Afifi, S. (2024). Generative AI in Improving Personalized Patient Care Plans: Opportunities and Barriers Towards Its Wider Adoption. *Applied Sciences (Basel, Switzerland)*, *14*(23), 10899. DOI: 10.3390/app142310899

Bakker, M. F., de Lange, S. V., Pijnappel, R. M., Mann, R. M., Peeters, P. H., Monninkhof, E. M., Emaus, M. J., Loo, C. E., Bisschops, R. H. C., Lobbes, M. B. I., de Jong, M. D. F., Duvivier, K. M., Veltman, J., Karssemeijer, N., de Koning, H. J., van Diest, P. J., Mali, W. P. T. M., van den Bosch, M. A. A. J., Veldhuis, W. B., & van Gils, C. H. (2019). Supplemental MRI screening for women with extremely dense breast tissue. *The New England Journal of Medicine*, *381*(22), 2091–2102. DOI: 10.1056/NEJMoa1903986 PMID: 31774954

Balbi, M., Mazzaschi, G., Leo, L., Dalla Tor, L. M., Milanese, G., Marrocchio, C., Silva, M., Mura, R., Favia, P., & Bocchialini, G.. (2025). Longitudinal changes of CT-radiomic and systemic inflammatory features predict survival in advanced non–small cell lung cancer patients treated with immune checkpoint inhibitors. *Journal of Thoracic Imaging*, *40*(1), e0801. DOI: 10.1097/RTI.0000000000000801

Ballester, P. J., & Carmona, J. (2021). Artificial intelligence for the next generation of precision oncology. *NPJ Precision Oncology*, *5*(1), 79. DOI: 10.1038/s41698-021-00216-w PMID: 34408248

Baltruschat, I., Steinmeister, L., Nickisch, H., Saalbach, A., Grass, M., Adam, G., Knopp, T., & Ittrich, H. (2021). Intelligent chest X-ray worklist prioritisation using artificial intelligence: A clinical workflow simulation. *European Radiology*, *31*(6), 3837–3845. DOI: 10.1007/s00330-020-07480-7 PMID: 33219850

Barnett, G. (2016). GWAS in radiogenomics [Dissertation, Cambridge University Hospitals NHS Trust, Department of Oncology, Cambridge, United Kingdom]. Cancer Letters. https://figshare.le.ac.uk/articles/conference_contribution/The_REQUITE_project_integrating_biomarkers_and_clinical_predictors_of_radiotherapy_side_effects/10214567/1/files/18418739.pdf

Barragán-Montero, A., Javaid, U., Valdés, G., Nguyen, D., Desbordes, P., Macq, B., Willems, S., Vandewinckele, L., Holmström, M., Löfman, F., Michiels, S., Souris, K., Sterpin, E., & Lee, J. A. (2021). Artificial intelligence and machine learning for medical imaging: A technology review. *Physica Medica*, *83*, 242–256. DOI: 10.1016/j.ejmp.2021.04.016

Barua, S., Islam, M. M., Yao, X., & Murase, K. (2014). MWMOTE—Majority weighted minority oversampling technique. *IEEE Transactions on Knowledge and Data Engineering*, *26*(2), 405–425. DOI: 10.1109/TKDE.2012.232

Batool, A., & Byun, Y.-C. (2024). Toward improving breast cancer classification using an adaptive voting ensemble learning algorithm. *IEEE Access : Practical Innovations, Open Solutions*, *12*, 12869–12882. DOI: 10.1109/ACCESS.2024.3356602

Batra, U., Nathany, S., Nath, S. K., Jose, J. T., Sharma, T., Pasricha, S., & Rawal, K. (2024). AI-based pipeline for early screening of lung cancer: Integrating radiology, clinical, and genomics data. *The Lancet Regional Health. Southeast Asia*, *24*, 100352. Advance online publication. DOI: 10.1016/j.lansea.2024.100352

Bejarano, A. (2023). The benefits of artificial intelligence in radiology: Transforming healthcare through enhanced diagnostics and workflow efficiency. *The Review of Contemporary Scientific and Academic Studies*, *3*(8), 1–4. DOI: 10.55454/rcsas.3.08.2023.005

Bengtsson, I., Smolders, A., Forsgren, A., Lomax, A., Weber, D. C., Fredriksson, A., & Albertini, F. (2024). Robust optimisation for contouring uncertainties in adaptive radiation therapy. 20th International Conference on the Use of Computers in Radiation Therapy, 1–4. https://www.iccr2024.org/papers/524476.pdf

Benzo, R. M., Gogineni, A., Tetrick, M. K., Singh, R., Washington, P., Fernandez, S., Paskett, E. D., Penedo, F. J., Ghazi, S., Osei, A., Clinton, S. K., Krok-Schoen, J., Weyrauch, S., & Addison, D. (2025). mHealth technologies in research studying cardiovascular health in cancer: A systematic review. *PLOS Digital Health*, *4*(9), e0001027. DOI: 10.1371/journal.pdig.0001027 PMID: 40996972

Bera, K., Katz, I., & Madabhushi, A. (2020). Reimagining T staging through artificial intelligence and machine learning image processing approaches in digital pathology. *JCO Clinical Cancer Informatics*, *4*(4), 1039–1050. DOI: 10.1200/CCI.20.00110 PMID: 33166198

Bera, K., Schalper, K. A., Rimm, D. L., Velcheti, V., & Madabhushi, A. (2019). Artificial intelligence in digital pathology—New tools for diagnosis and precision oncology. *Nature Reviews. Clinical Oncology*, *16*(11), 703–715. DOI: 10.1038/s41571-019-0252-y PMID: 31399699

Bhange, M., & Telange, D. (2025). Convergence of nanotechnology and artificial intelligence in the fight against liver cancer: A comprehensive review. *Discover. Oncology*, *16*(1), 77. Advance online publication. DOI: 10.1007/s12672-025-01821-y PMID: 39841330

Bhinder, B., Gilvary, C., Madukar, N. S., & Element, O. (2021). Artificial intelligence in cancer research and precision medicine. *Cancer Discovery*, *11*(4), 900–915.

Biccler, J. L. (2019). Statistical and machine learning methods for the dynamic prediction of prognosis in haematological malignancies [Doctoral dissertation, Aalborg University]. Aalborg Universitetsforlag. DOI: 10.5278/vbn.phd.med.00127

Biederer, J., Mirsadraee, S., Beer, M., Molinari, F., Hintze, C., Bauman, G., Both, M., Van Beek, E. J. R., Wild, J., & Puderbach, M. (2012). MRI of the lung (3/3)—Current applications and future perspectives. *Insights Into Imaging*, *3*(4), 373–386. DOI: 10.1007/s13244-011-0142-z

Biswas, S., & Hazra, R. (2022). State-of-the-art level set models and their performances in image segmentation: A decade review. *Archives of Computational Methods in Engineering*, *29*(4), 2019–2042. DOI: 10.1007/s11831-021-09646-y

Bi, W. L., Hosny, A., Schabath, M. B., Giger, M. L., Birkbak, N. J., Mehrtash, A., Allison, T., Arnaout, O., Abbosh, C., Dunn, I. F., Mak, R. H., Tamimi, R. M., Tempany, C. M., Swanton, C., Hoffmann, U., Schwartz, L. H., Gillies, R. J., Huang, R. Y., & Aerts, H. J. (2019). Artificial intelligence in cancer imaging: Clinical challenges and applications. *CA: a Cancer Journal for Clinicians*, *69*(2), 127–157. DOI: 10.3322/caac.21552 PMID: 30720861

Bizzego, A., Bussola, N., Chierici, M., Maggio, V., Francescatto, M., Cima, L., Cristoforetti, M., Jurman, G., & Furlanello, C. (2019). Evaluating reproducibility of AI algorithms in digital pathology with DAPPER. *PLoS Computational Biology*, *15*(3), e1006269. DOI: 10.1371/journal.pcbi.1006269 PMID: 30917113

Boldrini, L., Bibault, J.-E., Masciocchi, C., Shen, Y., & Bittner, M.-I. (2019). Deep Learning: A Review for the Radiation Oncologist. *Frontiers in Oncology*, *9*, 977. DOI: 10.3389/fonc.2019.00977 PMID: 31632910

Bongurala, A. R., Save, D., & Virmani, A. (2025). Progressive role of artificial intelligence in treatment decision-making in the field of medical oncology. *Frontiers in Medicine*, *12*, 1–5. DOI: 10.3389/fmed.2025.1533910 PMID: 40018354

Bordron, A., Rio, E., Badic, B., Miranda, O., Pradier, O., Hatt, M., Visvikis, D., Lucia, F., Schick, U., & Bourbonne, V. (2022). External Validation of a Radiomics Model for the Prediction of Complete Response to Neoadjuvant Chemoradiotherapy in Rectal Cancer. *Cancers (Basel)*, *14*(4), 1079. DOI: 10.3390/cancers14041079 PMID: 35205826

Bortolotto, C., Pinto, A., Brero, F., Messana, G., Cabini, R. F., Postuma, I., Robustelli Test, A., Stella, G. M., Galli, G., Mariani, M., Figini, S., Lascialfari, A., Filippi, A. R., Bottinelli, O. M., & Preda, L. (2024). CT and MRI radiomic features of lung cancer (NSCLC): Comparison and software consistency. *European Radiology Experimental*, *8*(1), 71. DOI: 10.1186/s41747-024-00468-8

Botlagunta, M., Botlagunta, M. D., Myneni, M. B., Lakshmi, D., Nayyar, A., Gullapalli, J. S., & Shah, M. A. (2023). Classification and diagnostic prediction of breast cancer metastasis on clinical data using machine learning algorithms. *Scientific Reports*, *13*(1), 1045. DOI: 10.1038/s41598-023-27548-w PMID: 36627367

Boubnovski Martell, M., Linton-Reid, K., Chen, M., & Aboagye, E. O. (2025). Radiomics for lung cancer diagnosis, management, and future prospects. *Clinical Radiology*, *86*, 106926. DOI: 10.1016/j.crad.2025.106926 PMID: 40344812

Bra, T. S. 2025 Lighthouse Challenge. (2025). *BraTS 2025 lighthouse challenge* [Data set]. The Cancer Imaging Archive. https://www.synapse.org/brats2025- Retrieved April 20, 2025

Bradley, S. H., Abraham, S., Callister, M. E. J., Grice, A., Hamilton, W. T., Rodriguez Lopez, R., Shinkins, B., & Neal, R. D. (2019). Sensitivity of chest X-ray for detecting lung cancer in people presenting with symptoms: A systematic review. *The British Journal of General Practice*, *69*(689), e827–e835. DOI: 10.3399/bjgp19X706853

Bray, F., Ferlay, J., Soerjomataram, I., Siegel, R. L., Torre, L. A., & Jemal, A. (2018). Global cancer statistics 2018: GLOBOCAN estimates of incidence and mortality worldwide for 36 cancers in 185 countries. *CA: a Cancer Journal for Clinicians*, *68*(6), 394–424. DOI: 10.3322/caac.21492

Bray, F., Laversanne, M., Sung, H., Ferlay, J., Siegel, R. L., Soerjomataram, I., & Jemal, A. (2024). Global cancer statistics 2022: GLOBOCAN estimates of incidence and mortality worldwide for 36 cancers in 185 countries. *CA: a Cancer Journal for Clinicians*, *74*(3), 229–263. DOI: 10.3322/caac.21834

Briggs, A., Fent, I., Brown, R., Hruby, G., Kneebone, A., & Booth, J. (2021). Individual disease site white paper (2.0 (Version 02.00.10) & Ethos Treatment Planning 1.0 (Version 01.00.10)). Adaptive Intelligence™ Consortium. https://filecache.mediaroom.com/mr5mr_varianmedicalaffairs/178507/download/AICBest%20Practices_Rectum.pdf

Byeon, K., Lim, J., Lee, J., Han, C., Bay, S., Park, G., & Kwak, J. T. (2025, January). Lightweight Look-ahead Multi-context Vision Transformer. In *2025 International Conference on Electronics, Information, and Communication (ICEIC)* (pp. 1-6). IEEE.

Camps, J., Jiménez-Franco, A., García-Pablo, R., Joven, J., & Arenas, M. (2025). Artificial intelligence-driven integration of multi-omics and radiomics: A new hope for precision cancer diagnosis and prognosis. *Biochimica et Biophysica Acta (BBA) -. Biochimica et Biophysica Acta. Molecular Basis of Disease, 1871*(6), 167841. DOI: 10.1016/j.bbadis.2025.167841 PMID: 40216368

Carlomagno, N., Incollingo, P., Tammaro, V., Peluso, G., Rupealta, N., Chiacchio, G., Sandoval Sotelo, M. L., Minieri, G., Pisani, A., Riccio, E., Sabbatini, M., Bracale, U. M., Calogero, A., Dodaro, C. A., & Santangelo, M. (2017). Diagnostic, Predictive, Prognostic, and Therapeutic Molecular Biomarkers in Third Millennium: A Breakthrough in Gastric Cancer. *BioMed Research International, 2017*, 1–11. DOI: 10.1155/2017/7869802 PMID: 29094049

Carriero, A., Gronhoff, L., Volginav, E., Basile, P., & Albera, M. (2024). Deep learning in breast cancer imaging: State of the art and recent advancement in early 2024. *Diagnostics (Basel), 14*(7), 848.

Carter, S. M., Rogers, W., Win, K. T., Frazer, H., Richards, B., & Houssami, N. (2020). The ethical, legal and social implications of using artificial intelligence systems in breast cancer care. *The Breast : Official Journal of the European Society of Mastology, 49*, 25–32. DOI: 10.1016/j.breast.2019.10.001

Chang, G., Chang, T., Pan, T., Clark, J. W.Jr, & Mawlawi, O. R. (2010). Joint correction of respiratory motion artifact and partial volume effect in lung/thoracic PET/CT imaging. *Medical Physics, 37*(12), 6221–6232. DOI: 10.1118/1.3512780

Chapla, D., Chorya, H. P., Ishfaq, L., Khan, A., Subrahmanyan, V. R., & Garg, S. (2024). An artificial intelligence (AI)-integrated approach to enhance early detection and personalized treatment strategies in lung cancer among smokers: A literature review. *Cureus, 16*(8). Advance online publication. DOI: 10.7759/cureus.66688

Chau, M. (2024). Ethical, legal, and regulatory landscape of artificial intelligence in Australian healthcare and ethical integration in radiography: A narrative review. *Journal of Medical Imaging and Radiation Sciences, 55*(4), 101733. DOI: 10.1016/j.jmir.2024.101733

Chawla, N. V., Bowyer, K. W., Hall, L. O., & Kegelmeyer, W. P. (2002). SMOTE: Synthetic minority over-sampling technique. *Journal of Artificial Intelligence Research, 16*, 321–357. DOI: 10.1613/jair.953

Chehade, A. H., Abdallah, N., Marion, J.-M., Oueidat, M., & Chauvet, P. (2022). Lung and colon cancer classification using medical imaging: A feature engineering approach. *Research Square*. DOI: 10.21203/rs.3.rs-1211832/v1

Cheng, C. H., & Shi, S. (2025). Artificial intelligence in cancer: Applications, challenges, and future perspectives. *Molecular Cancer, 24*(1), 274. DOI: 10.1186/s12943-025-02450-3 PMID: 41168799

Chen, Y.-H., Kan, K.-Y., Liu, S.-H., Lin, H.-H., & Lue, K.-H. (2023). Impact of respiratory motion on 18F-FDG PET radiomics stability: Clinical evaluation with a digital PET scanner. *Journal of Applied Clinical Medical Physics, 24*(12), e14200. DOI: 10.1002/acm2.14200

Cheung, H. M. C., & Rubin, D. (2021). Challenges and opportunities for artificial intelligence in oncological imaging. *Clinical Radiology, 76*(10), 728–736. DOI: 10.1016/j.crad.2021.03.009 PMID: 33902889

Chu, J. C. H. (2021). The role of artificial intelligence in radiation oncology. *International Journal of Radiation Oncology, Biology, Physics, 110*(3), 674–686.

Chukwunweike, J. N., Praise, A., & Bashirat, B. A. (2024). Harnessing Machine Learning for Cybersecurity: How Convolutional Neural Networks are Revolutionising Threat Detection and Data Privacy. *International Journal of Research Publication and Reviews, 5*(8), 3608–3617. DOI: 10.55248/gengpi.5.0824.2402

Cilla, S., Romano, C., Macchia, G., Pezzulla, D., Lepre, E., Buwenge, M., Donati, C. M., Galietta, E., Morganti, A. G., & Deodato, F. (2025). Radiomics-based explainable artificial intelligence to predict treatment response following lung stereotactic body radiation therapy. *The British Journal of Radiology, 98*(1175), tqaf043. Advance online publication. DOI: 10.1093/bjr/tqaf043

Cireşan, D. C., Giusti, A., Gambardella, L. M., & Schmidhuber, J. (2013). Mitosis detection in breast cancer histology images with deep neural networks. In *Medical Image Computing and Computer-Assisted Intervention* (pp. 411–418). DOI: 10.1007/978-3-642-40763-5_51

Cirolla, V. A., & Lora, O. (2024). Breast cancer between radiomics and adaptive radiotherapy. *International Journal of Contemporary Research in Multidisciplinary, 3*(4), 121–128. https://multiarticlesjournal.com/counter/d/3-4-34/IJCRM-2024-3-4-34.pdf

Clunie, D. A. (2001). DICOM structured reporting: An object model as an implementation boundary. In *Medical Imaging 2001: PACS and Integrated Medical Information Systems: Design and Evaluation* (Vol. 4323, pp. 207–215). DOI: 10.1117/12.435478

Coeckelbergh, M. (2020). Artificial intelligence, responsibility attribution, and a relational justification of explainability. *Science and Engineering Ethics*, *26*(4), 2051–2068. DOI: 10.1007/s11948-019-00146-8

Coudray, N., Ocampo, P. S., Sakellaropoulos, T., Narula, N., Snuderl, M., Fenyö, D., Moreira, A. L., Razavian, N., & Tsirigos, A. (2018). Classification and mutation prediction from non–small cell lung cancer histopathology images using deep learning. *Nature Medicine*, *24*(10), 1559–1567. DOI: 10.1038/s41591-018-0177-5 PMID: 30224757

Crosby, D., Bhatia, S., Brindle, K. M., Coussens, L. M., Dive, C., Emberton, M., Esener, S., Fitzgerald, R. C., Gambhir, S. S., Kuhn, P., Rebbeck, T. R., & Balasubramanian, S. (2022). Early detection of cancer. *Science*, *375*(6586), eaay9040. DOI: 10.1126/science.aay9040 PMID: 35298272

Cui, Q., Qiang, Z., Zhao, J., Qiang, Y., & Liao, X. (2017). A 3D segmentation method for pulmonary nodule image sequences based on supervoxels and multimodal data. *International Journal of Performability Engineering*, *13*(5), 682. DOI: 10.23940/ijpe.17.05.p12.682696

Cutillo, C. M., Sharma, K. R., Foschini, L., Kundu, S., Mackintosh, M., & Mandl, K. D. (2020). Machine intelligence in healthcare: Perspectives on trustworthiness, explainability, usability, and transparency. npj. *Digital Medicine*, *3*, 47.

Daghrir, J., Tlig, L., Bouchouicha, M., & Sayadi, M. (2020, September). Melanoma skin cancer detection using deep learning and classical machine learning techniques: A hybrid approach. In *the 5th International Conference on Advanced Technologies for Signal and Image Processing (ATSIP)* (pp. 1-5). IEEE. DOI: 10.1109/ATSIP49331.2020.9231544

Dai, B., Chen, R. C., Zhu, S. Z., & Zhang, W. W. (2018, December). Using random forest algorithm for breast cancer diagnosis. In *2018 International symposium on computer, consumer and control (IS3C)* (pp. 449-452). IEEE.

Dai, S., Lu, K., Dong, J., Zhang, Y., & Chen, Y. (2015). A novel approach of lung segmentation on chest CT images using graph cuts. *Neurocomputing*, *168*, 799–807. DOI: 10.1016/j.neucom.2015.05.044

Dankwa-Mullan, I., & Weeraratne, D. (2022). Artificial intelligence and machine learning technologies in cancer care: Addressing disparities, bias, and data diversity. *Cancer Discovery*, *12*(6), 1423–1427.

De Visschere, P. J. L., Vral, A., Perletti, G., Pattyn, E., Praet, M., Magri, V., & Villeirs, G. M. (2017). Multiparametric magnetic resonance imaging characteristics of normal, benign, and malignant conditions in the prostate. *European Radiology*, *27*(5), 2095–2109. DOI: 10.1007/s00330-016-4479-z

Debbadi, R. K., & Boateng, O. (2025). Developing intelligent automation workflows in Microsoft Power Automate by embedding deep learning algorithms for real-time process adaptation. *Int J Sci Res Arch*, *14*(2), 802–820. DOI: 10.30574/ijsra.2025.14.2.0449

Debbadi, R. K., & Boateng, O. (2025). Optimising end-to-end business processes by integrating machine learning models with UiPath for predictive analytics and decision automation. *Int J Sci Res Arch*, *14*(2), 778–796. DOI: 10.30574/ijsra.2025.14.2.0448

Deepak, S., & Ameer, P. M. (2021). Automated categorization of brain tumor from mri using cnn features and svm. *Journal of Ambient Intelligence and Humanized Computing*, *12*(8), 8357–8369. DOI: 10.1007/s12652-020-02568-w

DeFrank, J., & Luiz, A. (2022). AI-based personalised treatment recommendation for cancer patients. *Journal of Carcinogenesis*, *21*(2), 57–63. https://submissions.carcinogenesis.com/index.php/Carcinog/article/download/63/19/184

Dehmeshki, J., Amin, H., Valdivieso, M., & Ye, X. (2008). Segmentation of pulmonary nodules in thoracic CT scans: A region growing approach. *IEEE Transactions on Medical Imaging*, *27*(4), 467–480. DOI: 10.1109/TMI.2007.907555

Deist, T. M. (2019). Distributed learning and prediction modelling in radiation oncology [Doctoral dissertation, Maastricht University]. Proefschrift Maken Maastricht. DOI: 10.26481/dis.20190405td

Dembrower, K., Wåhlin, E., Liu, Y., Salim, M., Smith, K., Lindholm, P., Eklund, M., & Strand, F. (2020). Effect of artificial intelligence-based triaging of breast cancer screening mammograms on cancer detection and radiologist workload: A retrospective simulation study. *The Lancet. Digital Health*, *2*(9), e468–e474. DOI: 10.1016/S2589-7500(20)30185-0 PMID: 33328114

Dercle, L., Henry, T., Carré, A., Paragios, N., Deutsch, E., & Robert, C. (2021). Reinventing radiation therapy with machine learning and imaging bio-markers (radiomics): State-of-the-art, challenges and perspectives. Methods, 188, 44-60. https://hal.science/hal-04525175/file/S1046202319303184.pdf

Derevianko, A., Pizzoli, S. F. M., Pesapane, F., Rotili, A., Monzani, D., Grasso, R., Cassano, E., & Pravettoni, G. (2023). The use of artificial intelligence (AI) in the radiology field: What is the state of doctor–patient communication in cancer diagnosis? *Cancers (Basel), 15*(2), 470. DOI: 10.3390/cancers15020470 PMID: 36672417

Dheeba, J., Selvi, S. T., & Singh, N. A. (2011). Computer-aided detection of breast cancer on mammograms. *Journal of Biomedical Informatics, 44*(4), 640–647. PMID: 24509074

Dhillon, A., Singh, A., & Bhalla, V. K. (2023). A systematic review on biomarker identification for cancer diagnosis and prognosis in multi-omics: From computational needs to machine learning and deep learning. *Archives of Computational Methods in Engineering, 30*(2), 917–949. DOI: 10.1007/s11831-022-09821-9

Dhungel, N., Carneiro, G., & Bradley, A. P. (2015). Deep structured learning for mass segmentation from mammograms. In *IEEE International Conference on Image Processing* (pp. 2950–2954). DOI: 10.1109/ICIP.2015.7351343

Díaz, O., Rodríguez-Ruíz, A., & Sechopoulos, I. (2024). Artificial Intelligence for breast cancer detection: Technology, challenges, and prospects. *European Journal of Radiology, 175*, 111457.

Dipankar, P., Salazar, D., Dennard, E., Mohiyuddin, S., & Nguyen, Q. C. (2025). Artificial intelligence based advancements in nanomedicine for brain disorder management: An updated narrative review. *Frontiers in Medicine, 12*, 1599340. Advance online publication. DOI: 10.3389/fmed.2025.1599340 PMID: 40432717

Djahnine, A., Jupin-Delevaux, E., Nempont, O., Si-Mohamed, S. A., Craighero, F., Cottin, V., Douek, P., Popoff, A., & Boussel, L. (2024). Weakly-supervised learning-based pathology detection and localization in 3D chest CT scans. *Medical Physics, 51*(11), 8272–8282. DOI: 10.1002/mp.17302

Doi, K. (2007). Computer-aided diagnosis in medical imaging: Historical review, current status and future potential. *Computerized Medical Imaging and Graphics, 31*(4-5), 198–211.

Dorfner, F. J., Patel, J. B., Kalpathy-Cramer, J., Gerstner, E. R., & Bridge, C. P. (2025). A review of deep learning for brain tumor analysis in MRI. *NPJ Precision Oncology, 9*(1), 2. DOI: 10.1038/s41698-024-00789-2 PMID: 39753730

Dosovitskiy, A., Beyer, L., Kolesnikov, A., Weissenborn, D., Zhai, X., Unterthiner, T., . . . Houlsby, N. (2020). An image is worth 16x16 words: Transformers for image recognition at scale. *arXiv preprint arXiv:2010.11929.*

Du, Q., Baine, M., Bavitz, K., McAllister, J., Liang, X., Yu, H., Ryckman, J., Yu, L., Jiang, H., Zhou, S., Zhang, C., & Zheng, D. (2019). Radiomic feature stability across 4D respiratory phases and its impact on lung tumor prognosis prediction. *PLoS One*, *14*(5), e0216480. DOI: 10.1371/journal.pone.0216480

Elhaddad, M., & Hamam, S. (2024). AI-driven clinical decision support systems: An ongoing pursuit of potential. *Cureus*, *16*(4), 1–9. https://www.cureus.com/articles/244463-ai-driven-clinical-decision-support-systems-an-ongoing-pursuit-of-potential.pdf. DOI: 10.7759/cureus.57728 PMID: 38711724

El-Jammal, M., & Chung, C. (2025). Paving a Path to Clinical Impact with Radiomics: Enabling Reproducibility and Reach. *Cancer Research*, *85*(13), 2353–2355. DOI: 10.1158/0008-5472.CAN-25-2083 PMID: 40598943

Elkahwagy, D. M. A. S., Kiriacos, C. J., & Mansour, M. (2024). Logistic regression and other statistical tools in diagnostic biomarker studies. *Clinical & Translational Oncology*, *26*(9), 2172–2180. DOI: 10.1007/s12094-024-03413-8 PMID: 38530558

Elmore, J. G., Wells, C. K., Lee, C. H., Howard, D. H., & Feinstein, A. R. (1994). Variability in radiologists' interpretations of mammograms. *The New England Journal of Medicine*, *331*(22), 1493–1499.

El-Naqa, I., Yang, Y., Galatsanos, N. P., Nishikawa, R. M., & Wernick, M. N. (2002). A similarity learning approach to content-based image retrieval. *IEEE Transactions on Medical Imaging*, *23*(10), 1233–1244. DOI: 10.1109/TMI.2004.834601 PMID: 15493691

Elsayid, N. N., Aydaross Adam, E. I., Yousif Mahmoud, S. M., Saadeldeen, H., Nauman, M., Ahmed, T. A. A., & Awad Taha, A. I. (2025). The role of machine learning approaches in pediatric oncology: A systematic review. *Cureus*, *17*(1), e77524. DOI: 10.7759/cureus.77524 PMID: 39822251

Elter, M., & Horsch, A. (2009). CADx of mammographic masses and clustered microcalcifications: A review. *Medical Physics*, *36*(6), 2052–2068. DOI: 10.1118/1.3121511 PMID: 19610294

Erdur, A. C., Rusche, D., Scholz, D., Kiechle, J., Fischer, S., Llorián-Salvador, Ó., Buchner, J. A., Nguyen, M. Q., Etzel, L., Weidner, J., Metz, M.-C., Wiestler, B., Schnabel, J., Rueckert, D., Combs, S. E., & Peeken, J. C. (2025). Deep learning for autosegmentation for radiotherapy treatment planning: State-of-the-art and novel perspectives. *Strahlentherapie und Onkologie*, *201*(3), 236–254. DOI: 10.1007/s00066-024-02262-2 PMID: 39105745

Esteva, A., Chou, K., Yeung, S., Naik, N., Madani, A., Mottaghi, A., Liu, Y., Topol, E., Dean, J., & Socher, R. (2021). Deep learning-enabled medical computer vision. *NPJ Digital Medicine*, *4*(1), 5. DOI: 10.1038/s41746-020-00376-2

Esteva, A., Kuprel, B., Novoa, R. A., Ko, J., Swetter, S. M., Blau, H. M., & Thrun, S. (2017). Dermatologist-level classification of skin cancer with deep neural networks. *Nature*, *542*(7639), 115–118. DOI: 10.1038/nature21056 PMID: 28117445

Etli, D.. (2024). Generative AI and Patient Care: A Systematic Review Examining Applications, Limitations, and Future Directions for ChatGPT in Healthcare. *J. Qual. Healthc. Eco.*, *7*(1), 000361. DOI: 10.23880/jqhe-16000361

Fahami, M. A., Roshanzamir, M., Izadi, N. H., Keyvani, V., & Alizadehsani, R. (2021). Detection of effective genes in colon cancer: A machine learning approach. *Informatics in Medicine Unlocked*, *24*, 100605. DOI: 10.1016/j.imu.2021.100605

Fan, Y., Feigenberg, S. J., & Simone, C. B.II. (2025). Current and Future Applications of PET Radiomics in Radiation Oncology. *PET Clinics*, *20*(2), 185–193. DOI: 10.1016/j.cpet.2025.01.002 PMID: 39915189

Farasati Far, B. (2023). Artificial intelligence ethics in precision oncology: Balancing advancements in technology with patient privacy and autonomy. *Exploration of Targeted Anti-tumor Therapy*, *4*, 685–689. DOI: 10.37349/etat.2023.00160 PMID: 37720345

Febrianto, D. C., Soesanti, I., & Nugroho, H. A. (2020, March). Convolutional neural network for brain tumor detection. []. IOP Publishing.]. *IOP Conference Series. Materials Science and Engineering*, *771*(1), 012031. DOI: 10.1088/1757-899X/771/1/012031

Felder, R. M. (2021). Coming to terms with the black box problem: How to justify AI systems in health care. *The Hastings Center Report*, *51*(4), 38–45. DOI: 10.1002/hast.1248

Feng, X., Yang, J., Laine, A. F., & Angelini, E. D. (2017). Discriminative localization in CNNs for weakly-supervised segmentation of pulmonary nodules. In Medical Image Computing and Computer Assisted Intervention – *MICCAI 2017: 20th International Conference,* Quebec City, QC, Canada, September 11–13, 2017, *Proceedings, Part III* (pp. 568–576). Springer. DOI: 10.1007/978-3-319-66179-7_65

Feng, Y., Hao, P., Zhang, P., Liu, X., Wu, F., & Wang, H. (2023). Supervoxel based weakly-supervised multi-level 3D CNNs for lung nodule detection and segmentation. *Journal of Ambient Intelligence and Humanized Computing*, *14*(11), 1–11. DOI: 10.1007/s12652-018-01170-5

Ferlay, J., Ervik, M., Lam, F., Laversanne, M., Colombet, M., Mery, L., Piñeros, M., Znaor, A., Soerjomataram, I., & Bray, F. (2024). *Global Cancer Observatory: Cancer Today*. International Agency for Research on Cancer. https://gco.iarc.who.int/today

Fernandes, M. G. O., Dias, M., Santos, R., Ravara, S., Fernandes, P., Firmino-Machado, J., Antunes, J. P., Fernandes, O., Madureira, A., Hespanhol, V., Rodrigues, C., Vicente, C. A., Alves, S., Mendes, G., Ilgenfritz, R., Pinto, B. S., Alves, J., Saraiva, I., Bárbara, C., & Morais, A. (2024). Recommendations for the implementation of a national lung cancer screening program in Portugal: A consensus statement. *Pulmonology, 30*(6), 625–635. Advance online publication. DOI: 10.1016/j.pulmoe.2024.04.003

Ferro, A., Bottosso, M., Dieci, M. V., Scagliori, E., Miglietta, F., Aldegheri, V., Bonanno, L., Caumo, F., Guarneri, V., Griguolo, G., & Pasello, G. (2024). Clinical applications of radiomics and deep learning in breast and lung cancer: A narrative literature review on current evidence and future perspectives. *Critical Reviews in Oncology/Hematology*, *203*, 104479. DOI: 10.1016/j.critrevonc.2024.104479 PMID: 39151838

Filatov, D., & Yar, G. N. A. H. (2022). Brain tumor diagnosis and classification via pre-trained convolutional neural networks. *arXiv preprint arXiv:2208.00768*. DOI: 10.1101/2022.07.18.22277779

Filippi, C. G., Stein, J. M., Wang, Z., Bakas, S., Liu, Y., Chang, P. D., Lui, Y., Hess, C., Barboriak, D. P., Flanders, A. E., Wintermark, M., Zaharchuk, G., & Wu, O. (2023). Ethical Considerations and Fairness in the Use of Artificial Intelligence for Neuroradiology. *AJNR. American Journal of Neuroradiology*, *44*(11), 1242–1248. DOI: 10.3174/ajnr.A7963 PMID: 37652578

Fiorentino, G., Veniero, M., & Romano, C. (2023). Al powered cancer prediction, diagnosis and treatmeNt. *CEUR Workshop Proceedings*, *3486*, 1–6. https://ceur-ws.org/Vol-3486/153.pdf

Fitzgerald, R. C., Antoniou, A. C., Fruk, L., & Rosenfeld, N. (2022). The future of early cancer detection. *Nature Medicine*, *28*(4), 666–677. DOI: 10.1038/s41591-022-01746-x PMID: 35440720

Fletcher, J. W., Djulbegovic, B., Soares, H. P., Siegel, B. A., Lowe, V. J., Lyman, G. H., Coleman, R. E., Wahl, R., Paschold, J. C., Avril, N., Einhorn, L. H., Suh, W. W., Samson, D., Delbeke, D., Gorman, M., & Shields, A. F. (2008). Recommendations on the use of ^{18}F-FDG PET in oncology. *Journal of Nuclear Medicine*, *49*(3), 480–508. DOI: 10.2967/jnumed.107.047787

Fournier, L., Costaridou, L., Bidaut, L., Michoux, N., Lecouvet, F. E., De Geus-Oei, L.-F., Boellaard, R., Oprea-Lager, D. E., Obuchowski, N. A., Caroli, A., Kunz, W. G., Oei, E. H., O'Connor, J. P. B., Mayerhoefer, M. E., Franca, M., Alberich-Bayarri, A., Deroose, C. M., Loewe, C., Manniesing, R., & deSouza, N. M.European Society of Radiology. (2021). Incorporating radiomics into clinical trials: Expert consensus endorsed by the European Society of Radiology on considerations for data-driven compared to biologically driven quantitative biomarkers. *European Radiology, 31*(8), 6001–6012. DOI: 10.1007/s00330-020-07598-8 PMID: 33492473

Gamil, S., Zeng, F., Alrifaey, M., Asim, M., & Ahmad, N. (2024). An efficient AdaBoost algorithm for enhancing skin cancer detection and classification. *Algorithms, 17*(8), 353. DOI: 10.3390/a17080353

Garau, N., Paganelli, C., Summers, P., Choi, W., Alam, S., Lu, W., Fanciullo, C., Bellomi, M., Baroni, G., & Rampinelli, C. (2020). External validation of radiomics-based predictive models in low-dose CT screening for early lung cancer diagnosis. *Medical Physics, 47*(9), 4125–4136. DOI: 10.1002/mp.14308 PMID: 32488865

Garcia-Saiso, S., Marti, M., Pesce, K., Luciani, S., Mujica, O., Hennis, A., & D'Agostino, M. (2024). Artificial Intelligence as a Potential Catalyst to a More Equitable Cancer Care. *JMIR Cancer, 10*, e57276. DOI: 10.2196/57276 PMID: 39133537

Gaur, K., & Jagtap, M. M. (2022). Role of artificial intelligence and machine learning in prediction, diagnosis, and prognosis of cancer. *Cureus, 14*(11), e31008. DOI: 10.7759/cureus.31008 PMID: 36475188

George, Y., & Sahoo, A. (2020). Hybrid CNN–SVM model for breast cancer classification using ultrasound images. *Pattern Recognition Letters, 140*, 1–7.

Ghorbian, M., Ghorbian, S., & Ghobaei-Arani, M. (2025). Advancements in Machine Learning for Brain Tumor Classification and Diagnosis: A Comprehensive Review of Challenges and Future Directions. *Archives of Computational Methods in Engineering*, •••, 1–36. DOI: 10.1007/s11831-025-10340-6

Gierada, D. S., Black, W. C., Chiles, C., Pinsky, P. F., & Yankelevitz, D. F. (2020). Low-dose CT screening for lung cancer: Evidence from 2 decades of study. *Radiology. Imaging Cancer, 2*(2), e190058. DOI: 10.1148/rycan.2020190058

Gierlinger, M., Brandner, D., & Zagar, B. G. (2020). Multi-seed region growing algorithm for medical image segmentation. In Heizmann, M., & Längle, T. (Eds.), *Proceedings* (p. 267)., DOI: 10.58895/ksp/1000124383-21

Gillies, R. J., Kinahan, P. E., & Hricak, H. (2016). Radiomics: Images Are More than Pictures, They Are Data. *Radiology, 278*(2), 563–577. DOI: 10.1148/radiol.2015151169 PMID: 26579733

Gillies, R. J., & Schabath, M. B. (2020). Radiomics Improves Cancer Screening and Early Detection. *Cancer Epidemiology, Biomarkers & Prevention, 29*(12), 2556–2567. DOI: 10.1158/1055-9965.EPI-20-0075 PMID: 32917666

Giraud, P., Gasnier, A., El Ayachy, R., Kreps, S., Foy, J.-P., Durdux, C., Huguet, F., Burgun, A., & Bibault, J.-E. (2019). Radiomics and machine learning for radiotherapy in head and neck cancers. *Frontiers in Oncology, 9*, 174. Advance online publication. DOI: 10.3389/fonc.2019.00174 PMID: 30972291

Girvin, F., & Ko, J. P. (2008). Pulmonary nodules: Detection, assessment, and CAD. *AJR. American Journal of Roentgenology, 191*(4), 1057–1069. DOI: 10.2214/AJR.07.3472

Golden, N., Bhuvaneswari, E., & Venkatesan, R. (2025). A deep learning-driven multi-layer digital twin framework with IoT for precision oncology in cancer diagnosis. *Journal of Intelligent Systems and Internet of Things, 17*(01), 16–26. DOI: 10.54216/JISIoT.170102

Goldstraw, P., Chansky, K., Crowley, J., Rami-Porta, R., Asamura, H., Eberhardt, W. E. E., Nicholson, A. G., Groome, P., Mitchell, A., Bolejack, V., Goldstraw, P., Rami-Porta, R., Asamura, H., Ball, D., Beer, D. G., Beyruti, R., Bolejack, V., Chansky, K., Crowley, J., & Yokoi, K. (2016). The IASLC lung cancer staging project: Proposals for revision of the TNM stage groupings in the forthcoming (eighth) edition of the TNM classification for lung cancer. *Journal of Thoracic Oncology, 11*(1), 39–51. DOI: 10.1016/j.jtho.2015.09.009

Gonzalez, R. C. (2009). *Digital image processing*. Pearson Education India.

Gouda, W., Sama, N. U., Al-Waakid, G., Humayun, M., & Jhanjhi, N. Z. (2022, June). Detection of skin cancer based on skin lesion images using deep learning. [). MDPI.]. *Health Care, 10*(7), 1183. PMID: 35885710

Gould, M. K., Donington, J., Lynch, W. R., Mazzone, P. J., Midthun, D. E., Naidich, D. P., & Wiener, R. S. (2013). Evaluation of individuals with pulmonary nodules: When is it lung cancer? Diagnosis and management of lung cancer: American College of Chest Physicians evidence-based clinical practice guidelines. *Chest, 143*(5), e93S–e120S. DOI: 10.1378/chest.12-2351

Grahovac, M. (2023). Performance evaluation of in vivo predictive models built on conventional and probabilistic delineation-driven radiomic approaches in tumour patients [Doctoral thesis, Medical University of Vienna]. https://repositorium.meduniwien.ac.at/obvumwhs/content/titleinfo/11491791/full.pdf

Grant, R., Dowswell, T., Tomlinson, E., Brennan, P. M., Walter, F. M., Ben-Shlomo, Y., & Lawrie, T. A. (2020). Interventions to reduce the time to diagnosis of brain tumours. *Cochrane Database of Systematic Reviews*, 9. DOI: 10.1002/14651858.CD013564 PMID: 32901926

Großerueschkamp, F., Jütte, H., Gerwert, K., & Tannapfel, A. (2021). Advances in digital pathology: From artificial intelligence to label-free imaging. *Visceral Medicine*, *37*(6), 482–490. DOI: 10.1159/000518494 PMID: 35087898

Guo, Y., Li, N., Song, C., Yang, J., Quan, Y., & Zhang, H. (2025). Artificial intelligence-based automated breast ultrasound radiomics for breast tumor diagnosis and treatment: A narrative review. *Frontiers in Oncology*, *15*, 1578991. DOI: 10.3389/fonc.2025.1578991 PMID: 40406239

Gupta, V., & Bhavsar, A. (2019). Breast cancer histopathological image classification: A hybrid CNN and random forest approach. *Biomedical Signal Processing and Control*, *52*, 271–280.

Hage Chehade, A., Abdallah, N., Marion, J. M., Oueidat, M., & Chauvet, P. (2022). Lung and colon cancer classification using medical imaging: A feature engineering approach. *Physical and Engineering Sciences in Medicine*, *45*(3), 729–746. DOI: 10.1007/s13246-022-01139-x PMID: 35670909

Hajjar, M., Albaradei, S., & Aldabagh, G. (2024). Machine learning approaches in multi-cancer early detection. *Information (Basel)*, *15*(11), 627.

Hamano, J., Takeuchi, A., Keyaki, T., Nose, H., & Hayashi, K. (2024). Optimal machine learning models for developing prognostic predictions in patients with advanced cancer. *Cureus*, *16*(12), 1–8. DOI: 10.7759/cureus.76227 PMID: 39845249

Hameed Alsaedi, N. R., & Akay, M. F. (2025). Effective Breast Cancer Classification Using Deep MLP, Feature-Fused Autoencoder and Weight-Tuned Decision Tree. *Applied Sciences (Basel, Switzerland)*, *15*(13), 7213. DOI: 10.3390/app15137213

Han, H., Wang, W.-Y., & Mao, B.-H. (2005). Borderline-SMOTE: A new oversampling method in imbalanced data sets learning. In *Advances in intelligent computing* (pp. 878–887). DOI: 10.1007/11538059_91

Han, J., Kamber, M., & Pei, J. (2012). *Data mining: Concepts and. Techniques*. Morgan Kaufmann Publishers.

Han, K., Wang, Y., Chen, H., Chen, X., Guo, J., Liu, Z., Tang, Y., Xiao, A., Xu, C., Xu, Y., Yang, Z., Zhang, Y., & Tao, D. (2022). A survey on vision transformer. *IEEE Transactions on Pattern Analysis and Machine Intelligence*, *45*(1), 87–110. DOI: 10.1109/TPAMI.2022.3152247 PMID: 35180075

Hanna, M. G., Pantanowitz, L., Jackson, B., Palmer, O., Visweswaran, S., Pantanowitz, J., Deebajah, M., & Rashidi, H. H. (2025). Ethical and Bias Considerations in Artificial Intelligence/Machine Learning. *Modern Pathology*, *38*(3), 100686. DOI: 10.1016/j.modpat.2024.100686 PMID: 39694331

Hardavella, G., Frille, A., Sreter, K. B., Atrafi, F., Yousaf-Khan, U., Beyaz, F., Kyriakou, F., Bellou, E., Mullin, M. L., & Janes, S. M. (2024). Lung cancer screening: Where do we stand? *Breathe (Sheffield, England)*, *20*(2), 230190. Advance online publication. DOI: 10.1183/20734735.0190-2023

Harishbhai Tilala, M., Kumar Chenchala, P., Choppadandi, A., Kaur, J., Naguri, S., Saoji, R., & Devaguptapu, B. (2024). Ethical considerations in the use of artificial intelligence and machine learning in health care: A comprehensive review. *Cureus*, *16*(6), 1–8. DOI: 10.7759/cureus.62443 PMID: 39011215

Hashimoto, D. A., Rosman, G., Rus, D., & Meireles, O. R. (2018). Artificial Intelligence in Surgery: Promises and Perils. *Annals of Surgery*, *268*(1), 70–76. DOI: 10.1097/SLA.0000000000002693 PMID: 29389679

Hassan, Z. (2024). Application of Deep Learning in Cancer Prognosis: Predicting Tumour Progression, Recurrence, and Patient Outcomes Using Multi-Omics Data. *Journal of Biosciences and Innovations*, *1*(01), 44–53.

Heat, M., Bowyer, K., Kopans, D., Moore, R., & Kegelmeyer, P. (2000). The digital database for screening mammography. In *Digital Mammography–Proceedings of the 5th International Workshop on Digital Mammography (IWDM2000)* (pp. 212-218). Toronto.

He, J., Liu, N., & Zhao, L. (2025). New progress in imaging diagnosis and immunotherapy of breast cancer. *Frontiers in Immunology*, *16*, 1560257.

He, K., Zhang, X., Ren, S., & Sun, J. (2016). Deep residual learning for image recognition. In *Proceedings of the IEEE conference on computer vision and pattern recognition* (pp. 770-778).

Herbst, R. S., Morgensztern, D., & Boshoff, C. (2018). The biology and management of non-small cell lung cancer. *Nature*, *553*(7689), 446–454. DOI: 10.1038/nature25183

Hernández-Vázquez, N., Santos-Arce, S. R., Salido-Ruiz, R. A., Torres-Ramos, S., & Román-Godínez, I. (2024). Automatic cluster selection in K-means lung segmentation. In Flores Cuautle, J. d. J. A. (Eds.), *XLVI Mexican Conference on Biomedical Engineering (CNIB 2023)* (IFMBE Proceedings, Vol. 96). Springer, Cham. DOI: 10.1007/978-3-031-46933-6_17

Hertel, A., Kuru, M., Tollens, F., Tharmaseelan, H., Nörenberg, D., Rathmann, N., Schoenberg, S. O., & Froelich, M. F. (2024). Comparison of diagnostic accuracy of radiomics parameter maps and standard reconstruction for the detection of liver lesions in computed tomography. *Frontiers in Oncology*, *14*, 1444115. DOI: 10.3389/fonc.2024.1444115 PMID: 39435296

Hesso, I., Kayyali, R., Charalambous, A., Lavdaniti, M., Stalika, E., Ajami, T., Nabhani-Gebara, S., Boban, J., & Zacharias, L. (2023). Artificial Intelligence (AI) and Machine learning (ML) for optimising cancer imaging: A User Experience (UX) study. *JMIR Preprints*. DOI: 10.2196/preprints.52639

Hesso, I., Kayyali, R., Dolton, D. R., Joo, K., Zacharias, L., Charalambous, A., Lavdaniti, M., Stalika, E., Ajami, T., Acampa, W., Boban, J., & Nabhani-Gebara, S. (2023). Cancer care at the time of the fourth industrial revolution: An insight into healthcare professionals' perspectives on cancer care and artificial intelligence. *Radiation Oncology (London, England)*, *18*(1), 167. DOI: 10.1186/s13014-023-02351-z

Hirsch, L., Huang, Y., Makse, H. A., Martinez, D. F., Hughes, M., Eskreis-Winkler, S., Pinker, K., Morris, E. A., Parra, L. C., & Sutton, E. J. (2025). Early detection of breast cancer in MRI using AI. *Academic Radiology*, *32*(3), 1218–1225. DOI: 10.1016/j.acra.2024.10.014 PMID: 39482209

Hofmanninger, J., Prayer, F., Pan, J., Röhrich, S., Prosch, H., & Langs, G. (2020). Automatic lung segmentation in routine imaging is primarily a data diversity problem, not a methodology problem. *European Radiology Experimental*, *4*(1), 1–13. DOI: 10.1186/s41747-020-00173-2

Holzinger, A., Langs, G., Denk, H., Zatloukal, K., & Müller, H. (2019). Causability and explainability of artificial intelligence in medicine. *Wiley Interdisciplinary Reviews. Data Mining and Knowledge Discovery*, *9*(4), e1312. DOI: 10.1002/widm.1312

Hong, S., Hong, S., Oh, E., Lee, W. J., Jeong, W. K., & Kim, K. (2024). Development of a flexible feature selection framework in radiomics-based prediction modeling: Assessment with four real-world datasets. *Scientific Reports*, *14*(1), 29297. DOI: 10.1038/s41598-024-80863-8 PMID: 39592859

Horvat, N., Papanikolaou, N., & Koh, D.-M. (2024). Radiomics Beyond the Hype: A Critical Evaluation Toward Oncologic Clinical Use. *Radiology. Artificial Intelligence, 6*(4), e230437. DOI: 10.1148/ryai.230437 PMID: 38717290

Hosny, A., Parmar, C., Quackenbush, J., Schwartz, L. H., & Aerts, H. J. W. L. (2018). Artificial intelligence in radiology. *Nature Reviews. Cancer, 18*(8), 500–510. DOI: 10.1038/s41568-018-0016-5

Hosseini, F., Asadi, F., Emami, H., & Harari, R. E. (2023). Machine learning applications for early detection of oesophageal cancer: A systematic review. *BMC Medical Informatics and Decision Making, 23*(1), 124. DOI: 10.1186/s12911-023-02235-y PMID: 37460991

Houssami, N., Kirkpatrick-Jones, G., Noguchi, N., & Lee, C. I. (2019). Artificial Intelligence (AI) for the early detection of breast cancer: A scoping review to assess AI's potential in breast screening practice. *Expert Review of Medical Devices, 16*(5), 351–362. DOI: 10.1080/17434440.2019.1610387 PMID: 30999781

Huang, B., Tian, S., Zhan, N., Ma, J., Huang, Z., Zhang, C., Zhang, H., Ming, F., Liao, F., Ji, M., Zhang, J., Liu, Y., He, P., Deng, B., Hu, J., & Dong, W. (2021). Accurate diagnosis and prognosis prediction of gastric cancer using deep learning on digital pathological images: A retrospective multicentre study. *EBioMedicine, 73*, 73. DOI: 10.1016/j.ebiom.2021.103631 PMID: 34678610

Huang, D., Li, Z., Jiang, T., Yang, C., & Li, N. (2024). Artificial intelligence in lung cancer: Current applications, future perspectives, and challenges. *Frontiers in Oncology, 14*, 1486310. DOI: 10.3389/fonc.2024.1486310

Huang, J., Xiang, Y., Gan, S., Wu, L., Yan, J., Ye, D., & Zhang, J. (2025). Application of artificial intelligence in medical imaging for tumor diagnosis and treatment: A comprehensive approach. *Discover. Oncology, 16*(1), 1–23. DOI: 10.1007/s12672-025-03307-3 PMID: 40856916

Huang, L., Wu, X., You, J., Jin, Z., He, W., Sun, J., Shen, H., Liu, X., Yue, X., Cai, W., Zhang, S., & Zhang, B. (2025). Artificial Intelligence Can Predict Personalized Immunotherapy Outcomes in Cancer. *Cancer Immunology Research, 13*(7), 964–977. DOI: 10.1158/2326-6066.CIR-24-1270 PMID: 40499001

Huang, T.-C., Chou, K.-T., Wang, Y.-C., & Zhang, G. (2014). Motion freeze for respiration motion correction in PET/CT: A preliminary investigation with lung cancer patient data. *BioMed Research International, 2014*(1), 167491. DOI: 10.1155/2014/167491

Hu, Q., Yao, Y., Han, J., Yang, X., & Parton, J. (2024). Examining the existing usage gap of electronic health records in the United States: A study of National Health Survey. *SSM - Population Health, 25*, 101577. DOI: 10.1016/j.ssmph.2023.101577 PMID: 38094223

Hussain, S., Mubeen, I., Ullah, N., Shah, S. S. U. D., Khan, B. A., Zahoor, M., Ullah, R., Khan, F. A., & Sultan, M. A. (2022). Modern diagnostic imaging technique applications and risk factors in the medical field: A review. *BioMed Research International, 2022*(1), 5164970. DOI: 10.1155/2022/5164970 PMID: 35707373

Hussain, T., Shouno, H., Hussain, A., Hussain, D., Ismail, M., Mir, T. H., & Akhy, S. A. (2025). EFFResNet-ViT: A fusion-based convolutional and vision transformer model for explainable medical image classification. *IEEE Access : Practical Innovations, Open Solutions, 13*, 54040–54068. DOI: 10.1109/ACCESS.2025.3554184

Hyman, D. M., Taylor, B. S., & Baselga, J. (2017). Implementing genome-driven oncology. *Cell, 168*(4), 584–599. DOI: 10.1016/j.cell.2016.12.015

Ibrahim, A., Primakov, S., Beuque, M., Woodruff, H. C., Halilaj, I., Wu, G., Refaee, T., Granzier, R., Widaatalla, Y., Hustinx, R., Mottaghy, F. M., & Lambin, P. (2021). Radiomics for precision medicine: Current challenges, future prospects, and the proposal of a new framework. *Methods (San Diego, Calif.), 188*, 20–29. DOI: 10.1016/j.ymeth.2020.05.022 PMID: 32504782

Ijaz, M. F., & Wozniak, M. (2024). Editorial: Recent advances in deep learning and medical imaging for cancer treatment. *Cancers (Basel), 16*(4), 700.

Ilyas, Q. M., & Ahmad, M. (2021). An Enhanced Ensemble Diagnosis of Cervical Cancer: A Pursuit of Machine Intelligence Towards Sustainable Health. *IEEE Access : Practical Innovations, Open Solutions, 9*, 12374–12388. DOI: 10.1109/ACCESS.2021.3049165

Iqbal, A., Jaffar, M. A., & Jahangir, R. (2024). Enhancing Brain Tumour Multi-Classification Using Efficient-Net B0-Based Intelligent Diagnosis for Internet of Medical Things (IoMT) Applications. *Information (Basel), 15*(8), 489. DOI: 10.3390/info15080489

Isensee, F., Jaeger, P. F., Kohl, S. A., Petersen, J., & Maier-Hein, K. H. (2021). nnU-Net: A self-configuring method for deep learning-based biomedical image segmentation. *Nature Methods, 18*(2), 203–211. DOI: 10.1038/s41592-020-01008-z PMID: 33288961

Islam, M. M., Poly, T. N., Walther, B. A., Yeh, C. Y., Seyed-Abdul, S., Li, Y. C., & Lin, M. C. (2022). Deep learning for the diagnosis of oesophageal cancer in endoscopic images: A systematic review and meta-analysis. *Cancers (Basel), 14*(23), 5996. DOI: 10.3390/cancers14235996 PMID: 36497480

Itai, Y., Kim, H., Ishikawa, S., Katsuragawa, S., Ishida, T., Nakamura, K., & Yamamoto, A. (2005). Automatic segmentation of lung areas based on SNAKES and extraction of abnormal areas. In *Proceedings of the 17th IEEE International Conference on Tools with Artificial Intelligence (ICTAI 2005)* (pp. 5–10). DOI: 10.1109/ICTAI.2005.44

Jabin, I., & Rahman, M. M. (2021). Predicting lung cancer survivability: A machine learning regression model. Network Biology, 11(2), 68-81. http://www.iaees.org/publications/journals/nb/articles/2021-11(2)/predicting-lung-cancer-survivability.pdf

Jadwaa, S. K. (2022). X-ray lung image classification using a Canny edge detector. *Journal of Electrical and Computer Engineering, 2022*(1), 3081584. Advance online publication. DOI: 10.1155/2022/3081584

Jain, S. K., & Singh, S. (2007). A fuzzy logic-based approach for breast cancer diagnosis. *International Journal of Computer Science Issues, 4*(2), 32–36.

Jamal-Hanjani, M., Wilson, G. A., McGranahan, N., Birkbak, N. J., Watkins, T. B. K., Veeriah, S., Shafi, S., Johnson, D. H., Mitter, R., Rosenthal, R., Salm, M., Horswell, S., Escudero, M., Matthews, N., Rowan, A., Chambers, T., Moore, D. A., Turajlic, S., Xu, H., & Swanton, C. (2017). Tracking the evolution of non–small-cell lung cancer. *The New England Journal of Medicine, 376*(22), 2109–2121. DOI: 10.1056/NEJMoa1616288

Jeong, J., Kim, S., Pan, L., Hwang, D., Kim, D., Choi, J., Kwon, Y., Yi, P., Jeong, J., & Yoo, S. J. (2025). Reducing the workload of medical diagnosis through artificial intelligence: A narrative review. *Medicine, 104*(6), e41470. DOI: 10.1097/MD.0000000000041470 PMID: 39928829

Jha, A. K., Mithun, S., Sherkhane, U. B., Dwivedi, P., Puts, S., Osong, B., Traverso, A., Purandare, N., Wee, L., Rangarajan, V., & Dekker, A. (2023). Emerging role of quantitative imaging (radiomics) and artificial intelligence in precision oncology. *Exploration of Targeted Anti-tumor Therapy*, •••, 569–582. DOI: 10.37349/etat.2023.00153 PMID: 37720353

Jiang, P., Sinha, S., Aldape, K., Hannenhalli, S., Sahinalp, C., & Ruppin, E. (2022). Big data in basic and translational cancer research. *Nature Reviews. Cancer, 22*(11), 625–639. DOI: 10.1038/s41568-022-00502-0

Jiang, Z., & Li, P. (2024). DeepDR: A deep learning library for drug response prediction. *Bioinformatics (Oxford, England)*, *40*(12), btae688. Advance online publication. DOI: 10.1093/bioinformatics/btae688 PMID: 39558584

Jin, D., Harrison, A. P., Zhang, L., Yan, K., Wang, Y., Cai, J., & Lu, L. (2021). Artificial intelligence in radiology. In *Artificial Intelligence in Medicine* (pp. 265–289). Academic Press. DOI: 10.1016/B978-0-12-821259-2.00014-4

Jones, M. A., Islam, W., Faiz, R., Chen, X., & Zheng, B. (2022). Applying artificial intelligence technology to assist with breast cancer diagnosis and prognosis prediction. *Frontiers in Oncology*, *12*, 980793. DOI: 10.3389/fonc.2022.980793 PMID: 36119479

Jo, T., & Japkowicz, N. (2004). Class imbalances versus small disjuncts. *SIGKDD Explorations*, *6*(1), 40–49. DOI: 10.1145/1007730.1007737

Jumper, J., Evans, R., Pritzel, A., Green, T., Figurnov, M., Ronneberger, O., Tunyasuvunakool, K., Bates, R., Žídek, A., Potapenko, A., Bridgland, A., Meyer, C., Kohl, S. A. A., Ballard, A. J., Cowie, A., Romera-Paredes, B., Nikolov, S., Jain, R., Adler, J., & Hassabis, D. (2021). Highly accurate protein structure prediction with AlphaFold. *Nature*, *596*(7873), 583–589. DOI: 10.1038/s41586-021-03819-2 PMID: 34265844

Kakeda, S., Moriya, J., Sato, H., Aoki, T., Watanabe, H., Nakata, H., Oda, N., Katsuragawa, S., Yamamoto, K., & Doi, K. (2004). Improved detection of lung nodules on chest radiographs using a commercial computer-aided diagnosis system. *AJR. American Journal of Roentgenology*, *182*(2), 505–510. DOI: 10.2214/ajr.182.2.1820505

Kann, B. H., Hosny, A., & Aerts, H. J. W. L. (2021). *Artificial intelligence for clinical oncology. Cell*. Elsevier.

Karim, M. R., Comet, L. M., Shajalal, M., Beyan, O. D., Rebholz-Schuhmann, D., & Decker, S. (2023). From large language models to knowledge graphs for biomarker discovery in cancer. *arXiv preprint arXiv:2310.08365*.

Kavitha, M. S., Shanthini, J., & Sabitha, R. (2019). ECM-CSD: An efficient classification model for cancer stage diagnosis in CT lung images using FCM and SVM techniques. *Journal of Medical Systems*, *43*(3), 73. Advance online publication. DOI: 10.1007/s10916-019-1190-z

Khalid, A., Mehmood, A., Alabrah, A., Alkhamees, B. F., Amin, F., AlSalman, H., & Choi, G. S. (2023). Breast cancer detection and prevention using machine learning. *Diagnostics (Basel)*, *13*(19), 3113.

Khalsan, M., Machado, L. R., Al-Shamery, E. S., Ajit, S., Anthony, K., Mu, M., & Agyeman, M. O. (2022). A survey of machine learning approaches applied to gene expression analysis for cancer prediction. *IEEE Access : Practical Innovations, Open Solutions*, *10*, 27522–27534. DOI: 10.1109/ACCESS.2022.3146312

Khandaker, S., & Almanuin, , M. AIslam, , M. MHossain, , KHassan Melon, , M. MJaved, , M. S. (2024). Unveiling early detection and prevention of cancer: Machine learning and deep learning approaches. *Education Administration: Theory and Practice*, *30*(5), 14814–14828.

Khandezamin, Z., Naderan, M., & Rashti, M. J. (2020). Detection and classification of breast cancer using logistic regression feature selection and GMDH classifier. *Journal of Biomedical Informatics*, *111*, 103591.

Khansari, N. (2024). AI machine learning improves personalised cancer therapies. *The Australasian Medical Journal*, *17*(2), 1166–1173. DOI: 10.21767/AMJ.2024.4019

Kido, S., Kidera, S., Hirano, Y., Mabu, S., Kamiya, T., Tanaka, N., Suzuki, Y., Yanagawa, M., & Tomiyama, N. (2022). Segmentation of lung nodules on CT images using a nested three-dimensional fully connected convolutional network. *Frontiers in Artificial Intelligence*, *5*, 782225. DOI: 10.3389/frai.2022.782225

Klein, C., Zeng, Q., Arbaretaz, F., Devêvre, E., Calderaro, J., Lomenie, N., & Maiuri, M. C. (2021). Artificial intelligence for solid tumour diagnosis in digital pathology. *British Journal of Pharmacology*, *178*(21), 4291–4315. DOI: 10.1111/bph.15633 PMID: 34302297

Kodete, C. S., Saradhi, D. V., Suri, V. K., Varma, P. B. S., Tirumanadham, N. S. K. M. K., & Shariff, V. (2024). Boosting lung cancer prediction accuracy through advanced data processing and machine learning models. In *Proceedings of the 2024 4th International Conference on Sustainable Expert Systems (ICSES)* (pp. 1107–1114). IEEE. DOI: 10.1109/ICSES63445.2024.10763338

Kourou, K., Exarchos, K. P., Papaloukas, C., Sakaloglou, P., Exarchos, T., & Fotiadis, D. I. (2021). Title. *Computational and Structural Biotechnology Journal*, *19*, 5546–5555.

Kourou, K., Exarchos, T. P., Exarchos, K. P., Karamouzis, M. V., & Fotiadis, D. I. (2015). Machine learning applications in cancer prognosis and prediction. *Computational and Structural Biotechnology Journal*, *13*, 8–17. DOI: 10.1016/j.csbj.2014.11.005 PMID: 25750696

Krishnamurthy, S., Narasimhan, G., & Rengasamy, U. (2016). A level set evolution morphology-based segmentation of lung nodules and false nodule elimination by 3D centroid shift and frequency domain DC constant analysis. *International Journal of u- and e-Service. Science and Technology*, *9*(1), 187–198. DOI: 10.14257/ijunesst.2016.9.10.18

Kristoffersen, A. E., Wider, B., Nilsen, J. V., Bjelland, M., Mora, D. C., Nordberg, J. H., Broderstad, A. R., Nakandi, K., & Stub, T. (2022). Prevalence of late and long-term effects of cancer (treatment) and use of complementary and alternative medicine in Norway. *BMC Complementary Medicine and Therapies*, *22*(1), 322. DOI: 10.1186/s12906-022-03790-z PMID: 36471296

Kubeyev, A., Giorni, A., Sivasubramaniam, P., Silva, L., Laurie, J., Foster, M., Griffiths, M., & Asghar, U. (2023). A prognostic machine learning model for early breast cancer which combines clinical and genetic data in patients treated with neo/adjuvant chemotherapy. Concr. https://concr.co/ASSETS/files/AACR-OS-Breast-Cancer.pdf

Kuhn, M., & Johnson, K. (2013). *Applied predictive modeling*. Springer.

Kumar, A. (2024). AI driven precision oncology: Predictive biomarker discovery and personalised treatment optimisation using genomic data. *International Journal of Advance Research Publication and Reviews*, *1*(3), 21–39. https://ijarpr.com/uploads/V1ISSUE3/IJARPR0104.pdf. DOI: 10.55248/gengpi.5.0224.0421

Kumar, D., Pawar, P. P., Gonaygunta, H., Nadella, G. S., Meduri, K., & Singh, S. (2024). Machine learning's role in personalised medicine & treatment optimisation. *World Journal of Advanced Research and Reviews*, *21*(02), 1675–1686. DOI: 10.30574/wjarr.2024.21.2.0641

Kumar, N., Verma, R., Sharma, S., Bhargava, S., Vahadane, A., & Sethi, A. (2017). A dataset and a technique for generalized nuclear segmentation for computational pathology. *IEEE Transactions on Medical Imaging*, *36*(7), 1550–1560. DOI: 10.1109/TMI.2017.2677499 PMID: 28287963

Kumar, V., Gu, Y., Basu, S., Berglund, A., Eschrich, S. A., Schabath, M. B., Forster, K., Aerts, H. J. W. L., Dekker, A., Fenstermacher, D., Goldgof, D. B., Hall, L. O., Lambin, P., Balagurunathan, Y., Gatenby, R. A., & Gillies, R. J. (2012). Radiomics: The process and the challenges. *Magnetic Resonance Imaging*, *30*(9), 1234–1248. DOI: 10.1016/j.mri.2012.06.010

Kurniawan, M. H., Handiyani, H., Nuraini, T., Hariyati, R. T. S., & Sutrisno, S. (2024). A systematic review of artificial intelligence-powered (AI-powered) chatbot intervention for managing chronic illness. *Annals of Medicine*, *56*(1), 2302980. DOI: 10.1080/07853890.2024.2302980 PMID: 38466897

Lagree, A., Shiner, A., Alera, M. A., Fleshner, L., Law, E., Law, B., Lu, F.-I., Dodington, D., Gandhi, S., Slodkowska, E. A., Shenfield, A., Jerzak, K. J., Sadeghi-Naini, A., & Tran, W. T. (2021). Assessment of digital pathology imaging biomarkers associated with breast cancer histologic grade. *Current Oncology (Toronto, Ont.)*, *28*(6), 4298–4316. DOI: 10.3390/curroncol28060366 PMID: 34898544

Lamare, F., Fayad, H., Fernandez, P., & Visvikis, D. (2015). Local respiratory motion correction for PET/CT imaging: Application to lung cancer. *Medical Physics*, *42*(10), 5903–5912. DOI: 10.1118/1.4930251

Lambin, P., Leijenaar, R. T. H., Deist, T. M., Peerlings, J., de Jong, E. E. C., van Timmeren, J., Sanduleanu, S., Larue, R. T. H. M., Even, A. J. G., Jochems, A., van Wijk, Y., Woodruff, H., van Soest, J., Lustberg, T., Roelofs, E., van Elmpt, W., Dekker, A., Mottaghy, F. M., Wildberger, J. E., & Walsh, S. (2017). Radiomics: The bridge between medical imaging and personalized medicine. *Nature Reviews. Clinical Oncology*, *14*(12), 749–762. DOI: 10.1038/nrclinonc.2017.141

Laury, A. R., Blom, S., Ropponen, T., Virtanen, A., & Carpén, O. M. (2021). Artificial intelligence-based image analysis can predict outcome in high-grade serous carcinoma via histology alone. *Scientific Reports*, *11*(1), 19165. DOI: 10.1038/s41598-021-98480-0 PMID: 34580357

Lavanya, M., Arivalagan, M., Princye, P. H., Sivasubramanian, S., & Madhu, S. (2020). A review on lung nodule segmentation techniques for nodule detection. In *2020 4th International Conference on Electronics, Communication and Aerospace Technology (ICECA)* (pp. 1423–1428). IEEE. DOI: 10.1109/ICECA49313.2020.9297387

Layaq, S., & Manjula, B. (2020). A recapitulation of imbalanced data. *International Journal of Innovative Technology and Exploring Engineering*, *9*(3), 452–455. DOI: 10.35940/ijitee.B8120.019320

LeCun, Y., Bengio, Y., & Hinton, G. (2015). Deep learning. *Nature*, *521*(7553), 436–444. DOI: 10.1038/nature14539

Lee, S.-H., Cho, H., Lee, H. Y., & Park, H. (2019). Clinical impact of variability on CT radiomics and suggestions for suitable feature selection: A focus on lung cancer. *Cancer Imaging; the Official Publication of the International Cancer Imaging Society*, *19*(1), 1–12. DOI: 10.1186/s40644-019-0239-z

Lei, M., Varghese, B., Hwang, D., Cen, S., Lei, X., Desai, B., Azadikhah, A., Oberai, A., & Duddalwar, V. (2021). Benchmarking various radiomic toolkit features while applying the Image Biomarker Standardization Initiative toward clinical translation of radiomic analysis. *Journal of Digital Imaging*, *34*(5), 1156–1170. DOI: 10.1007/s10278-021-00506-6

Li, B., Chen, Q., Peng, G., Guo, Y., Chen, K., Tian, L. F., Ou, S., & Wang, L. (2016). Segmentation of pulmonary nodules using adaptive local region energy with probability density function-based similarity distance and multi-features clustering. *Biomedical Engineering Online*, *15*(1), 49. DOI: 10.1186/s12938-016-0164-3

Li, N., Peng, E., & Liu, F. (2025). Prediction of lymph node metastasis in cervical cancer patients using AdaBoost machine learning model: Analysis of risk factors. *American Journal of Cancer Research*, *15*(3), 1158–1173. DOI: 10.62347/UMKG8609 PMID: 40226481

Li, S., Deng, Y.-Q., Zhu, Z.-L., Hua, H.-L., & Tao, Z.-Z. (2021). A Comprehensive Review on Radiomics and Deep Learning for Nasopharyngeal Carcinoma Imaging. *Diagnostics (Basel)*, *11*(9), 1523. DOI: 10.3390/diagnostics11091523 PMID: 34573865

Li, S., & Zhou, B. (2022). A review of radiomics and genomics applications in cancers: The way towards precision medicine. *Radiation Oncology (London, England)*, *17*(1), 217. DOI: 10.1186/s13014-022-02192-2

Li, T., Li, Y., Zhu, X., He, Y., Wu, Y., Ying, T., & Xie, Z. (2023). Artificial intelligence in cancer immunotherapy: Applications in neoantigen recognition, antibody design and immunotherapy response prediction. *Seminars in Cancer Biology*, *91*, 50–69. DOI: 10.1016/j.semcancer.2023.02.007 PMID: 36870459

Litjens, G., Kooi, T., Bejnordi, B. E., Setio, A. A. A., Ciompi, F., Ghafoorian, M., & Sánchez, C. I. (2017). A survey on deep learning in medical image analysis. *Medical Image Analysis*, *42*, 60–88.

Liu, R. (2024). Towards developing an AI-powered digital twin modeling framework for personalised radiotherapy. Midwest Radiation Oncology Symposium, University of Nebraska Medical Center. https://www.unmc.edu/cce/_archived/2024/live/radonc/attendee-info/sat13_liu.pdf

Liu, H., Geng, F., Guo, Q., Zhang, C., & Zhang, C. (2018). A fast weakly-supervised pulmonary nodule segmentation method based on modified self-adaptive FCM algorithm. *Soft Computing*, *22*(12), 3983–3995. DOI: 10.1007/s00500-017-2608-5

Liu, H., Zhang, C. M., Su, Z. Y., Wang, K., & Deng, K. (2015). Research on a pulmonary nodule segmentation method combining fast self-adaptive FCM and classification. *Computational and Mathematical Methods in Medicine*, *2015*(1), 185726. DOI: 10.1155/2015/185726

Liu, R., Rizzo, S., Wang, L., Chaudhary, N., Maund, S., Garmhausen, M. R., McGough, S., Copping, R., & Zou, J. (2024). Characterizing mutation-treatment effects using clinico-genomics data of 78,287 patients with 20 types of cancers. *Nature Communications*, *15*(1), 10884. DOI: 10.1038/s41467-024-55251-5 PMID: 39738052

Liu, S., Sun, Q., & Ren, X. (2023). Novel strategies for cancer immunotherapy: Counter-immunoediting therapy. *Journal of Hematology & Oncology*, *16*(1), 38. DOI: 10.1186/s13045-023-01430-8

Liu, X., Zhang, J., Zhou, J., He, Y., Xu, Y., Zhang, Z., Cao, G., Miao, H., Chen, Z., Zhao, Y., Jin, X., & Wang, M. (2022). Multi-modality radiomics nomogram based on DCE-MRI and ultrasound images for benign and malignant breast lesion classification. *Frontiers in Oncology*, *12*, 992509. DOI: 10.3389/fonc.2022.992509 PMID: 36531052

Liu, Y., Bai, P., Li, C., & Zhao, Y. (2018). A novel level set model originated from fuzzy connectedness guided initial contours. In *Proceedings of the 2018 IEEE 3rd International Conference on Image, Vision and Computing (ICIVC)* (pp. 288–293). IEEE. DOI: 10.1109/ICIVC.2018.8492772

Liu, Z., Peng, J., Guo, X., Chen, S., & Liu, L. (2024). Breast cancer classification method based on improved VGG16 using mammography images. *Journal of Radiation Research and Applied Sciences*, *17*(2), 100885. DOI: 10.1016/j.jrras.2024.100885

Liu, Z., Zhang, X.-Y., Shi, Y.-J., Wang, L., Zhu, H.-T., Tang, Z., Wang, S., Li, X.-T., Tian, J., & Sun, Y.-S. (2017). Radiomics analysis for evaluation of pathological complete response to neoadjuvant chemoradiotherapy in locally advanced rectal cancer. *Clinical Cancer Research*, *23*(23), 7253–7262. DOI: 10.1158/1078-0432.CCR-17-1038

Li, X., Li, B., Liu, F., Yin, H., & Zhou, F. (2020). Segmentation of pulmonary nodules using a GMM fuzzy C-means algorithm. *IEEE Access : Practical Innovations, Open Solutions*, *8*, 37541–37556. DOI: 10.1109/ACCESS.2020.2968936

Li, Y., Sadée, C. Y., Carrillo-Perez, F., Selby, H. M., Thieme, A. H., & Gevaert, O. (2024). A 3D lung lesion variational autoencoder. *Cell Reports Methods*, *4*(2), 100695. DOI: 10.1016/j.crmeth.2024.100695

Lopez-Beltran, A., Henriques, V., Cimadamore, A., Santoni, M., Cheng, L., Gevaert, T., Blanca, A., Massari, F., Scarpelli, M., & Montironi, R. (2018). The Identification of Immunological Biomarkers in Kidney Cancers. *Frontiers in Oncology*, *8*, 456. Advance online publication. DOI: 10.3389/fonc.2018.00456 PMID: 30450335

Lu, L., Tan, Y., Schwartz, L. H., & Zhao, B. (2015). Hybrid detection of lung nodules on CT scan images. *Medical Physics*, *42*(9), 5042–5505. DOI: 10.1118/1.4927573

Luo, Y., Chen, S., & Valdes, G. (2020). Machine learning for radiation outcome modeling and prediction. *Medical Physics*, *47*(5), e178–e184. DOI: 10.1002/mp.13570 PMID: 32418338

Lu, S.-C., Swisher, C. L., Chung, C., Jaffray, D., & Sidey-Gibbons, C. (2023). On the importance of interpretable machine learning predictions to inform clinical decision making in oncology. *Frontiers in Oncology*, *13*, 1129380. DOI: 10.3389/fonc.2023.1129380 PMID: 36925929

Lu, T., Fang, Y., Liu, H., Chen, C., Li, T., Lu, M., & Song, D. (2024). Comparison of machine learning and logic regression algorithms for predicting lymph node metastasis in patients with Gastric Cancer: A two-Center Study. *Technology in Cancer Research & Treatment*, *23*. DOI: 10.1177/15330338231222331 PMID: 38190617

Lu, Y., Shi, X. Q., Zhao, X., Song, D., & Li, J. (2019). Value of computer software for assisting sonographers in the diagnosis of Thyroid Imaging Reporting and Data System grade 3 and 4 thyroid space-occupying lesions. *Journal of Ultrasound in Medicine*, *38*(12), 3291–3300. DOI: 10.1002/jum.15065 PMID: 31237716

Machine Learning Repository, U. C. I. (n.d.). *Breast cancer Wisconsin (diagnostic) dataset*. https://archive.ics.uci.edu/dataset/17/breast+cancer+wisconsin+diagnostic

Mackin, D., Fave, X., Zhang, L., Yang, J., Jones, A. K., Ng, C. S., & Court, L. (2018). Correction: Harmonizing the pixel size in retrospective computed tomography radiomics studies. *PLoS One*, *13*(1), e0191597. DOI: 10.1371/journal.pone.0191597

MacMahon, H., Naidich, D. P., Goo, J. M., Lee, K. S., Leung, A. N. C., Mayo, J. R., Mehta, A. C., Ohno, Y., Powell, C. A., Prokop, M., Rubin, G. D., Schaefer-Prokop, C. M., Travis, W. D., Van Schil, P. E., & Bankier, A. A. (2017). Guidelines for management of incidental pulmonary nodules detected on CT images: From the Fleischner Society 2017. *Radiology*, *284*(1), 228–243. DOI: 10.1148/radiol.2017161659

Magnin, C. Y., Lauer, D., Ammeter, M., & Gote-Schniering, J. (2025). From images to clinical insights: An educational review on radiomics in lung diseases. *Breathe (Sheffield, England)*, *21*(1), 230225. DOI: 10.1183/20734735.0225-2023 PMID: 40104259

Majumder, S., Katz, S., Kontos, D., & Roshkovan, L. (2023). State of the art: Radiomics and radiomics-related artificial intelligence on the road to clinical translation. *BJR|Open, 6*(1), tzad004. DOI: 10.1093/bjro/tzad004

Maniaci, A., Lavalle, S., Gagliano, C., Lentini, M., Masiello, E., Parisi, F., Iannella, G., Cilia, N. D., Salerno, V., Cusumano, G., & La Via, L. (2024). The Integration of Radiomics and Artificial Intelligence in Modern Medicine. *Life (Chicago, Ill.), 14*(10), 1248. DOI: 10.3390/life14101248 PMID: 39459547

Manikandan, T., & Bharathi, N. (2011). Lung cancer diagnosis from CT images using fuzzy inference system. In V. V. Das & N. Thankachan (Eds.), *Computational Intelligence and Information Technology* (CCIS, Vol. 250). Springer, Berlin, Heidelberg. DOI: 10.1007/978-3-642-25734-6_110

Manjula, B., & Layaq, S. (2022). An integrated approach to reduce class imbalance. In *Intelligent systems* (Lecture Notes in Networks and Systems, Vol. 431, pp. 381–392). Springer. DOI: 10.1007/978-981-19-0901-6_35

Manjula, B., & Layaq, S. (2022). An innovative oversampling method for imbalanced data reduction. *Advanced Engineering Science, 54*(1), 891–899.

Manjula, B., & Layaq, S. (2023). A new method for imbalanced data reduction using data-based under sampling. In *Proceedings of the 5th International Conference on Soft Computing & Signal Processing* (pp. 243–250). DOI: 10.1007/978-981-19-8669-7_22

Mantrala, S., Ginter, P. S., Mitkari, A., Joshi, S., Prabhala, H., Ramachandra, V., Kini, L., Idress, R., D'Alfonso, T. M., Fineberg, S., Jaffer, S., Sattar, A. K., Chagpar, A. B., Wilson, P., Singh, K., Harigopal, M., & Koka, D. (2022). Concordance in breast cancer grading by artificial intelligence on whole slide images compares with a multi-institutional cohort of breast pathologists. *Archives of Pathology & Laboratory Medicine, 146*(11), 1369–1377. DOI: 10.5858/arpa.2021-0299-OA PMID: 35271701

Manzari, O. N., Ahmadabadi, H., Kashiani, H., Shokouhi, S. B., & Ayatollahi, A. (2023). MedViT: A robust vision transformer for generalized medical image classification. *Computers in Biology and Medicine, 157*, 106791. DOI: 10.1016/j.compbiomed.2023.106791 PMID: 36958234

Mao, Y. J., Lim, H. J., Ni, M., Yan, W. H., Wong, D. W. C., & Cheung, J. C. W. (2022). Breast tumour classification using ultrasound elastography with machine learning: A systematic scoping review. *Cancers (Basel), 14*(2), 367. DOI: 10.3390/cancers14020367 PMID: 35053531

Maqsood, S., Damaševičius, R., & Maskeliūnas, R. (2022). Multimodal brain tumour detection using deep neural networks and multiclass SVM. *Medicina, 58*(8), 1090. DOI: 10.3390/medicina58081090 PMID: 36013557

Maroni, R., Massat, N. J., Parmar, D., Dibden, A., Cuzick, J., Sasieni, P. D., & Duffy, S. W. (2021). A case-control study to evaluate the impact of the breast screening programme on mortality in England. *British Journal of Cancer, 124*(4), 736–743. DOI: 10.1038/s41416-020-01163-2 PMID: 33223536

Martin, P., Holloway, L., Metcalfe, P., Koh, E.-S., & Brighi, C. (2022). Challenges in Glioblastoma Radiomics and the Path to Clinical Implementation. *Cancers (Basel), 14*(16), 3897. DOI: 10.3390/cancers14163897 PMID: 36010891

Martucci, M., Russo, R., Schimperna, F., D'Apolito, G., Panfili, M., Grimaldi, A., Perna, A., Ferranti, A. M., Varcasia, G., Giordano, C., & Gaudino, S. (2023). Magnetic resonance imaging of primary adult brain tumors: State of the art and future perspectives. *Biomedicines, 11*(2), 364. DOI: 10.3390/biomedicines11020364 PMID: 36830900

Maurya, S., Tiwari, S., Mothukuri, M. C., Tangeda, C. M., Nandigam, R. N. S., & Addagiri, D. C. (2023). A review on recent developments in cancer detection using machine learning and deep learning models. *Biomedical Signal Processing and Control, 80*, 104398. DOI: 10.1016/j.bspc.2022.104398

Maurya, S., Tiwari, S., Mothukuri, M. C., Tangeda, C. M., Nandigam, R. N. S., & Addagiri, D. C. (2023). Title. *Biomedical Signal Processing and Control, 80*, 104398.

Mayerhoefer, M. E., Materka, A., Langs, G., Häggström, I., Szczypiński, P., Gibbs, P., & Cook, G. (2020). Introduction to Radiomics. *Journal of Nuclear Medicine, 61*(4), 488–495. DOI: 10.2967/jnumed.118.222893 PMID: 32060219

Mayuri, A. V. R., Rashmi, V., Das, B., Mandal, A., & Neelakandan, S. (2023). Artificial neural network (ANN) with Chan–Vese (CV) algorithm-based plant disease detection and classification. In *Proceedings of the 2023 International Conference on Applied Intelligence and Sustainable Computing (ICAISC)* (pp. 1–6). IEEE. DOI: 10.1109/ICAISC58445.2023.10199472

McIlhagga, W. (2011). The Canny edge detector revisited. *International Journal of Computer Vision, 91*(3), 251–261. DOI: 10.1007/s11263-010-0392-0

Meenalochini, G., & Ramkumar, S. (2024). A deep learning-based breast cancer classification system using mammograms. *Journal of Electrical Engineering & Technology, 19*(4), 2637–2650. DOI: 10.1007/s42835-023-01747-x

Mehmood, A., Gulzar, Y., Ilyas, Q. M., Jabbari, A., Ahmad, M., & Iqbal, S. (2023). SBXception: A Shallower and Broader Xception Architecture for Efficient Classification of Skin Lesions. *Cancers (Basel), 15*(14), 3604. DOI: 10.3390/cancers15143604 PMID: 37509267

Meier-Schroers, M., Homsi, R., Skowasch, D., Buermann, J., Zipfel, M., Schild, H. H., & Thomas, D. (2018). Lung cancer screening with MRI: Results of the first screening round. *Journal of Cancer Research and Clinical Oncology*, *144*(1), 117–125. DOI: 10.1007/s00432-017-2521-4

Miles, K. (2020). Radiomics for personalised medicine: The long road ahead. *British Journal of Cancer*, *122*(7), 929–930. DOI: 10.1038/s41416-019-0699-8 PMID: 31937924

Miteva, M. D. (2025). Artificial intelligence in radiogenomics: Innovations for supporting diagnosis, treatment decisions, and prognostication in oncology [Doctoral dissertation, Sofia University St. Kliment Ohridski]. https://www.uni-sofia.bg/index.php/eng/layout/set/print/content/download/333402/2148902/version/2/file/Abstract_Mariya_Miteva_EN.pdf

Mohammed, M. A., Lakhan, A., Abdulkareem, K. H., & Garcia-Zapirain, B. (2023). A hybrid cancer prediction based on multi-omics data and reinforcement learning, state action reward state action (SARSA). *Computers in Biology and Medicine*, *154*, 106617. DOI: 10.1016/j.compbiomed.2023.106617 PMID: 36753981

Mohammed, S., & Malhotra, N. (2025). Ethical and regulatory challenges in machine learning-based healthcare systems: A review of implementation barriers and future directions. BenchCouncil Transactions on Benchmarks. *Standards and Evaluations*, *5*(1), 100215. DOI: 10.1016/j.tbench.2025.100215

Molina-Aguilar, C., & Robles-Espinoza, C. D. (2023). Tackling the lack of diversity in cancer research. *Disease Models & Mechanisms*, *16*(9), dmm050275. Advance online publication. DOI: 10.1242/dmm.050275 PMID: 37681401

Morgado, R. L. M. (2024). Robust automatic planning for stereotactic body radiation therapy [Doctoral dissertation, Faculty of Sciences and Technology of the University of Coimbra]. https://estudogeral.uc.pt/retrieve/275228/Dissertacao_MIEF_RitaMorgado_vPosDefesa_30_07_2024.pdf

Moy, S., Irannejad, M., Manning, S. J., Farahani, M., Ahmed, Y., Gao, E., Prabhune, R., Lorenz, S., Mirza, R., & Klinger, C. (2024). Patient Perspectives on the Use of Artificial Intelligence in Health Care: A Scoping Review. *Journal of Patient-Centered Research and Reviews*, *11*(1), 51–62. DOI: 10.17294/2330-0698.2029 PMID: 38596349

Musa, I. H., Zamit, I., Okeke, M., Akintunde, T. Y., & Musa, T. H. (2021). Artificial Intelligence and Machine Learning in Oncology: Historical Overview of Documents Indexed in the Web of Science Database. EJMO, 5(3), 239–248. https://www.ejmo.org/pdf/Artificial%20Intelligence%20and%20Machine%20Learning%20in%20Oncology%20Historical%20Overview%20of%20Documents%20Indexed%20in%20the%20Web%20of%20Science%20Database-24856.pdf

Musulin, J., Štifanić, D., Zulijani, A., Ćabov, T., Dekanić, A., & Car, Z. (2021). An enhanced histopathology analysis: An AI-based system for multiclass grading of oral squamous cell carcinoma and segmenting of epithelial and stromal tissue. *Cancers (Basel), 13*(8), 1784. DOI: 10.3390/cancers13081784 PMID: 33917952

Najar Najafi, N., Hajihassani, H., & Azimzadeh Irani, M. (2025). The Impact of Artificial Intelligence on Cancer Diagnosis and Treatment: A Review. *Cancer Informatics, 24,* 11769351251371273. DOI: 10.1177/11769351251371273 PMID: 40979169

Nanni, L., Brahnam, S., & Lumini, A. (2012). A very high performing system to discriminate tissues in histopathology images. *Expert Systems with Applications, 39*(12), 10465–10470.

Nardone, V., Reginelli, A., Rubini, D., Gagliardi, F., Del Tufo, S., Belfiore, M. P., Boldrini, L., Desideri, I., & Cappabianca, S. (2024). Delta radiomics: An updated systematic review. *La Radiologia Medica, 129*(8), 1197–1214. DOI: 10.1007/s11547-024-01853-4 PMID: 39017760

National Brain Tumor Society. (2023). *Brain tumor facts.* National Brain Tumor Society. https://braintumor.org/brain-tumors/about-brain-tumors/brain-tumor-facts/

National Comprehensive Cancer Network. (2024). *NCCN Clinical Practice Guidelines in Oncology (NCCN Guidelines): Lung cancer screening* (Version 1.2024) https://www.nccn.org/professionals/physician_gls/pdf/lung_screening.pdf *(Accessed July 10, 2025)*

National Lung Screening Trial Research Team. (2011). Reduced lung-cancer mortality with low-dose computed tomographic screening. *The New England Journal of Medicine, 365*(5), 395–409. DOI: 10.1056/NEJMoa1102873

National Lung Screening Trial Research Team. (2011). The National Lung Screening Trial: Overview and study design. *Radiology, 258*(1), 243–253. DOI: 10.1148/radiol.10091808

Ng, W. W., Hu, J., Yeung, D. S., Yin, S., & Roli, F. (2015). Diversified sensitivity-based undersampling for imbalance classification problems. *IEEE Transactions on Cybernetics, 45*(11), 2402–2412. DOI: 10.1109/TCYB.2014.2372060 PMID: 25474818

Nickparvar, M. (2020). *Brain tumor MRI dataset [Data set].* Kaggle. https://www.kaggle.com/datasets/masoudnickparvar/brain-tumor-mri-dataset- Retrieved May 15, 2025.

Nishikawa, R. M. (2007). Computer-aided detection and diagnosis in breast imaging. *Breast Imaging, 30*(1), 1–10.

Nishikawa, R. M. (2007). Computer-aided detection and diagnosis in breast imaging: A review. *Breast Imaging, 30*(1), 1–10.

Niu, C., Lyu, Q., Carothers, C. D., Kaviani, P., Tan, J., Yan, P., Kalra, M. K., Whitlow, C. T., & Wang, G. (2025). Medical multimodal multitask foundation model for lung cancer screening. *Nature Communications, 16*(1), 1523. DOI: 10.1038/s41467-025-56822-w

Noury, H., Rahdar, A., Romanholo Ferreira, L. F., & Jamalpoor, Z. (2025). AI-driven innovations in smart multifunctional nanocarriers for drug and gene delivery: A mini-review. *Critical Reviews in Oncology/Hematology, 210*, 104701. DOI: 10.1016/j.critrevonc.2025.104701 PMID: 40086770

O'Connor, S. D., & Bhalla, M. (2021). Should artificial intelligence tell radiologists which study to read next? *Radiology. Artificial Intelligence, 3*(2), e210009. DOI: 10.1148/ryai.2021210009 PMID: 33939773

O'Shea, R., Manickavasagar, T., Horst, C., Hughes, D., Cusack, J., Tsoka, S., Cook, G., & Goh, V. (2023). Weakly supervised segmentation models as explainable radiological classifiers for lung tumour detection on CT images. *Insights Into Imaging, 14*(195), 195. Advance online publication. DOI: 10.1186/s13244-023-01542-2

Observer Research Foundation. (n.d.). *Rising breast cancer in India: Challenges and opportunities.* https://www.orfonline.org/expert-speak/rising-breast-cancer-in-india-challenges-and-opportunities

Ofek, N., Rokach, L., Stern, R., & Shabtai, A. (2017). Fast-CBUS: A fast clustering-based undersampling method. *Neurocomputing, 243*, 88–102. DOI: 10.1016/j.neucom.2017.03.011

Ogundokun, R. O., Owolawi, P. A., Tu, C., & van Wyk, E. (2025). Autoencoder-Assisted Stacked Ensemble Learning for Lymphoma Subtype Classification: A Hybrid Deep Learning and Machine Learning Approach. *Tomography : a Journal for Imaging Research, 11*(8), 91. DOI: 10.3390/tomography11080091 PMID: 40863882

Olawade, D. B., Clement David-Olawade, A., Adereni, T., Egbon, E., Teke, J., & Boussios, S. (2025). Integrating AI into cancer immunotherapy—A narrative review of current applications and future directions. *Diseases (Basel, Switzerland), 13*(1), 24. DOI: 10.3390/diseases13010024 PMID: 39851488

Oneda, E., Abu Hilal, M., & Zaniboni, A. (2020). Biliary tract cancer: Current medical treatment strategies. *Cancers (Basel), 12*(5), 1237. DOI: 10.3390/cancers12051237

Orrantia-Borunda, E., Anchondo-Nuñez, P., Acuña-Aguilar, L. E., Gómez-Valles, F. O., & Ramírez-Valdespino, C. A. (2022). Subtypes of breast cancer. *Breast Cancer (Tokyo, Japan)*. PMID: 36122153

Osareh, A., & Shadgar, B. (2010). A computer-aided diagnosis system for breast cancer using SVM-based feature selection. *International Journal of Computer Theory and Engineering, 2*(6), 883–887.

Osei-Afriyie, S., Addae, A. K., Oppong, S., Amu, H., Ampofo, E., & Osei, E. (2021). Breast cancer awareness, risk factors and screening practices among future health professionals in Ghana: A cross-sectional study. *PLoS One, 16*(6), e0253373. DOI: 10.1371/journal.pone.0253373 PMID: 34166407

Oudkerk, M., Devaraj, A., Vliegenthart, R., Henzler, T., Prosch, H., Heussel, C. P., Bastarrika, G., Sverzellati, N., Mascalchi, M., Delorme, S., Baldwin, D. R., Callister, M. E., Becker, N., Heuvelmans, M. A., Rzyman, W., Infante, M. V., Pastorino, U., Pedersen, J. H., Paci, E., & Field, J. K. (2017). European position statement on lung cancer screening. *The Lancet. Oncology, 18*(12), e754–e766. DOI: 10.1016/S1470-2045(17)30861-6

Păcuraru, I.-M., Chirvase, C.-S., & Tiriteu, Ş.-I. (2025). The role of artificial intelligence in personalised medicine: Advancements, challenges, and future perspectives. *Business Excellence and Management, 15*(1), 59–60. DOI: 10.24818/beman/2025.15.1-05

Painuli, D., Bhardwaj, S., & köse, U. (2022). Recent advancement in cancer diagnosis using machine learning and deep learning techniques: A comprehensive review. *Computers in Biology and Medicine, 146*, 105580. DOI: 10.1016/j.compbiomed.2022.105580 PMID: 35551012

Pantelaios, D., Theofilou, P. A., Tzouveli, P., & Kollias, S. (2024, May). Hybrid CNN-ViT models for medical image classification. In *2024 IEEE international symposium on biomedical imaging (ISBI)* (pp. 1-4). IEEE. DOI: 10.1109/ISBI56570.2024.10635205

Park, S., & Kim, J. (2024). Explainability of deep neural networks for brain tumor detection. *arXiv preprint arXiv:2410.07613.*

Parmar, C., Grossmann, P., Bussink, J., Lambin, P., & Aerts, H. J. W. L. (2015). Machine learning methods for quantitative radiomic biomarkers. *Scientific Reports*, *5*(1), 13087. DOI: 10.1038/srep13087

Parmar, C., Grossmann, P., Rietveld, D., Rietbergen, M. M., Lambin, P., & Aerts, H. J. W. L. (2015). Radiomic Machine-Learning Classifiers for Prognostic Biomarkers of Head and Neck Cancer. *Frontiers in Oncology*, *5*. Advance online publication. DOI: 10.3389/fonc.2015.00272 PMID: 26697407

Parmar, C., Leijenaar, R. T. H., Grossmann, P., Rios Velazquez, E., Bussink, J., Rietveld, D., Rietbergen, M. M., Haibe-Kains, B., Lambin, P., & Aerts, H. J. W. L. (2015). Radiomic feature clusters and prognostic signatures specific for lung and head & neck cancer. *Scientific Reports*, *5*(1), 11044. DOI: 10.1038/srep11044

Partin, A., Brettin, T. S., Zhu, Y., Narykov, O., Clyde, A., Overbeek, J., & Stevens, R. L. (2023). Deep learning methods for drug response prediction in cancer: Predominant and emerging trends. *Frontiers in Medicine*, *10*, 1086097. Advance online publication. DOI: 10.3389/fmed.2023.1086097 PMID: 36873878

Pauly, R., & Schwartz, C. E. (2019). The future of clinical diagnosis: Moving functional genomics approaches to the bedside. *Advances in Molecular Pathology*, *2*(1), 13–19. DOI: 10.1016/j.yamp.2019.08.001

Pei, Q., Luo, Y., Chen, Y., Li, J., Xie, D., & Ye, T. (2022). Artificial intelligence in clinical applications for lung cancer: Diagnosis, treatment and prognosis. [CCLM]. *Clinical Chemistry and Laboratory Medicine*, *60*(12), 1974–1983. DOI: 10.1515/cclm-2022-0291

Prasad, V. (2016). Perspective: The precision-oncology illusion. *Nature*, *537*(7619), S63. DOI: 10.1038/537S63a

Prelaj, A., Miskovic, V., Zanitti, M., Trovo, F., Genova, C., Viscardi, G., Rebuzzi, S. E., Mazzeo, L., Provenzano, L., Kosta, S., Favali, M., Spagnoletti, A., Castelo-Branco, L., Dolezal, J., Pearson, A. T., Lo Russo, G., Proto, C., Ganzinelli, M., Giani, C., & Pedrocchi, A. L. G. (2024). Artificial intelligence for predictive biomarker discovery in immuno-oncology: A systematic review. *Annals of Oncology : Official Journal of the European Society for Medical Oncology*, *35*(1), 29–65. DOI: 10.1016/j.annonc.2023.10.125 PMID: 37879443

Prencipe, B., Delprete, C., Garolla, E., Corallo, F., Gravina, M., Natalicchio, M. I., Buongiorno, D., Bevilacqua, V., Altini, N., & Brunetti, A. (2023). An explainable radiogenomic framework to predict mutational status of KRAS and EGFR in lung adenocarcinoma patients. *Bioengineering (Basel, Switzerland)*, *10*(7), 747. DOI: 10.3390/bioengineering10070747

Preti, L. M., Ardito, V., Compagni, A., Petracca, F., & Cappellaro, G. (2024). Implementation of machine learning applications in health care organisations: Systematic review of empirical studies. *Journal of Medical Internet Research*, *26*, e55897. https://www.jmir.org/2024/1/e55897/PDF. DOI: 10.2196/55897 PMID: 39586084

Prusa, J., Khoshgoftaar, T. M., Dittman, D. J., & Napolitano, A. (2015). Using random undersampling to alleviate class imbalance on tweet sentiment data. In *IEEE International Conference on Information Reuse and Integration* (pp. 197–202). DOI: 10.1109/IRI.2015.39

Qin, Z. Z., Sander, M. S., Rai, B., Titahong, C. N., Sudrungrot, S., Laah, S. N., Adhikari, L. M., Carter, E. J., Puri, L., Codlin, A. J., & Creswell, J. (2019). Using artificial intelligence to read chest radiographs for tuberculosis detection: A multi-site evaluation of the diagnostic accuracy of three deep learning systems. *Scientific Reports*, *9*(1), 15000. DOI: 10.1038/s41598-019-51503-3 PMID: 31628424

Quang, L. T., Baek, B. H., Yoon, W., Kim, S. K., & Park, I. (2024). Comparison of Normalization Techniques for Radiomics Features From Magnetic Resonance Imaging in Predicting Histologic Grade of Meningiomas. *Investigative Magnetic Resonance Imaging*, *28*(2), 61. DOI: 10.13104/imri.2024.0010

Quinlan, J. R. (1993). *C4.5: Programs for machine learning*. Morgan Kaufmann.

Quraishi, M. I. (2022). Radiomics-Guided Precision Medicine Approaches for Colorectal Cancer. *Frontiers in Oncology*, *12*, 872656. DOI: 10.3389/fonc.2022.872656 PMID: 35756680

Rahman, A., Hayat, M., Iqbal, N., Alarfaj, F. K., Alkhalaf, S., & Alturise, F. (2025). Enhanced MRI brain tumor detection using deep learning in conjunction with explainable AI SHAP based diverse and multi feature analysis. *Scientific Reports*, *15*(1), 29411. DOI: 10.1038/s41598-025-14901-4 PMID: 40790336

Rajakumari, R., & Kalaivani, L. (2022). Breast Cancer Detection and Classification Using Deep CNN Techniques. *Intelligent Automation & Soft Computing*, *32*(2).

Rajatha, & Ashoka, D. V. (2025). EffiViT:: Hybrid CNN-Transformer for Retinal Imaging.

Rakha, E. A., Vougas, K., & Tan, P. H. (2022). Digital technology in diagnostic breast pathology and immunohistochemistry. *Pathobiology*, *89*(5), 334–342. DOI: 10.1159/000521149 PMID: 34969036

Rathore, S., Niazi, T., Iftikhar, M. A., & Chaddad, A. (2020). Glioma grading via machine learning analysis of digital pathology images. *Cancers (Basel)*, *12*(3), 578. DOI: 10.3390/cancers12030578 PMID: 32131409

Razzaghi, P., Abbasi, K., Shirazi, M., & Rashidi, S. (2022). Multimodal brain tumor detection using multimodal deep transfer learning. *Applied Soft Computing*, *129*, 109631. DOI: 10.1016/j.asoc.2022.109631

Ren, H., Zhou, L., Liu, G., Peng, X., Shi, W., Xu, H., Shan, F., & Liu, L. (2020). An unsupervised semi-automated pulmonary nodule segmentation method based on enhanced region growing. *Quantitative Imaging in Medicine and Surgery*, *10*(1), 233–242. DOI: 10.21037/qims.2019.12.02

Riaz, I. B., Khan, M. A., & Osterman, T. J. (2025). Artificial intelligence across the cancer care continuum. *Cancer*, *131*(16), e70050. DOI: 10.1002/cncr.70050 PMID: 40810209

Ribli, D., Horváth, A., Unger, Z., Pollner, P., & Csabai, I. (2018). Detecting and classifying lesions in mammograms with deep learning. *Scientific Reports*, *8*(1), 4165. DOI: 10.1038/s41598-018-22437-z PMID: 29545529

Rizzo, S., Botta, F., Raimondi, S., Origgi, D., Fanciullo, C., Morganti, A. G., & Bellomi, M. (2018). Radiomics: The facts and the challenges of image analysis. *European Radiology Experimental*, *2*(1), 1–8. DOI: 10.1186/s41747-018-0068-z

Rocha, J., Cunha, A., & Mendonça, A. M. (2020). Conventional filtering versus U-Net based models for pulmonary nodule segmentation in CT images. *Journal of Medical Systems*, *44*(4), 81. DOI: 10.1007/s10916-020-1541-9

Rodriguez, J. P. M., Rodriguez, R., Silva, V. W. K., Kitamura, F. C., Corradi, G. C. A., de Marchi, A. C. B., & Rieder, R. (2022). Artificial intelligence as a tool for diagnosis in digital pathology whole slide images: A systematic review. *Journal of Pathology Informatics, 13*, 100138. DOI: 10.1016/j.jpi.2022.100138 PMID: 36268059

Ronneberger, O., Fischer, P., & Brox, T. (2015, October). U-net: Convolutional networks for biomedical image segmentation. In *International Conference on Medical image computing and computer-assisted intervention* (pp. 234-241). Cham: Springer international publishing. DOI: 10.1007/978-3-319-24574-4_28

Roy, R., Banerjee, P., & Chowdhury, A. S. (2020). A level set based unified framework for pulmonary nodule segmentation. *IEEE Signal Processing Letters, 27*, 1465–1469. DOI: 10.1109/LSP.2020.3016563

Rudin, C. (2019). Stop explaining black box machine learning models for high stakes decisions and use interpretable models instead. *Nature Machine Intelligence, 1*(5), 206–215. DOI: 10.1038/s42256-019-0048-x

Russo, L., Charles-Davies, D., Bottazzi, S., Sala, E., & Boldrini, L. (2024). Radiomics for clinical decision support in radiation oncology. *Clinical Oncology, 36*(8), e269–e281. DOI: 10.1016/j.clon.2024.03.003 PMID: 38548581

Sachdeva, R. K., Bathla, P., Rani, P., Lamba, R., Ghantasala, G. P., & Nassar, I. F. (2024). A novel K-nearest neighbor classifier for lung cancer disease diagnosis. *Neural Computing & Applications, 36*(35), 22403–22416. DOI: 10.1007/s00521-024-10235-w

Sahiner, B., Chan, H.-P., Petrick, N., Helvie, M. A., Goodsitt, M. M., & Hadjiiski, L. (1996). Classification of mass and normal breast tissue on digital mammograms. *Medical Physics, 23*(7), 1065–1075.

Samal, B. R., Loers, J. U., Vermeirssen, V., & De Preter, K. (2022). Opportunities and challenges in interpretable deep learning for drug sensitivity prediction of cancer cells. *Frontiers in Bioinformatics, 2*, 1036963. Advance online publication. DOI: 10.3389/fbinf.2022.1036963 PMID: 36466148

Samathoti, P., Kumarachari, R. K., Bukke, S. P. N., Rajasekhar, E. S. K., Jaiswal, A. A., & Eftekhari, Z. (2025). The role of nanomedicine and artificial intelligence in cancer health care: Individual applications and emerging integrations—a narrative review. *Discover. Oncology, 16*(1), 697. Advance online publication. DOI: 10.1007/s12672-025-02469-4 PMID: 40338421

Samek, W., Wiegand, T., & Müller, K.-R. (2017). Explainable artificial intelligence: Understanding, visualizing and interpreting deep learning models. *arXiv Preprint*, arXiv:1708.08296. https://doi.org//arXiv.1708.08296DOI: 10.48550

Sangaraju, V. V. (2025). AI and Data Privacy in Healthcare: Compliance with HIPAA, GDPR, and emerging regulations. *International Journal of Emerging Trends in Computer Science and Information Technology*, 67-74.

Sarvamangala, D. R., & Kulkarni, R. V. (2022). Convolutional neural networks in medical image understanding: A survey. *Evolutionary Intelligence*, *15*(1), 1–22. DOI: 10.1007/s12065-020-00540-3 PMID: 33425040

Sasikumar, P., Cherukuvada, S., Balmurugan, P., Anand, P. V., Brindasri, S., & Nareshkumar, R. (2024, May). An Efficient Brain tumor classification using CNN and transfer learning. In *2024 International Conference on Advances in Computing, Communication and Applied Informatics (ACCAI)* (pp. 1-5). IEEE. DOI: 10.1109/ACCAI61061.2024.10602391

Satushe, V., Vyas, V., Metkar, S., & Singh, D. P. (2025). AI in MRI brain tumor diagnosis: A systematic review of machine learning and deep learning advances (2010–2025). *Chemometrics and Intelligent Laboratory Systems*, *263*, 105414. DOI: 10.1016/j.chemolab.2025.105414

Schaefer-Prokop, C., Neitzel, U., Venema, H. W., Uffmann, M., & Prokop, M. (2008). Digital chest radiography: An update on modern technology, dose containment and control of image quality. *European Radiology*, *18*(9), 1818–1830. DOI: 10.1007/s00330-008-0948-3

Schmidt, M. E., Goldschmidt, S., Hermann, S., & Steindorf, K. (2022). Late effects, long-term problems and unmet needs of cancer survivors. *International Journal of Cancer*, *151*(8), 1280–1290. DOI: 10.1002/ijc.34152 PMID: 35657637

Seeram, E. (2015). *Computed tomography: Physical principles, clinical applications, and quality control* (4th ed.). Elsevier.

Shaikh, F. J., & Rao, D. S. (2022). Prediction of cancer disease using machine learning approach. *Materials Today: Proceedings*, *50*, 40–47.

Shamsara, E., & Shamsara, J. (2020). Bio-informatics analysis of the genes involved in the extension of prostate cancer to adjacent lymph nodes by supervised and unsupervised machine learning methods: The role of SPAG1 and PLEKHF. *Genomics*, *112*(5), 3871–3882.

Shao, J., Feng, J., Li, J., Liang, S., Li, W., & Wang, C. (2023). Novel tools for early diagnosis and precision treatment based on artificial intelligence. *Chinese Medical Journal Pulmonary and Critical Care Medicine*, *01*(03), 148–160. DOI: 10.1016/j.pccm.2023.05.001 PMID: 39171128

Sharma, V. (2023). Automating complex healthcare workflows with AI and RPA: A new era of efficiency. [IJLRP]. *International Journal of Leading Research Publication*, *4*(2), 1–8. https://www.ijlrp.com/papers/2023/1/1249.pdf

Shirzad, M., Shaban, M., Mohammadzadeh, V., Rahdar, A., Fathi-karkan, S., Hoseini, Z. S., Najafi, M., Kharaba, Z., & Aboudzadeh, M. A. (2025). Artificial Intelligence-Assisted Design of Nanomedicines for Breast Cancer Diagnosis and Therapy: Advances, Challenges, and Future Directions. *BioNanoScience*, *15*(3), 354. Advance online publication. DOI: 10.1007/s12668-025-01980-w

Shi, Y., Fan, H., Li, L., Hou, Y., Qian, F., Zhuang, M., & Fei, S. (2024). The value of machine learning approaches in the diagnosis of early gastric cancer: A systematic review and meta-analysis—World. *Journal of Surgical Oncology*, *22*(1), 40. PMID: 38297303

Shmatko, A., Ghaffari Laleh, N., Gerstung, M., & Kather, J. N. (2022). Artificial intelligence in histopathology: Enhancing cancer research and clinical oncology. *Nature Cancer*, *3*(9), 1026–1038. DOI: 10.1038/s43018-022-00436-4 PMID: 36138135

Singh, M. P., & Keche, Y. N. (2025). Ethical integration of artificial intelligence in healthcare: Narrative review of global challenges and strategic solutions. *Cureus*, *17*(5), 1–16. DOI: 10.7759/cureus.84804 PMID: 40568260

Singla, N., & Singla, S. (2020). Harnessing Big Data with Machine Learning in Precision Oncology. *Kidney Cancer Journal : Official Journal of the Kidney Cancer Association*, *18*(3), 83–84. http://www.kidney-cancer-journal.com/pdf/KCJ_nirmish.pdf PMID: 33163139

Song, F., Song, X., Feng, Y., Fan, G., Sun, Y., Zhang, P., Li, J., Liu, F., & Zhang, G. (2023). Radiomics feature analysis and model research for predicting histopathological subtypes of non-small cell lung cancer on CT images: A multi-dataset study. *Medical Physics*, *50*(7), 4351–4365. DOI: 10.1002/mp.16233

Spaanderman, D. J., Hakkesteegt, S. N., Hanff, D. F., Schut, A. R. W., Schiphouwer, L. M., Vos, M., Messiou, C., Doran, S. J., Jones, R. L., Hayes, A. J., Nardo, L., Abdelhafez, Y. G., Moawad, A. W., Elsayes, K. M., Lee, S., Link, T. M., Niessen, W. J., Van Leenders, G. J. L. H., Visser, J. J., & Starmans, M. P. A. (2024). Multicenter external validation of an automated method segmenting and differentiating atypical lipomatous tumors from lipomas using radiomics and deep-learning on MRI. *EClinicalMedicine*, *76*, 102802. DOI: 10.1016/j.eclinm.2024.102802 PMID: 39351025

Spanhol, F. A., Oliveira, L. S., Petitjean, C., & Heutte, L. (2016). A dataset for breast cancer histopathological image classification. *IEEE Transactions on Biomedical Engineering*, *63*(7), 1455–1462. DOI: 10.1109/TBME.2015.2496264 PMID: 26540668

Stefano, A. (2024). Challenges and limitations in applying radiomics to PET imaging: Possible opportunities and avenues for research. *Computers in Biology and Medicine*, *179*, 108827. DOI: 10.1016/j.compbiomed.2024.108827 PMID: 38964244

Street, W. N., Wolberg, W. H., & Mangasarian, O. L. (1993). Nuclear feature extraction for breast tumor diagnosis. *IS&T/SPIE Proceedings, 1905*, 861–870.

Sung, H., Ferlay, J., Siegel, R. L., Laversanne, M., Soerjomataram, I., Jemal, A., & Bray, F. (2021). Global cancer statistics 2020: GLOBOCAN estimates of incidence and mortality worldwide for 36 cancers in 185 countries. *CA: a Cancer Journal for Clinicians*, *71*(3), 209–249. DOI: 10.3322/caac.21660

Sutton, R. T., Pincock, D., Baumgart, D. C., Sadowski, D. C., Fedorak, R. N., & Kroeker, K. I. (2020). An overview of clinical decision support systems: Benefits, risks, and strategies for success. *NPJ Digital Medicine*, *3*(1), 17. DOI: 10.1038/s41746-020-0221-y PMID: 32047862

Suzuki, K. (2017). Computer-aided detection of lung cancer. In Arimura, H. (Ed.), *Image-based computer-assisted radiation therapy* (pp. 9–40). Springer., DOI: 10.1007/978-981-10-2945-5_2

Swanson, K., Wu, E., Zhang, A., Alizadeh, A. A., & Zou, J. (2023). From patterns to patients: Advances in clinical machine learning for cancer diagnosis, prognosis, and treatment. *Cell*, *186*(9), 1772.

Taha, A. A., & Hanbury, A. (2015). Metrics for evaluating 3D medical image segmentation: Analysis, selection, and tool. *BMC Medical Imaging*, *15*(1), 1–28. DOI: 10.1186/s12880-015-0068-x

Tandon, R., Agrawal, S., Rathore, N. P. S., Mishra, A. K., & Jain, S. K. (2024). A systematic review of deep learning-based automated cancer diagnosis models. *Journal of Cellular and Molecular Medicine*, *28*(6), e18144. DOI: 10.1111/jcmm.18144 PMID: 38426930

Tan, M., & Le, Q. (2021, July). Efficientnetv2: Smaller models and faster training. In *International conference on machine learning* (pp. 10096-10106). PMLR.

Tan, M., & Le, Q. V. (2019). *EfficientNet: Rethinking model scaling for convolutional neural networks*. In *Proceedings of the 36th International Conference on Machine Learning (ICML 2019)* (Vol. 97, pp. 6105–6114).

Tembhurne, J. V., Hebbar, N., Patil, H. Y., & Diwan, T. (2023). Skin cancer detection using an ensemble of machine learning and deep learning techniques. *Multimedia Tools and Applications*, *82*(18), 27501–27524. DOI: 10.1007/s11042-023-14697-3

Thaha, M. M., Kumar, K. P. M., Murugan, B. S., Dhanasekeran, S., Vijayakarthick, P., & Selvi, A. S. (2019). Brain tumor segmentation using convolutional neural networks in MRI images. *Journal of Medical Systems*, *43*(9), 294. DOI: 10.1007/s10916-019-1416-0 PMID: 31342192

Tharwat, M., Sakr, N. A., El-Sappagh, S., Soliman, H., Kwak, K. S., & Elmogy, M. (2022). Colon cancer diagnosis based on machine learning and deep learning: Modalities and analysis techniques. *Sensors (Basel)*, *22*(23), 9250. DOI: 10.3390/s22239250 PMID: 36501951

Theriault-Lauzier, P., Cobin, D., Tastet, O., Langlais, E. L., Taji, B., Kang, G., Chong, A.-Y., So, D., Tang, A., & Gichoya, J. W.. (2024). A responsible framework for applying artificial intelligence on medical images and signals at the point-of-care: The PACSAI platform. *The Canadian Journal of Cardiology*, *40*(10), 1828–1840. Advance online publication. DOI: 10.1016/j.cjca.2024.05.025

Thirumalaisamy, S., Thangavilou, K., Rajadurai, H., Saidani, O., Alturki, N., Mathivanan, S. K., Jayagopal, P., & Gochhait, S. (2023). Breast cancer classification using synthesized deep learning model with metaheuristic optimization algorithm. *Diagnostics (Basel)*, *13*(18), 2925. DOI: 10.3390/diagnostics13182925 PMID: 37761292

Topol, E. J. (2019). High-performance medicine: The convergence of human and artificial intelligence. *Nature Medicine*, *25*(1), 44–56. DOI: 10.1038/s41591-018-0300-7

Tran, K. A., Kondrashova, O., Bradley, A., Williams, E. D., Pearson, J. V., & Waddell, N. (2021). Deep learning in cancer diagnosis, prognosis and treatment selection. *Genome Medicine*, *13*(1), 152. DOI: 10.1186/s13073-021-00968-x PMID: 34579788

Tran, W. T., Sadeghi-Naini, A., Lu, F. I., Gandhi, S., Meti, N., Brackstone, M., Rakovitch, E., & Curpen, B. (2021). Computational radiology in breast cancer screening and diagnosis using artificial intelligence. *Canadian Association of Radiologists Journal, 72*(1), 98–108. DOI: 10.1177/0846537120949974 PMID: 32865001

Travis, W. D., Asamura, H., Bankier, A. A., Beasley, M. B., Detterbeck, F., Flieder, D. B., Goo, J. M., MacMahon, H., Naidich, D., Nicholson, A. G., ... (2016). The IASLC lung cancer staging project: Proposals for coding T categories for subsolid nodules and assessment of tumor size in part-solid tumors in the forthcoming eighth edition of the TNM classification of lung cancer. *Journal of Thoracic Oncology, 11*(8), 1204–1223. DOI: 10.1016/j.jtho.2016.03.025

Travis, W. D., Brambilla, E., Nicholson, A. G., Yatabe, Y., Austin, J. H. M., Beasley, M. B., Chirieac, L. R., Dacic, S., Duhig, E., Flieder, D. B., Geisinger, K., Hirsch, F. R., Ishikawa, Y., Kerr, K. M., Noguchi, M., Pelosi, G., Powell, C. A., Tsao, M. S., & Wistuba, I. (2015). The 2015 World Health Organization classification of lung tumors: Impact of genetic, clinical, and radiologic advances since the 2004 classification. *Journal of Thoracic Oncology*, *10*(9), 1243–1260. DOI: 10.1097/JTO.0000000000000630

Trebeschi, S., Drago, S. G., Birkbak, N. J., Kurilova, I., Călin, A. M., Delli Pizzi, A., Lalezari, F., Lambregts, D. M. J., Rohaan, M. W., Parmar, C., Rozeman, E. A., Hartemink, K. J., Swanton, C., Haanen, J. B A G., Blank, C. U., Smit, E. F., Beets-Tan, R. G. H., & Aerts, H. J. W. L. (2019). Predicting response to cancer immunotherapy using noninvasive radiomic biomarkers. *Annals of Oncology : Official Journal of the European Society for Medical Oncology*, *30*(6), 998–1004. DOI: 10.1093/annonc/mdz108

Tsimberidou, A. M., Fountzilas, E., Nikanjam, M., & Kurzrock, R. (2020). Review of precision cancer medicine: Evolution of the treatment paradigm. *Cancer Treatment Reviews*, *86*, 102019. DOI: 10.1016/j.ctrv.2020.102019

Tunali, I., Gillies, R. J., & Schabath, M. B. (2021). Application of radiomics and artificial intelligence for lung cancer precision medicine. *Cold Spring Harbor Perspectives in Medicine*, *11*(8), a039537. DOI: 10.1101/cshperspect.a039537

Tunçel, N. (2021). Adaptive radiotherapy from past to future frontiers. *International Journal of Radiology & Radiation Therapy*, *8*(2), 81–84. https://avesis.akdeniz.edu.tr/yayin/1be4388d-be5d-477b-a818-97d75a92f181/adaptive-radiotherapy-from-past-to-future-frontiers/document.pdf. DOI: 10.15406/ijrrt.2021.08.00298

Ugemuge, P. K., Khandalkar, G. G., & Ingle, R. G. (2024). Artificial intelligence could be the personalised treatment strategy for cancer. *International Journal of Pharmaceutical Quality Assurance*, *15*(2), 1017–1022. https://impactfactor.org/PDF/IJPQA/15/IJPQA,Vol15,Issue2,Article72.pdf. DOI: 10.25258/ijpqa.15.2.72

Unterrainer, M., Eze, C., Ilhan, H., Marschner, S., Roengvoraphoj, O., Schmidt-Hegemann, N.-S., Walter, F., Kunz, W. G., af Rosenschöld, P. M., & Jeraj, R.. (2020). Recent advances of PET imaging in clinical radiation oncology. *Radiation Oncology (London, England)*, *15*(1), 1–15. DOI: 10.1186/s13014-020-01519-1

Vaka, A. R., Soni, B., & Reddy, S. (2020). Breast cancer detection by leveraging Machine Learning. *ICT Express*, *6*(4), 320–324.

Vamathevan, J., Clark, D., Czodrowski, P., Dunham, I., Ferran, E., Lee, G., Li, B., Madabhushi, A., Shah, P., Spitzer, M., & Zhao, S. (2019). Applications of machine learning in drug discovery and development. *Nature Reviews. Drug Discovery*, *18*(6), 463–477. DOI: 10.1038/s41573-019-0024-5 PMID: 30976107

Van der Velden, B. H., Kuijf, H. J., Gilhuijs, K. G., & Viergever, M. A. (2022). Explainable artificial intelligence (XAI) in deep learning-based medical image analysis. *Medical Image Analysis*, *79*, 102470. DOI: 10.1016/j.media.2022.102470

Van Leeuwen, K. G., de Rooij, M., Schalekamp, S., van Ginneken, B., & Rutten, M. J. (2022). How does artificial intelligence in radiology improve efficiency and health outcomes? *Pediatric Radiology*, *52*(11), 1–7. DOI: 10.1007/s00247-021-05114-8 PMID: 34117522

van Leeuwen, K. G., de Rooij, M., Schalekamp, S., van Ginneken, B., & Rutten, M. J. (2024). Clinical use of artificial intelligence products for radiology in the Netherlands between 2020 and 2022. *European Radiology*, *34*(1), 348–354. DOI: 10.1007/s00330-023-09991-5 PMID: 37515632

Van Timmeren, J. E., Cester, D., Tanadini-Lang, S., Alkadhi, H., & Baessler, B. (2020). Radiomics in medical imaging—"How-to" guide and critical reflection. *Insights Into Imaging*, *11*(1), 91. DOI: 10.1186/s13244-020-00887-2 PMID: 32785796

Varlamova, E. V., Butakova, M. A., Semyonova, V. V., Soldatav, S. A., Poltavskiy, A. V., Kit, O. I., & Soldatov, A. V. (2024). Machine learning meets cancer. *Cancers (Basel)*, *16*(6), 1100.

Vellido, A. (2020). The importance of interpretability and visualization in machine learning for applications in medicine and health care. *Neural Computing & Applications*, *32*(24), 18069–18083. DOI: 10.1007/s00521-019-04051-w

Vemula, C., Chavva, P., Battu, U., Vemulapalli, S., Prasad, K. V., & Kannaiah, S. K. (2024, May). Revolutionizing Breast Cancer Diagnosis: Insights from KNN and SVM Models in Machine Learning. In *2024 5th International Conference for Emerging Technology (INCET)* (pp. 1-9). IEEE.

Verma, B., McLeod, P., & Klevansky, A. (2010). Classification of benign and malignant patterns in digital mammograms for the diagnosis of breast cancer. *Expert Systems with Applications*, *37*(4), 3344–3351.

Vindhya, J., Pooja, C., Dongre, M. H., Gowrishankar, S., Srinivasa, A. H., & Veena, A. (2023). Skin Lesion Classification Using Machine Learning. In *Inventive Computation and Information Technologies Proceedings of ICICIT, 2022*, 385–397.

Visibelli, A. (2022). Machine learning in Bioinformatics: Novel approaches to Precision Medicine, Life Sciences and Healthcare [Doctoral dissertation, University of Siena]. https://tesidottorato.depositolegale.it/bitstream/20.500.14242/87419/1/phd_unisi_085878.pdf

Viswanathan, V. S., Toro, P., Corredor, G., Mukhopadhyay, S., & Madabhushi, A. (2022). The state of the art for artificial intelligence in lung digital pathology. *The Journal of Pathology*, *257*(4), 413–429. DOI: 10.1002/path.5966 PMID: 35579955

Vo, D. M., Nguyen, N. Q., & Lee, S. W. (2019). Classification of breast cancer histology images using incremental boosting convolution networks. *Information Sciences*, *482*, 123–138. DOI: 10.1016/j.ins.2018.12.089

Vuong, D. (2021). Radiomics as biomarker in multi-modality treatment of locally advanced non-small cell lung cancer [Doctoral dissertation, Universität Zürich]. https://www.zora.uzh.ch/id/eprint/211927/1/Dissertation_Vuong_2021.pdf

Wahl, R. L., Jacene, H., Kasamon, Y., & Lodge, M. A. (2009). From RECIST to PERCIST: Evolving considerations for PET response criteria in solid tumors. *Journal of Nuclear Medicine*, *50*(Suppl. 1), 122S–150S. DOI: 10.2967/jnumed.108.057307

Wang, C. W., Khalil, M. A., & Firdi, N. P. (2022). A survey on deep learning for precision oncology. *Diagnostics (Basel)*, *12*(6), 1489. DOI: 10.3390/diagnostics12061489 PMID: 35741298

Wang, C., Lye, X., Kaalia, R., Kumar, P., & Rajapakse, J. C. (2022). Deep learning and multi-omics approach to predict drug responses in cancer. *BMC Bioinformatics*, *22*(S10), 632. Advance online publication. DOI: 10.1186/s12859-022-04964-9 PMID: 36443676

Wang, H., Zheng, B., Yoon, S. W., & Ko, H. S. (2018). A support vector machine-based ensemble algorithm for breast cancer diagnosis. *European Journal of Operational Research, 267*(2), 687–699.

Wang, J., Cheng, Y., Guo, C., & Tamura, S. (2015). A new pulmonary nodules detection scheme utilizing region grow and adaptive fuzzy c-means clustering. *Journal of Medical Imaging and Health Informatics, 5*(8), 1941–1946. DOI: 10.1166/jmihi.2015.1674

Wang, L., Lu, Q., Li, R., Harrison, T. B., Jia, H., Huang, M., Dowst, H., Zhang, R., Badr, H., Fan, J. W., & Liu, H. (2025). Understanding Cancer Survivorship Care Needs Using Amazon Reviews: Content Analysis, Algorithm Development, and Validation Study. *JMIR Cancer, 11*, e71102. DOI: 10.2196/71102 PMID: 40986859

Waqas, A., Tripathi, A., Ramachandran, R. P., Stewart, P., & Rasool, G. (2024). Multimodal data integration for oncology in the era of deep neural networks: A review. https://arxiv.org/pdf/2303.06471

Waqas, A., Tripathi, A., Ramachandran, R. P., Stewart, P., & Rasool, G. (2024). Multimodal Data Integration for Oncology in the Era of Deep Neural Networks: A Review. *Frontiers in Artificial Intelligence, 7*, 1408843. DOI: 10.3389/frai.2024.1408843 PMID: 39118787

Wei, B., Li, L., Feng, Y., Liu, S., Fu, P., & Tian, L. (2024). Exploring prognostic biomarkers in pathological images of colorectal cancer patients via deep learning. *The Journal of Pathology. Clinical Research, 10*(6), e70003. Advance online publication. DOI: 10.1002/2056-4538.70003 PMID: 39343999

Wen, Y., Ma, L., & Ju, C. (2023). Recent insights into the pathogenesis and therapeutic targets of chronic liver diseases. *eGastroenterology, 1*(2), e100020. DOI: 10.1136/egastro-2023-100020 PMID: 38074919

Willemink, M. J., Koszek, W. A., Hardell, C., Wu, J., Fleischmann, D., Harvey, H., Folio, L. R., Summers, R. M., Rubin, D. L., & Lungren, M. P. (2020). Preparing medical imaging data for machine learning. *Radiology, 295*(1), 4–15. DOI: 10.1148/radiol.2020192224

Wilson, R., & Devaraj, A. (2017). Radiomics of pulmonary nodules and lung cancer. *Translational Lung Cancer Research, 6*(1), 86–91. DOI: 10.21037/tlcr.2017.01.04

Wong, A. N. N., He, Z., Leung, K. L., To, C. C. K., Wong, C. Y., Wong, S. C. C., Yoo, J. S., Chan, C. K. R., Chan, A. Z., Lacambra, M. D., & Yeung, M. H. Y. (2022). Current developments of artificial intelligence in digital pathology and its future clinical applications in gastrointestinal cancers. *Cancers (Basel)*, *14*(15), 3780. DOI: 10.3390/cancers14153780 PMID: 35954443

World Health Organization. (2024, February 1). *Global cancer burden growing amidst mounting need for services.* https://www.who.int/news/item/01-02-2024-global-cancer-burden-growing--amidst-mounting-need-for-services

Wu, J., & Hicks, C. (2021). Breast cancer type classification using machine learning. *Journal of Personalized Medicine*, *11*(2), 61. DOI: 10.3390/jpm11020061 PMID: 33498339

Wulczyn, E., Steiner, D. F., Xu, Z., Sadhwani, A., Wang, H., Flament, I., Mermel, C. H., Chen, P.-H. C., Liu, Y., & Stumpe, M. C. (2020). Deep learning-based survival prediction for multiple cancer types using histopathology images. *PLoS One*, *15*(6), e0233678. DOI: 10.1371/journal.pone.0233678 PMID: 32555646

Xia, T. (2023). Radiogenomics framework for associating medical image features with tumour genetic characteristics [Doctoral dissertation, The University of Sydney]. https://core.ac.uk/download/pdf/590715623.pdf

Xie, Q., Li, Y., He, N., Ning, M., Ma, K., Wang, G., Lian, Y., & Zheng, Y. (2022). Unsupervised domain adaptation for medical image segmentation by disentanglement learning and self-training. *IEEE Transactions on Medical Imaging*, *43*(1), 4–14. DOI: 10.1109/TMI.2022.3192303

Xu, Z., Wang, X., Zeng, S., Ren, X., Yan, Y., & Gong, Z. (2021). Applying artificial intelligence for cancer immunotherapy. *Acta Pharmaceutica Sinica. B*, *11*(11), 3393–3405. DOI: 10.1016/j.apsb.2021.02.007 PMID: 34900525

Yadav, M., Lee, J., Kim, H., Lee, S., Um, T., Lee, S., Djunadi, T. A., Chung, L. I.-Y., Yu, J., Rodrigues, D., Gennaro, N., Kim, L., Nam, M., Kim, Y., Hong, I., Jang, J., Kang, G., Cho, A., Velichko, Y., & Chae, Y. K. (2024). Pre-treatment CT radiomics for predicting immunotherapy response in non-small cell lung cancer (NSCLC): RECIST vs. irRECIST criteria. *Journal of Clinical Oncology*, *42*(16, Suppl), e20613. DOI: 10.1200/JCO.2024.42.16_suppl.e20613

Yang, F., Zhang, J., Zhou, L., Xia, W., Zhang, R., Wei, H., Feng, J., Zhao, X., Jian, J., Gao, X., & Yuan, S. (2022). CT-based radiomics signatures can predict the tumor response of non-small cell lung cancer patients treated with first-line chemotherapy and targeted therapy. *European Radiology*, *32*(3), 1538–1547. DOI: 10.1007/s00330-021-08277-y

Yang, H.-H., Wang, F.-E., Sun, C., Huang, K.-C., Chen, H.-W., Chen, Y., Chen, H.-C., Liao, C.-Y., Kao, S.-H., & Wang, Y.-C. F.. (2021). Leveraging auxiliary information from EMR for weakly supervised pulmonary nodule detection. In Medical Image Computing and Computer Assisted Intervention – *MICCAI 2021: 24th International Conference,* Strasbourg, France, September 27–October 1, 2021, *Proceedings, Part VII* (pp. 251–261). Springer. DOI: 10.1007/978-3-030-87234-2_24

Yang, M., Shi, L., Huang, T., Li, G., Shao, H., Shen, Y., Zhu, J., & Ni, B. (2023). Value of contrast-enhanced magnetic resonance imaging-T2WI-based radiomic features in distinguishing lung adenocarcinoma from lung squamous cell carcinoma with solid components ≥ 8 mm. *Journal of Thoracic Disease, 15*(2), 635–648. DOI: 10.21037/jtd-23-142

Yao, I. Z., Dong, M., & Hwang, W. Y. K. (2025). Deep Learning Applications in Clinical Cancer Detection: A Review of Implementation Challenges and Solutions. *Mayo Clinic Proceedings. Digital Health, 3*(3), 100253. DOI: 10.1016/j.mcpdig.2025.100253 PMID: 40822144

Yeghiazaryan, V., & Voiculescu, I. (2015). *An overview of current evaluation methods used in medical image segmentation* (Tech. Rep. RR-15-08, pp. 22). Department of Computer Science, Oxford, UK.

Yen, S.-J., & Lee, Y.-S. (2009). Cluster-based under-sampling approaches for imbalanced data distributions. *Expert Systems with Applications, 36*(3), 5718–5727. DOI: 10.1016/j.eswa.2008.06.108

Ying, W., Cunxi, C., Tong, J., & Xinhe, X. (2009). Segmentation of regions of interest in lung CT images based on 2-D Otsu optimized by genetic algorithm. In *2009 Chinese Control and Decision Conference* (pp. 5185–5189). IEEE. DOI: 10.1109/CCDC.2009.5195024

Yousefi, B., Jahani, N., LaRiviere, M. J., Cohen, E., Hsieh, M.-K., Luna, J. M., Chitalia, R. D., Thompson, J. C., Carpenter, E. L., Katz, S. I., ... (2019). Correlative hierarchical clustering-based low-rank dimensionality reduction of radiomics-driven phenotype in non-small cell lung cancer. In *Medical Imaging 2019: Imaging Informatics for Healthcare, Research, and Applications* (Vol. 10954, pp. 278–285). SPIE. DOI: 10.1117/12.2515609

Yousif, M., van Diest, P. J., Laurinavicius, A., Rimm, D., van der Laak, J., Madabhushi, A., & Pantanowitz, L. (2022). Artificial intelligence applied to breast pathology. *Virchows Archiv*, •••, 1–19. PMID: 34791536

Yurttakal, A. H., Erbay, H., İkizceli, T., & Karaçavuş, S. (2020). Detection of breast cancer via deep convolutional neural networks using MRI images. *Multimedia Tools and Applications*, *79*(21), 15555–15573. DOI: 10.1007/s11042-019-7479-6

Zarei, M., Sotoudeh Paima, S., McCabe, C., Abadi, E., & Samei, E. (2024). A physics-informed deep neural network for harmonization of CT images. *IEEE Transactions on Biomedical Engineering*, *71*(12), 3494–3504. Advance online publication. DOI: 10.1109/TBME.2024.3428399

Zhang, W., Huang, H., Wang, L., Lehmann, B. D., & Chen, S. X. (2025). An Integrative Multi-Omics Random Forest Framework for Robust Biomarker Discovery. bioRxiv, 2025-03.

Zhang, B., Shi, H., & Wang, H. (2023). Machine learning and artificial intelligence in cancer prognosis, prediction and treatment selection: A critical approach. *Journal of Multidisciplinary Healthcare*, *16*, 1779–1791.

Zhang, H., Chen, Y., & Li, F. (2021). Predicting Anticancer Drug Response With Deep Learning Constrained by Signaling Pathways. *Frontiers in Bioinformatics*, *1*, 639349. Advance online publication. DOI: 10.3389/fbinf.2021.639349 PMID: 36303766

Zhang, L., Gopalakrishnan, V., Lu, L., Summers, R. M., Moss, J., & Yao, J. (2018). Self-learning to detect and segment cysts in lung CT images without manual annotation. In *Proceedings of the 2018 IEEE 15th International Symposium on Biomedical Imaging (ISBI 2018)* (pp. 1100–1103). DOI: 10.1109/ISBI.2018.8363763

Zhang, R., Hong, M., Cai, H., Liang, Y., Chen, X., Liu, Z., Wu, M., Zhou, C., Bao, C., Wang, H., Yang, S., & Hu, Q. (2023). Predicting the pathological invasiveness in patients with a solitary pulmonary nodule via Shapley additive explanations interpretation of a tree-based machine learning radiomics model: A multicenter study. *Quantitative Imaging in Medicine and Surgery*, *13*(12), 7828–7845. DOI: 10.21037/qims-23-615

Zhang, W., Zhang, X., Zhao, J., Qiang, Y., Tian, Q., & Tang, X. (2017). A segmentation method for lung nodule image sequences based on superpixels and density-based spatial clustering of applications with noise. *PLoS One*, *12*(9), e0184290. DOI: 10.1371/journal.pone.0184290

Zhang, Y., Oikonomou, A., Wong, A., Haider, M. A., & Khalvati, F. (2017). Radiomics-based prognosis analysis for non-small cell lung cancer. *Scientific Reports*, *7*(1), 46349. DOI: 10.1038/srep46349

Zhang, Y.-P., Zhang, X.-Y., Cheng, Y.-T., Li, B., Teng, X.-Z., Zhang, J., Lam, S., Zhou, T., Ma, Z.-R., Sheng, J.-B., Tam, V. C. W., Lee, S. W. Y., Ge, H., & Cai, J. (2023). Artificial intelligence-driven radiomics study in cancer: The role of feature engineering and modeling. *Military Medical Research*, *10*(1), 22. DOI: 10.1186/s40779-023-00458-8 PMID: 37189155

Zheng, J., Yan, Z., Wang, R., Xiao, H., Chen, Z., Ge, X., Li, Z., Liu, Z., Yu, H., Liu, H., Wang, G., Yu, P., Fu, J., Zhang, G., Zhang, J., Liu, B., Huang, Y., Deng, H., Wang, C., & Liang, H. (2025). NeoPred: Dual-phase CT AI forecasts pathologic response to neoadjuvant chemo-immunotherapy in NSCLC. *Journal for Immunotherapy of Cancer*, *13*(5), e011773. DOI: 10.1136/jitc-2025-011773 PMID: 40449955

Zhong, J., Liu, X., Hu, Y., Xing, Y., Ding, D., Ge, X., Song, Y., Wang, S., Chen, L., Zhu, Y., Lu, W., Zhang, H., & Yao, W. (2024). Robustness of quantitative diffusion metrics from four models: A prospective study on the influence of scan-rescans, voxel size, coils, and observers. *Journal of Magnetic Resonance Imaging*, *60*(4), 1470–1483. DOI: 10.1002/jmri.29192

Zhou, A., Ma, Y., Ji, W., Zong, M., Yang, P., Wu, M., & Liu, M. (2023). Multi-head attention-based two-stream EfficientNet for action recognition. *Multimedia Systems*, *29*(2), 487–498. DOI: 10.1007/s00530-022-00961-3

Zhou, A., Yousem, D. M., & Alvin, M. D. (2018). Cost-Effectiveness Analysis in Radiology: A Systematic Review. *Journal of the American College of Radiology*, *15*(11), 1536–1546. DOI: 10.1016/j.jacr.2018.06.018 PMID: 30057243

Zhou, J., Wen, Y., Ding, R., Liu, J., Fang, H., Li, X., Zhao, K., & Wan, Q. (2024). Radiomics signature based on robust features derived from diffusion data for differentiation between benign and malignant solitary pulmonary lesions. *Cancer Imaging; the Official Publication of the International Cancer Imaging Society*, *24*(1), 14. DOI: 10.1186/s40644-024-00660-4

Zhovannik, I. (2022). Pitfalls of image biomarker analysis in radiation oncology [Doctoral dissertation, Radboud University Nijmegen]. https://repository.ubn.ru.nl/bitstream/handle/2066/289611/289611.pdf?sequence=1#page=133

Zuo, Y., Liu, Q., Li, N., Li, P., Fang, Y., Bian, L., Zhang, J., & Song, S. (2024). Explainable 18F-FDG PET/CT radiomics model for predicting EGFR mutation status in lung adenocarcinoma: A two-center study. *Journal of Cancer Research and Clinical Oncology*, *150*(10), 469. DOI: 10.1007/s00432-024-05998-7

Zwanenburg, A., Vallières, M., Abdalah, M. A., Aerts, H. J. W. L., Andrearczyk, V., Apte, A., Ashrafinia, S., Bakas, S., Beukinga, R. J., Boellaard, R., Bogowicz, M., Boldrini, L., Buvat, I., Cook, G. J. R., Davatzikos, C., Depeursinge, A., Desseroit, M.-C., Dinapoli, N., Dinh, C. V., & Löck, S. (2020). The image biomarker standardization initiative: Standardized quantitative radiomics for high-throughput image-based phenotyping. *Radiology*, *295*(2), 328–338. DOI: 10.1148/radiol.2020191145

About the Contributors

Manvi Mishra is the Associate Professor and Head of the department of Computer Science & Engineering at Shri Ram Murti Smarak College of Engineering Technology and Research, Bareilly, India. With 19 years of academic experience, she holds a Bachelor's in Information Technology (2006) and a Master's with honors in Software Engineering (2011) from Dr. A.P.J. Abdul Kalam Technical University, Lucknow. She earned her Ph.D. in Computer Science and Engineering from the same institution. Her research interests span Artificial Intelligence, Machine Learning, Radiological/Medical Image Processing, Cryptography and Network Security, Data Compression, and Software Engineering. Dr. Mishra has presented her work at national and international conferences and published in reputed journals. She is a member of IEI, CSI, and IEEE. Her accolades include the Bharat Vikas Award (2017), Young Woman Educator and Researcher Award (2021), and Woman Power India Award (2024), honoring her contributions to teaching, research, and social impact.

Piyush Kumar is a distinguished Radiation Oncologist at Shri Ram Murti Smarak Institute of Medical Sciences, India, with over 18 years of academic and research experience. His expertise focuses on brain tumors, head and neck cancers, esophagus cancer, and cervix cancer. A prolific researcher, he has guided 21 theses and co-guided 40, published 80 papers in national and international journals, and contributed to books such as "Gynecological Malignancies – A Handbook for Post Graduates". He is the Founding Editor-in-Chief of the SRMS Journal of Medical Sciences and has edited the institute's quarterly newsletter Medivision since 2010. Awarded prestigious fellowships including: AROI–Dr. Reddy's Overseas Fellowship (2014) AROI-Nucletron Overseas Fellowship (2009) Parwati Devi Gold Medal for Best Paper (2005) DST & CSIR Travel Grant (2007) for presenting research in Singapore. His work aims to improve cancer treatment, including dosimetric analysis of IMRT to reduce oral mucositis in head and neck cancers. Key Contributions:

187+ PG paper presentations guided Editor & academic leader in oncology research Award-winning researcher advancing radiation therapy.

Himanshi Khattar has completed M.B.B.S, MD,DNB Radiation Oncology, Fellowship in Diabetes Mellitus and CCEPC. Her Thesis was Dosimetric Analysis and Clinical correlation of Brachial plexus in Head and Neck cancers treated with Intensity modulated radiotherapy. Research Area: Her Research Areas are Head and Neck cancer, Artificial Intelligence. Breast cancer Number of Published papers: She has several published papers in and international journal such as: Khattar H, Kumar P, Navitha S. Delineation of Oral Mucosa as a Pseudo-Organ-at-Risk May Lead to a Decrease in the Incidence of Oral Mucositis: A Dosimetric Analysis of Intensity-Modulated Radiation Therapy Plans in Head and Neck Cancers. Cureus. 2022 Mar 31;14(3). Perspective of Recent Advances in Medical Research Vol. 12 Dosimetric Analysis of IMRT Plans in Head and Neck Cancers to Evaluate the Probability to Decrease Oral Mucositis. Special Award: She achieved Neil joseph Fellowship award in National AROICON 2022.and Age<35 yrs in National AROICON 2023.

Mohammad Zubair Khan is a distinguished Professor in the Faculty of Computer and Information Systems, Islamic University of Madinah, Saudi Arabia. Recognized as one of the World's Top 2% Scientists by Stanford University in 2023, he has made significant contributions to the fields of Machine Learning, Artificial Intelligence, Medical Image Processing, Cybersecurity, and High-Performance Computing. With over 19 years of teaching and research experience, Dr. Khan has supervised numerous Ph.D. and Master's theses, published 100+ peer-reviewed articles in high-impact journals (including IEEE Access, Engineering Applications of AI, and Neurocomputing), and holds 7 patents. His research projects, funded by Saudi Arabia's Ministry of Education and other institutions, focus on IoT, healthcare technology, and secure communication systems. An IEEE Senior Member and active participant in academic administration, Dr. Khan has served as Head of Department, ABET/NCAAA committee member, and curriculum designer. He is also a sought-after keynote speaker and guest lecturer. Education: Ph.D. in Computer Science & IT (MJP Rohilkhand University, India) M.Tech in Computer Science (UP Technical University, India) MCA (MJP Rohilkhand University, India)

***

Roba Mohammad Alhahshmiy Alamir is an AI and Data Science researcher, Data Developer, and Analyst, holding an M.Sc. in Computer Science from Taibah University. Her research focuses on federated learning, edge–cloud image processing, cybersecurity, and deep learning applications. She has published in leading international journals, including ACM, MDPI Systems, and the International Journal of Computers and Informatics.

Anirban Bose received his B. Tech degree in Instrumentation Engineering from Haldia Institute of Technology, India in 2002 and M. Tech in Control System Engineering from IIT Kharagpur, India in 2006. He received his Ph.D. degree in Engineering (Information Technology) from Indian Institute of Engineering Science and Technology, Shibpur (formerly known as Bengal Engineering and Science University, Shibpur), India in 2019. He is now working as an Assistant Professor in the Dept. of Computer Science and Engineering at Dr. B. C. Roy Engineering College, Durgapur, India since July, 2006. His research interests include Digital Image Watermarking and Secret Sharing, Compressed Sensing, Medical Image Processing, Image Denoising, Machine Learning, Deep Learning, Time Series Analysis. He has published 13 research papers in International Journals and Conference Proceedings. He received IEEE Young Professional Best paper award in Computational Intelligence, Communications, and Business Analytics (CICBA) – 2017. Recently, he has organized a workshop titled as "Basics of Python" conducted jointly by IIT Bombay and FOSSEE at Dr. B. C. Roy Engineering College, Durgapur.

Bappaditya Das is an Assistant Professor in the Computer Science and Engineering department at Dr. B.C. Roy Engineering College, Durgapur, West Bengal, India. He holds a PhD in Computer Science and Engineering. He received his B.Tech. and M.Tech. degrees in Computer Science and Engineering from the University of Calcutta, West Bengal, India, in 2001 and 2007, respectively. He completed his B.Sc. in Physics (Hons) from the University of Calcutta, West Bengal, India 1998. He received the National Award under National Scholarship Scheme (1998-99), MHRD, Government of India, for his exceptional academic performance. He has authored and co-authored more than 15 research articles in international journals and conferences with more than 180 citations. He is a life member of The Institution of Engineers (India), Computer Society of India (CSI) and Fellow Member of Scholars Academic and Scientific Society. His research interests include machine learning, computer vision, deep learning, image processing, and WSN.

Qazi Mudassar Ilyas received his Ph.D. in Information and Communication Engineering from Huazhong University of Science and Technology, China, in 2005, after completing his BS and MS from the University of Agriculture, Faisalabad, Pakistan. He has over two decades of teaching and research experience across Pakistan, Saudi Arabia, and Brunei Darussalam. Dr. Ilyas has held academic positions at leading institutions including GIK Institute, the University of the Punjab, and COMSATS University in Pakistan. He served at King Faisal University, Saudi

Arabia, from 2010 to 2025, where he contributed to international accreditation and academic quality initiatives in addition to teaching and research. Currently, he is an Associate Professor of AI at Universiti Islam Sultan Sharif Ali (UNISSA), Brunei Darussalam. His research focuses on machine learning, knowledge management, information retrieval, and generative AI. He has published widely in reputed journals and continues to explore the intersection of AI, education, and Islamic values in higher education.

Ayman Noor is an Assistant Professor in the Department of Computer Science, Madinah branch at Taibah University, Saudi Arabia. Dr. Noor is currently HoD of Computer Science. His research interests include Cloud and Edge Computing, Monitoring Performance, the Internet of Things, Artificial Intelligence, and Blockchain. Dr. Noor received his Ph.D. from the School of Computing Science, Newcastle University, United Kingdom in 2021. He earned a Master of Science in Computer and Information Science from Gannon University, Pennsylvania, United States of America in 2013. Contact him at anoor@taibahu.edu.sa

Talal H. Noor is an assistant professor in the College of Computer Science and Engineering – Yanbu branch and director of the IT research center (NOOR) at Taibah University, Saudi Arabia. His research interests include Services Computing, Security and Privacy, Trust Management, Social Computing, and Human Computer Interaction. Noor received a PhD in computer science from the University of Adelaide, Australia. He is a member of IEEE. Contact him at tnoor@taibahu.edu.sa.

Liyakathunisa Syed is an Associate Professor at the College of Computer Science and Engineering, Taibah University, Al Madinah Al Munawwarah, Saudi Arabia. She earned her Ph.D. in Computer Science from Visvesvaraya Technological University, India. Her research focuses on Artificial Intelligence, Computer Vision, Machine Learning, Deep Learning, and Big Data Analytics, with applications in healthcare, medical imaging, smart cities, agriculture, environmental monitoring, and social media analysis. She has authored over 60 peer-reviewed publications in leading SCI/SCOPUS-indexed journals, conferences, and edited volumes.

Index

P

R

S

T

www.ingramcontent.com/pod-product-compliance
Lightning Source LLC
LaVergne TN
LVHW080908300926
849162LV00003B/599
9798337343129